Radiographic Positioning AND Related Anatomy Workbook AND Laboratory Manual

VOLUME 2

FIFTH EDITION

Radiographic Positioning AND Related Anatomy

Workbook AND Laboratory Manual

VOLUME 2
Chapters 14-24

Kenneth L. Bontrager, MA, RT(R)
John P. Lampignano, M.Ed., RT(R) (CT)

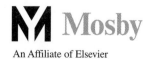

Mosby

An Affiliate of Elsevier

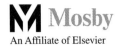

Mosby

An Affiliate of Elsevier

Executive Editor: Jeanne Wilke
Developmental Editor: Jennifer Moorhead
Project Manager: Linda McKinley
Production Editor: Rich Barber
Designer: Julia Ramirez
Cover Art: Amy Buxton

Mosby

11830 Westline Industrial Drive
St. Louis, Missouri 63146

Printed in the United States of America

International Standard Book Number
0-323-0143-64

04 GW/KPT 9 8 7 6 5 4

Acknowledgments

I am pleased to acknowledge and recognize those persons who have made significant contributions to the fifth edition of this student workbook and laboratory manual.

I first want to thank **John P. Lampignano,** MS, RT(R) (CT), who as coauthor expanded the objectives for each chapter and submitted first drafts of additional questions for the new sections of the textbook. John is a very qualified and effective educator and has put a lot of effort and energy into this project. Thank you, John, for your excellent contributions.

I want to thank **David Hall,** MS, RT(R) for his careful and meticulous review and proofing of all chapters of this manuscript. Not only did he make corrections, but he also made valuable suggestions for improving the clarity of the information being presented.

I also thank **Jeanne Rowland, Jennifer Moorhead,** and **Rich Barber** of the Mosby staff for their help and support in the preparation of this manuscript.

David Hall and **Cindy Murphy,** ACR, also reviewed, made suggestions, and proofed the more than 1200 questions in the computerized test bank, which is available as an ancillary to these workbooks and the textbook. Thank you, Dave and Cindy, for the significant time and effort you invested in this project. Both John Lampignano and I greatly appreciate your valuable contributions.

Last and most important, I want to thank my wife, **Mary Lou,** for organizing our rough composition of questions and answers, along with the associated illustrations, into an orderly and easy-to-follow format.

KLB

I would like to thank **Ken Bontrager** for his patience and dedication in developing my skills as a writer. I've been honored to work with him over the past two editions. **Jennifer Moorhead,** our developmental editor, deserves praise for her dedication and vision in coordinating this project. She kept us on task and focused but always with a smile and a gentle word.

I would like to thank the diagnostic medical imaging faculty and clinical instructors at GateWay Community College who provide a shining example of excellence each and every day for our students and community. To my students—past, present, and future—you have made teaching a rewarding experience! Without you, I would never have had the courage to write a single word. Finally, to my close friend, **Jerry Olson,** who taught me everything about radiography and many things about life—you have made my life richer and more worthwhile.

My family—**Deborah, Daniel,** and **Molly**—provide me with the greatest joy of all. I look at each of you and realize that I'm the luckiest person alive. Thank you for your love and support for the past 25 years. This book is dedicated to each of you.

JPL

Preface

The success of the first four editions of this workbook and the accompanying textbook, along with the associated audiovisual materials, is demonstrated by the many schools of radiologic technology throughout the United States, Canada, and other countries that have been using all or parts of these instructional media for more than 25 years.

New to This Edition

New illustrations and **expanded questions** have been added to reflect all the new content added to the fifth edition of *Textbook of Radiographic Positioning and Related Anatomy.* The use of visuals in these review exercises not only increases comprehension but also increases retention, because most individuals retain information most effectively through visual images.

The **detailed laboratory activities** have been updated, and the positioning question and answer exercises have been expanded with less emphasis on rote memory recall. More **situational questions** involving **clinical applications** have been added. These questions aid in the understanding of positioning principles and of which anatomical structures are best demonstrated on which projections. The clinical situational questions added to each chapter require students to think through and understand how application of this positioning information relates to specific clinical examples.

Pathology questions have been added to help students understand why they are performing specific exams and how exposure factors may be affected.

Critique exercises have been reorganized to be consistent with the new format of radiographic critique descriptions in the textbook.

Included in the positioning chapters of both the textbook and these workbooks are new sections on **geriatric** and **pediatric considerations, alternative modalities and procedures,** and **pathologic indications.** As in the textbook, entirely new sections added to the workbook include **venipuncture, digital radiography, bone densitometry, sialography,** and **hysterosalpingography.** Introductions to **nuclear medicine, radiation oncology,** and **ultrasound imaging** have also been added.

How to Work with the Textbook and the Workbook and Laboratory Manuals

This fifth edition of the student workbook and laboratory manual is organized to be in complete agreement with the fifth edition of the *Textbook of Radiographic Positioning and Related Anatomy.* Each chapter in the textbook has a corresponding chapter in the workbook-manuals to reinforce and supplement the information presented in the main text.

The most effective way to use this workbook-manual is for the student to complete the workbook chapter exercises immediately after reading and studying corresponding chapters in the textbook. To use both the student's and the instructor's time most effectively, this study should be done **before** the classroom presentation. The instructor can therefore spend more time in both the classroom and laboratory on problem areas and answering questions and less time on the fundamentals of anatomy and positioning, which students should already have learned.

Ancillaries

A **computerized test bank** (CTB) is available to instructors who use the textbook in their classrooms. The test bank features more than 1200 questions and 60 images. Some of these questions originally appeared as the Final Evaluation Exams in the Instructor's Manual in previous editions, but they have been expanded and fully revised into registry-type questions for the test bank. These questions can be used as final evaluation exams for each chapter, or they can be used to create custom exams.

Also available for the first time is an **electronic image collection** (EIC), which features more than 2000 images that are fully coordinated with the fifth edition textbook and workbooks. The fourth edition slide set contains 1780 slides and includes the two-volume Instructor's Manual with lecture notes and thumbnail prints of each slide.

Contents

Volume 2

Volume 1

Student Instructions

The following information will show you how correctly using this workbook and the accompanying textbook will help you master radiographic anatomy and positioning.

This course becomes the core of all your studies and your work as a radiographer. **This is one course that you must master.** You cannot become a proficient radiographer by marginally passing this course. Therefore please read these instructions carefully **before** beginning Chapter 1.

Objectives

Study the list of objectives carefully so that you will understand what you must know and be able to do after you complete each chapter.

Learning Exercises

These exercises are the focal point of this workbook-laboratory manual. Using them correctly will help you learn and remember the important information presented in each chapter of the textbook. To maximize the benefits from each exercise, **follow the correct six-step order of activities** as outlined next:

Chapter 1   Textbook and Workbook

Chapter 1 is a comprehensive introduction that prepares you for the remaining chapters of this positioning course. It is divided into six sections in both the textbook and this workbook. Your instructor may assign specific sections of this chapter at various times during your study of radiographic positioning and/or procedures. Read and study these sections in the textbook first, and then complete the corresponding review exercise in this workbook before taking that portion of the self-test.

Chapters 2 to 24

PART I

Step 1.   **A. Textbook:** Carefully read and learn the **radiographic anatomy** section of each chapter. Include the anatomic reviews on labeled radiographs provided in each chapter of the textbook. Pay particular attention to those items in **bold type** and to the **summary review boxes** where provided.

Step 2.   **B. Workbook:** Complete **Part I** of the review exercises on **radiographic anatomy.** Do **not** look up the answers in the textbook or look at the answer sheet until you have answered as many of the questions as you can. Then refer to the textbook and/or the answer sheet and correct or complete those questions you missed. Reread those sections of the textbook in which you could not answer questions. Textbook page numbers are provided next to each review exercise in this workbook.

PART II

Step 3.   **A. Textbook:** Carefully read and study Part II on **radiographic positioning.** Note the general **positioning considerations, alternate modalities,** and **pathologic indications** for each chapter. This is followed by the specific positioning pages, which include **pathology demonstrated; technical factors;** and the **dose ranges** of skin, midline, and specific organ doses where provided. Pay particular attention to dose comparisons between different techniques, or anteroposterior (AP) versus posteroanterior (PA) projections. Learn the **specific positioning steps,** the **central ray location and angle,** and the four-part **radiographic criteria** for each projection or position.

Step 4.   **B. Workbook:** Complete **Part II** of the review exercises, which include **technical considerations and positioning.** Also included is a section on **problem solving for technical and positioning errors.** As before, complete as many of the questions as you can before looking up the answers in the textbook or checking the answers on the answer sheet.

   The last review exercise covers **radiographic critique questions** in the workbook. This challenging section is based on the critique radiographs at the end of chapters in the textbook. These important exercises will help you make the transition from factual knowledge to application and will help you prepare for clinical experience. **Compare each critique radiographs that demonstrate errors with correctly positioned radiographs in that chapter of the textbook** and see if you can determine which radiographic criteria points could be improved and which are repeatable errors. Students who complete these exercises successfully will be ahead of those students who don't attempt them before coming to the classroom. The instructor will then explain and clarify those repeatable and non-repeatable errors on each radiograph.

PART III

Step 5.   **Workbook – Laboratory Activity:** These exercises must be performed in a radiographic laboratory using a phantom and/or a student (without making exposure) with an energized radiographic unit and illuminators for viewing radiographs. Arrange for a time when you can use your radiographic laboratory or a diagnostic radiographic room in a clinic setting.

   This is one of the most important aspects of this learning series and should not be neglected or underemphasized. Students frequently have difficulty transferring the information they have learned about positioning to effective use in a clinical setting. Therefore you must carry out the laboratory activities as described in each chapter. Your instructors and/or lab assistants will assist you as needed in these exercises.

   Each radiograph taken of the phantom and/or other radiographs provided by your instructor should be evaluated as described in your lab manual. Critique and evaluate each radiograph for errors of less-than-optimal positioning or exposure factors based on radiographic criteria provided in the textbook. Also, with the help of your instructor, learn how to discriminate between less-than-optimal, but passable radiographs, and those that need to be repeated. This generally requires additional experience and practice before you can make these judgments without assistance from a supervising technologist or radiologist.

Step 6. Self-Test

   You should **take the self-test only after you have completed all of the preceding steps.** Treat the self-test like an actual exam. After you have completed it, compare your answers with the answer sheet at the end of this workbook. If your score is less than 90% to 95%, you should go back and review the textbook again; pay special attention to the areas you missed before you take the final chapter evaluation exam provided by your instructor.

   Warning: Statistics prove that students who diligently complete all the exercises described in this section will invariably get higher grades in their positioning courses and will perform better in the clinical setting than those who don't. **Avoid the temptation of taking shortcuts.** If you bypass some of these exercises or just fill in the answers from the answer sheets, your instructors will know by your grade and by your clinical performance that you have taken these shortcuts. Most importantly, you will know that you are not doing your best and you will have difficulty competing with better prepared technologists in the job market when you graduate.

   Go to it and enjoy the feeling of satisfaction and success that only comes when you know you're doing your best!

CHAPTER 14

Upper Gastrointestinal System

Radiographic procedures involving the administration of some form of contrast medium are described in the next four chapters. These include common procedures, which may comprise 20% to 30% of the radiology department case load. You will likely be performing these examinations early in your clinical training. If you learn and understand the fundamentals provided in these next four chapters, combined with clinical experience, you will soon become a proficient radiographer of these organ systems.

CHAPTER OBJECTIVES

After you have completed **all** the activities of this chapter, you will be able to:

_____ 1. List the major organs of the upper gastrointestinal system and specific accessory organs.

_____ 2. List the three primary functions of the digestive system.

_____ 3. List three divisions of the pharynx.

_____ 4. Identify the anatomic location, function, and features of the esophagus, stomach, and duodenum.

_____ 5. Identify the effect of body position on the distribution of air and contrast media in the stomach.

_____ 6. Describe the impact of body habitus on the position and shape of the stomach.

_____ 7. Using drawings and radiographs, identify specific anatomy of the upper gastrointestinal system.

_____ 8. Identify differences between mechanical digestion and chemical digestion.

_____ 9. Identify the contrast media, patient preparation, room preparation, and the fluoroscopic procedure for an esophagram and an upper gastrointestinal series.

_____ 10. List and define the specific pathologic indications and contraindications for an esophagram and upper GI series.

_____ 11. Match specific types of pathology to the correct radiographic appearances and signs.

_____ 12. Describe specific breathing maneuvers and positioning techniques used to detect esophageal reflux.

_____ 13. List the basic and special positions or projections for the esophagram and upper gastrointestinal (GI) series to include, size and type of image receptor, central ray location, direction and angulation of the central ray, and anatomy best demonstrated.

_____ 14. Identify which anatomy is best demonstrated with specific projections of an esophagram and upper GI series.

_____ 15. List patient dose ranges for skin, midline, and gonads for specific projections of an esophagram and upper GI series.

_____ 16. Given various hypothetical situations, identify the correct modification of a position and/or exposure factors to improve the radiographic image.

POSITIONING AND FILM CRITIQUE

_____ 1. Using a peer, position for basic and special projections for the esophagram and upper GI series.

_____ 2. Critique and evaluate esophagram and upper GI series radiographs based on the four divisions of radiographic criteria: (1) structures shown, (2) position, (3) collimation and CR, and (4) exposure criteria.

_____ 3. Distinguish between acceptable and unacceptable esophagram and upper GI series radiographs that result from exposure factors, motion, collimation, positioning, or other errors.

Learning Exercises

Complete the following review exercises after reading the associated pages in the textbook as indicated by each exercise. Answers to each review exercise are given at the end of the review exercises.

PART I: Radiographic Anatomy, Digestion, and Body Habitus

REVIEW EXERCISE A: Radiographic Anatomy of the Upper Gastrointestinal System
(see textbook pp. 442-448)

1. List the seven major components of the alimentary canal:

    A. _____   E. _____

    B. _____   F. _____

    C. _____   G. _____

    D. _____

2. List the four accessory organs of digestion:

    A. _____   C. _____

    B. _____   D. _____

3. What are the three primary functions of the digestive system?

    A. _____

    B. _____

    C. _____

4. What two terms refer to a radiographic examination of the pharynx and esophagus?

    _____ or _____

5. Which term describes the radiographic study of the distal esophagus, stomach, and duodenum?

    _____

6. The three pairs of salivary glands that are accessory organs of digestion associated with the mouth are:

    A. _____

    B. _____

    C. _____

7. The act of swallowing is called _____ .

8. List the three divisions of the pharynx:

    A. _____   B. _____   C. _____

9. What structures create the two indentations seen along the lateral border of the esophagus?

   A. _____   B. _____

10. List the three structures that pass through the diaphragm.

    A. _____   B. _____   C. _____

11. What part of the upper GI tract is a common site for ulcer disease? _____

12. What term describes the junction between the duodenum and jejunum? _____
    (This is a significant reference point in small bowel studies.)

13. The C-loop of the duodenum and pancreas are _____ (intraperitoneal or retroperitoneal)
    structures?

14. Name the following structures of the mouth and pharynx (Fig. 14-1):

    A. _____

    B. _____

    C. _____

    D. _____

    E. _____

    F. _____

    G. _____

    H. _____

    I. _____

    J. _____

    K. _____

    L. _____

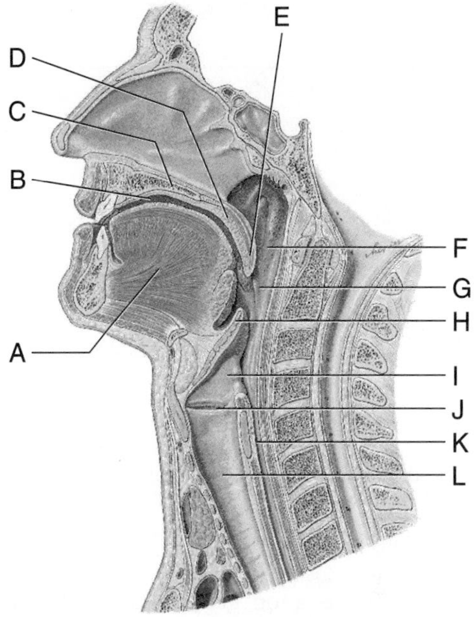

Fig. 14-1 Structures of the mouth and pharynx.

15. Identify the correct body position for each of the following drawings of the stomach filled with air and barium (Fig.
    14-2) (erect, prone, or supine) Barium = white, Air = black.

    A. _____   B. _____   C. _____

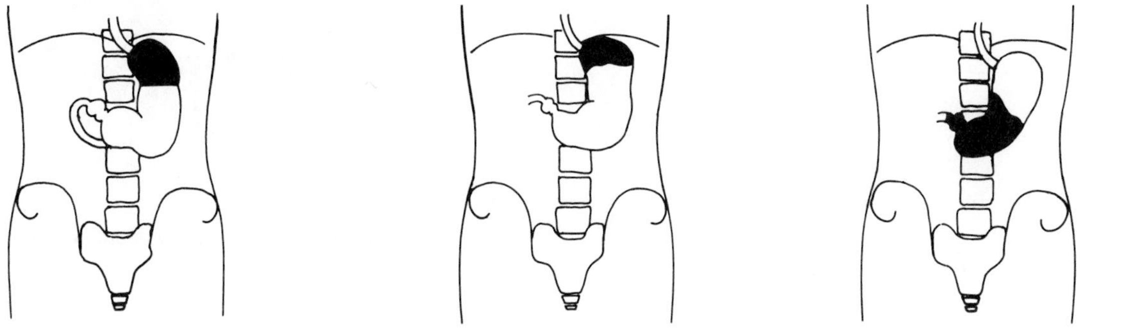

Fig. 14-2 Body position identification based on stomach filled with air or barium.

16. True/False: The body of the stomach curves inferiorly and posteriorly from the fundus.

17. Identify the parts labeled on Fig. 14-3:

A. _____

B. _____

C. _____

D. _____
     (formed by rugae along lesser curvature)

E. _____

F. _____

G. _____

H. _____

I. _____

J. _____
     (abdominal segment of esophagus)

K. _____

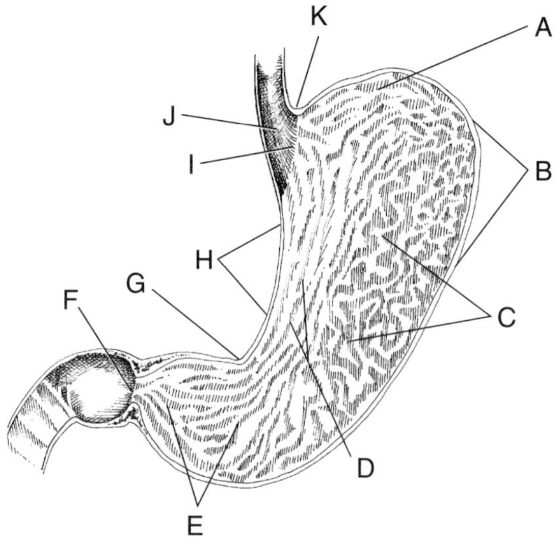

Fig. 14-3 Sectional anatomy of the stomach.

18. The three main subdivisions of the stomach are:

A. _____   B. _____   C. _____

19. The division of the stomach labeled "E" is divided into two parts, which are _____ and

_____ .

20. The correct term for "gastric folds" of the stomach is _____ .

21. Identify the parts labeled on Fig. 14-4:

A. _____

B. _____

C. _____

D. _____

E. _____

F. _____

G. _____

H. Region of _____

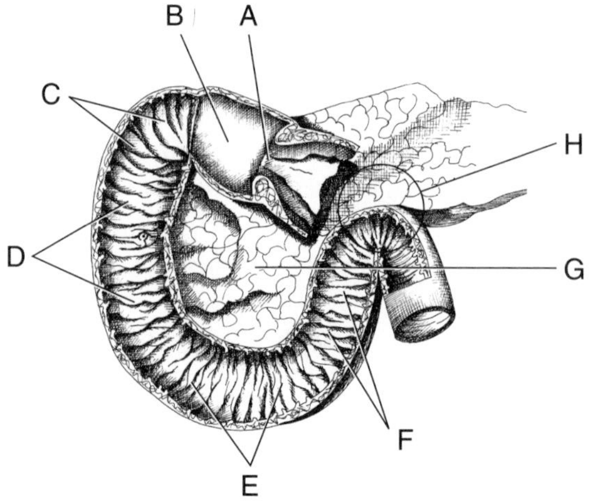

Fig. 14-4 Anatomy of the duodenum and pancreas.

22. Name the two anatomic structures implicated in the phrase "romance of the abdomen" illustrated in Fig. 14-4.

    A. _____   B. _____

23. Identify the gastrointestinal structures labeled on Fig. 14-5:

    A. _____

    B. _____

    C. _____

    D. _____

    E. _____

    F. _____

    G. _____

    H. _____

    I. _____

    J. _____

    K. _____

    L. _____

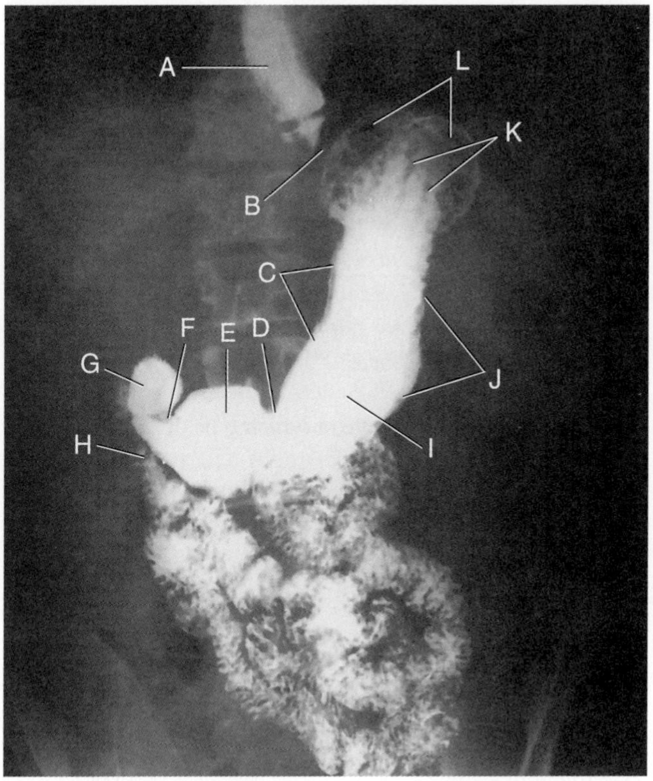

Fig. 14-5 Radiograph of gastrointestinal structures.

REVIEW EXERCISE B: Mechanical and Chemical Digestion and Body Habitus (see textbook pp. 419-421)

1. True/False: Mechanical digestion includes movements of all the gastrointestinal tract.

2. Peristaltic activity is *not* found in the following structure:
    A. Pharynx   C. Stomach
    B. Esophagus   D. Small intestine

3. Stomach contents are churned into a semifluid mass called _____ .

4. A churning or mixing activity present in the small bowel is called _____ .

5. List the three classes of substances that are ingested and need to be chemically digested.

    A. _____   B. _____   C. _____

6. Biological catalysts that speed up the process of digestion are called _____ .

7. List the end products of digestion of the following classes of foods:

    A. Carbohydrates _____

    B. Lipids _____

    C. Proteins _____

8. List the liquid substance that aids in digestion and is manufactured in the liver and stored in the gallbladder.

   _____

9. Absorption primarily takes place in the (A), _____ although some substances are absorbed

   through the lining of the (B) _____ .

10. _____ is a substance that is not an enzyme but serves to emulsify fats.

11. Of the three primary food substances listed in question 7, the digestion of which one begins in the mouth?

    _____

12. Any residues of digestion or unabsorbed digestive products are eliminated from the _____
    as a component of feces.

13. Peristalsis is an example of which type of digestion? _____

14. Which term describes food once it is mixed with gastric secretions in the stomach? _____

15. A high and transverse stomach would be found in a(n) _____ patient.
    A. Hypersthenic   C. Hyposthenic
    B. Sthenic   D. Asthenic

16. A J-shaped stomach more vertical and lower in the abdomen with the duodenal bulb at the level of L3-4 would be

    found in a _____ patient.
    A. Hypersthenic   C. Hyposthenic/asthenic
    B. Sthenic   D. None of the above

17. On the average, how much will abdominal organs drop in the erect position? _____

18. Name the two abdominal organs most dramatically affected, in relation to location, by body habitus:

    A. _____   B. _____

19. Would the fundus of the stomach be more superior or more inferior when one takes in a deep breath?

    _____ Why? _____

20. Match the types of mechanical digestion that occur in each of the following anatomical sites (each anatomical site may
    have more than one type of digestion).

ANATOMICAL SITES		TYPES OF MECHANICAL DIGESTION	
_____	1. Oral cavity	A.	Mastication
_____	2. Pharynx	B.	Deglutition
_____	3. Esophagus	C.	Peristalsis
_____	4. Stomach	D.	Mixing
_____	5. Small intestine	E.	Rhythmic segmentation

PART II: Radiographic Positioning

REVIEW EXERCISE C: Contrast Media, Fluoroscopy, and Pathologic Indications and Contraindications for
Upper Gastrointestinal Studies (see textbook pp. 452-468)

1. True/False: With the use of digital fluoroscopy, the number of post-fluoroscopy radiographs ordered has greatly diminished.

2. What is the most common form of positive contrast medium used for studies of the gastrointestinal system?

   _____

3. Another term for a negative contrast medium is _____ .

4. What types of crystals are most commonly used to produce carbon dioxide gas as a negative contrast medium for

   gastrointestinal studies? _____

5. Is a mixture of barium sulfate a suspension or a solution? _____

6. True/False: Barium sulfate never dissolves in water.

7. True/False: Certain salts of barium are poisonous to humans, so barium contrast studies require a pure sulfate salt of barium for human consumption during GI studies.

8. What is the ratio of water to barium for a thin mixture of barium sulfate? _____

9. What is the chemical symbol for barium sulfate? _____

10. When is the use of barium sulfate contraindicated? _____

11. What patient condition would prevent the use of a water-soluble contrast media for an upper GI?

    _____

12. What is the major advantage for using a double-contrast media technique for esophagrams and upper GIs?

    _____

13. The speed with which barium sulfate passes through the GI tract is called gastric _____ .

14. What is the purpose of the gas with a double contrast media technique?

    _____

15. Image intensification:

    A. The photospot or cine images, such as recorded on 105 mm film, are taken from the _____
       (input or output) side of the image intensifier?

    B. Conventional spot cassette taken on 18 x 24 cm (8 x 10 in.) cassettes are taken from the _____
       (input or output) side of the image intensifier?

    C. Which of the images in A or B above is the brighter image? _____

    D. How many times brighter is the fluoro image when enhanced or brightened by the image intensifier? _____

16. What device found beneath the radiographic table when correctly positioned greatly reduces scatter from the fluoro-scopic x-ray tube?

    A. Lead skirt   B. Lead drape   C. Bucky slot shield   D. Fluoroscopy tube shield

17. How is the device referred to in question 16 activated or placed in its correct position for fluoroscopy?

    _____

18. What is the major benefit in using a compression paddle during an upper GI study?

    A. Reduces exposure to the patient   C. Reduces exposure to arms and hands of radiologist

    B. Reduces exposure to the eyes of radiologist   D. Reduces exposure to the torso of radiologist

19. During an upper GI fluoroscopy procedure, if the technologist stands directly beside the radiologist next to the pa-tient's head and shoulders (see textbook, p. 56, zone C in Fig. 166), how much radiation would the technologist re-ceive to the lead apron at waist level during each fluoro exam if the radiologist averaged 5 minutes of fluoroscopy exposure per patient? (Hint: determine exposure dose range in mR/min in zone C and multiply by 5 minutes.)

    _____

20. Where is the best place for the technologist to stand during an upper GI procedure, and how much exposure would he or she receive in that position with 5 minutes of fluoroscopy?

    _____

21. List the six advantages or unique features and capabilities of digital fluoroscopy over conventional fluoro recording systems:

    A. _____

    B. _____

    C. _____

    D. _____

    E. _____

    F. _____

22. What is another term describing intermittent "road mapping" when used in digital fluoroscopy?

    _____

23. Match the following definitions or statements to the correct pathologic indication for the esophagram:

    _____ A. Difficulty in swallowing   1. Achalasia

    _____ B. Replacement of normal squamous epithelium with columnar   2. Zenker's diverticulum
             -epithelium
    _____ C. May lead to esophagitis   3. Esophageal varices

    _____ D. May be secondary to cirrhosis of the liver   4. Carcinoma of esophagus

    _____ E. Large outpouching of the esophagus   5. Barrett's esophagus

    _____ F. Also called *cardiospasm*   6. Esophageal reflux

    _____ G. Most common form is adenocarcinoma   7. Dysphagia

24. Match the following definitions or statements to the correct pathologic indication for the upper GI series:

_____ A. Blood in vomit	1. Hiatal hernia
_____ B. Inflammation of lining of stomach	2. Gastric carcinoma
_____ C. Blind outpouching of the mucosal wall	3. Bezoar
_____ D. Undigested material trapped in stomach	4. Hematemesis
_____ E. Synonymous with gastric or duodenal ulcer	5. Gastritis
_____ F. Portion of stomach protruding through diaphragmatic opening	6. Perforating ulcer
_____ G. Only 5% of ulcers lead to this form of ulcer	7. Peptic ulcer
_____ H. Double contrast upper GI is the gold standard for diagnosing this condition	8. Diverticulae

25. Match the following pathologic conditions or diseases to the correct radiographic appearance:

_____ A. Its presence indicates a possible sliding hiatal hernia	1. Ulcers
_____ B. Speckled appearance of gastric mucosa	2. Hiatal hernia
_____ C. "Wormlike" appearance of esophagus	3. Achalasia
_____ D. Stricture of esophagus	4. Zenker's diverticulum
_____ E. Gastric bubble above diaphragm	5. Schatzke's ring
_____ F. Irregular filling defect within stomach	6. Gastritis
_____ G. Enlarged recess in proximal esophagus	7. Esophageal varices
_____ H. "Halo" sign during upper GI	8. Gastric carcinoma

REVIEW EXERCISE D: Patient Preparation and Positioning for Esophagram and Upper Gastrointestinal Study (see textbook pp. 427-445)

1. What does the acronym NPO stand for and what does it mean?

   _____

2. True/False: The patient must be NPO 4 to 6 hours before an esophagram.

3. True/False: The esophagram usually begins with fluoroscopy with the patient in the erect position.

4. What materials may be used for swallowing to aid in the diagnosis of radiolucent foreign bodies in the esophagus?

   _____

5. List the four tests that may be performed to detect esophageal reflux:

   A. _____   C. _____

   B. _____   D. _____

6. A breathing technique in which the patient takes in a deep breath and bears down is called the

_____

7. What position is the patient usually placed in during the water test? _____

8. The compression paddle is sometimes used by the radiologist during an esophagram to better visualize the

_____ region.

9. What type of contrast media should be used if the patient has a history of bowel perforation?

_____

10. What is the minimum amount of time that the patient should be NPO before an upper GI?

_____

11. Why should cigarette and gum chewing be restricted before an upper GI?

_____

12. Why should the technologist review the patient's chart before the beginning of an upper GI?
    A. Identify any known allergies   C. Look for pertinent clinical history
    B. Ensure that the proper study has been ordered   D. All of the above

13. In which hand does the patient usually hold the barium cup during the start of an upper GI? _____

14. List the recommended dosages of barium sulfate during an upper GI for each of the following pediatric age groups:

    Newborn to 1 year: _____

    1 to 3 years: _____

    3 to 10 years: _____

    Over 10 years: _____

15. What is the name of the special adapter attached to a syringe to deliver contrast media through a nasogastric tube?

_____

16. Which one of the following imaging modalities is an alternative to an esophagram in detecting esophageal varices?
    A. Nuclear medicine   C. Sonography
    B. Computed tomography   D. None of the above

17. Gastric emptying studies are performed using:
    A. Intraesophageal sonography   C. Magnetic resonance
    B. Radionuclides   D. Computed tomography

18. Why is the RAO preferred over the LAO for an esophagram?

_____

19. How much obliquity should be used for the RAO projection of the esophagus?

_____

20. Which optional position should be performed to demonstrate the upper esophagus located between the shoulders?

_____

21. Which aspect of the GI tract is best demonstrated with an RAO position during an upper GI?

   A. Fundus of stomach   C. Body of stomach

   B. Pylorus of stomach and C-loop   D. Fourth (ascending) portion of duodenum

22. How much obliquity should be used for the RAO position during an upper GI?

   A. 30 to 35°   C. 40 to 70°

   B. 15 to 20°   D. 10 to 15°

23. What is the average kVp range for an esophagram and upper GI when using barium sulfate (without double-contrast study)?

_____

24. Which aspect of the upper GI tract will be filled with barium with the PA projection (prone position)?

_____

25. What is the purpose of the PA axial projection for the hypersthenic patient during an upper GI?

_____

26. What CR angle is used for the PA axial projection?

   A. 10 to 15° caudad   C. 35 to 45° cephalad

   B. 20 to 25° cephalad   D. 60 to 70° cephalad

27. Which projection taken during an upper GI will best demonstrate the retrogastric space?

   A. RAO   C. LPO

   B. Lateral   D. PA

28. A double contrast upper GI requires a slightly **higher** or **lower kVp** compared with a single contrast medium study?

_____

29. The female gonadal dose range for a well-collimated RAO projection of the upper GI procedure is:

   A. 10 to 15 mrad   C. 200 to 500 mrad

   B. 50 to 100 mrad   D. 600 to 1000 mrad

30. The upper GI series usually begins with the table and patient in the _____ position.

31. The five most common basic or routine projections for an upper GI series are (not counting a possible AP scout image):

   A. _____   C. _____   E. _____

   B. _____   D. _____

32. The three most common basic or routine projections for an esophagram are:

    A. _____   B. _____   C. _____

33. The major parts of the stomach on an average patient are usually confined to which abdominal quadrant?

    _____

34. Most of the duodenum is usually found to which side of the midline on an average patient? Right or left?

    _____

35. True/False: Respiration should be suspended during inspiration for upper GI radiographic projections.

REVIEW EXERCISE E: Problem Solving for Technical and Positioning Errors (see textbook pp. 461-478)

1. **Situation:** A radiograph of an RAO projection taken during an esophagram demonstrates incomplete filling of the esophagus with barium. What can the technologist do to ensure better filling of the esophagus during the repeat exposure?

    _____

    _____

2. **Situation:** A series of radiographs taken during an upper GI reveal that the stomach mucosa is not well visualized. The following factors were used during this positioning routine: high-speed screens, Bucky, 40 in. (102 cm) SID, 80 kVp, 30 mAs, and 300 ml of barium sulfate ingested during the procedure. Which exposure factor should be changed to produce a more diagnostic study?

    _____

    _____

3. **Situation:** A radiograph taken during an upper GI reveals that the anatomical side marker is missing. The technologist is unsure whether it is a recumbent AP or PA projection. The fundus of the stomach is filled with barium. Which position does this radiograph represent?

    _____

    _____

4. **Situation:** A radiograph of an RAO projection taken during an upper GI reveals that the duodenal bulb is not well demonstrated and not profiled. The RAO was a 45° oblique performed on a hypersthenic-type patient. What positioning modification needs to be made to produce a better image of the duodenal bulb?

    _____

    _____

5. **Situation:** A radiograph of an upper GI was taken, but the student technologist is unsure of the position. The radiograph demonstrates that the fundus is filled with barium, but the duodenal bulb is air-filled and seen in profile. Which position does this radiograph represent?

    _____

    _____

6. **Situation:** A patient with a clinical history of hiatal hernia comes to the radiology department. Which procedure should be performed on this patient to rule out this condition?

   _____

7. **Situation:** A patient with a possible lacerated duodenum enters the emergency room. The physician orders an upper GI to determine the extent of the injury. What type of contrast media should be used for this examination?

   _____

   _____

8. **Situation:** A patient with a fish bone stuck in his esophagus enters the emergency room. What modification to a standard esophagram may be needed to locate the foreign body?

   _____

   _____

9. **Situation:** An upper GI is being performed on a thin, asthenic-type patient. Due to room scheduling conflicts, this patient was brought into your room for the overhead follow-up images after the upper GI fluoro is completed. Where would you center the CR and the 11 x 14 in. (30 x 35 cm) image receptor to ensure that you included the stomach and duodenal regions?

   _____

   _____

10. **Situation:** A patient with a clinical history of a possible bezoar comes to the radiology department. What is a bezoar, and what radiographic study should be performed to demonstrate this condition?

    _____

    _____

11. **Situation:** A radiograph of an RAO position taken during an esophagram reveals that the esophagus is superimposed over the vertebral column. What positioning error led to this radiographic outcome?

    _____

    _____

12. **Situation:** A PA projection taken during an upper GI series performed on an infant reveals that the body and pylorus of the stomach are superimposed. What modification needs to be employed during the repeat exposure to separate these two regions?

    _____

    _____

    _____

PART III: Laboratory Exercises (see textbook pp. 469-478)

You must gain experience in positioning each part of the esophagram and upper GI procedures before performing the following exams on actual patients. You can get experience in positioning and radiographic evaluation of these projections by performing exercises using radiographic phantoms and practicing on other students (although you will not be taking actual exposures).

LABORATORY EXERCISE A: Radiographic Evaluation

1. Evaluate and critique the radiographs produced during the previous experiments, additional radiographs of esophagrams, and upper GI procedures provided by your instructor. Evaluate each position for the following points. (Check off when completed.):

_____ Evaluate the completeness of the study. (Are all the pertinent anatomic structures included on the radiograph?)

_____ Evaluate for positioning or centering errors (e.g., rotation, off centering).

_____ Evaluate for correct exposure factors and possible motion. (Are the density and contrast of the images acceptable?)

_____ Determine whether markers and an acceptable degree of collimation and/or area shielding are visible on the images.

LABORATORY EXERCISE B: Physical Positioning

On another person, simulate performing all basic and special projections of the upper GI as follows: (Check off each when completed satisfactorily.) Include the following six steps as described in the textbook.

Step 1. Appropriate size and type of image receptor holder with correct markers
Step 2. Correct CR placement and centering of part to CR and/or image receptor
Step 3. Accurate collimation
Step 4. Area shielding of patient where advisable
Step 5. Use of proper immobilizing devices when needed
Step 6. Approximate correct exposure factors, breathing instructions where applicable, and "making" exposure

Projections	Step 1	Step 2	Step 3	Step 4	Step 5	Step 6
• RAO esophagram	_____	_____	_____	_____	_____	_____
• Left lateral esophagram	_____	_____	_____	_____	_____	_____
• AP (PA) esophagram	_____	_____	_____	_____	_____	_____
• LAO esophagram	_____	_____	_____	_____	_____	_____
• Soft tissue lateral esophagram	_____	_____	_____	_____	_____	_____
• RAO upper GI	_____	_____	_____	_____	_____	_____
• PA upper GI	_____	_____	_____	_____	_____	_____
• Right lateral upper GI	_____	_____	_____	_____	_____	_____
• LPO upper GI	_____	_____	_____	_____	_____	_____
• AP upper GI	_____	_____	_____	_____	_____	_____

Answers to Review Exercises

Review Exercise A: Radiographic Anatomy of the Upper Gastrointestinal System

1. A. Mouth
   B. Pharynx
   C. Esophagus
   D. Stomach
   E. Small intestine
   F. Large intestine
   G. Anus
2. A. Salivary glands
   B. Pancreas
   C. Liver
   D. Gallbladder
3. A. Intake and digestion of food
   B. Absorption of digested food particles
   C. Elimination of solid waste products
4. Esophagram or barium swallow
5. Upper gastrointestinal series (UGI) or upper GI
6. A. Parotid
   B. Sublingual
   C. Submandibular
7. Deglutition
8. A. Nasopharynx
   B. Oropharynx
   C. Laryngopharynx
9. A. Aortic arch
   B. Left primary bronchus
10. A. Esophagus
    B. Inferior vena cava
    C. Aorta
11. Duodenal bulb or cap
12. Duodenojejunal flexure (suspensory ligament or ligament of Trietz)
13. Retroperitoneal or behind peritoneum
14. A. Tongue
    B. Oral cavity (mouth)
    C. Hard palate
    D. Soft palate
    E. Uvula
    F. Nasopharynx
    G. Oropharynx
    H. Epiglottis
    I. Laryngopharynx
    J. Larynx
    K. Esophagus
    L. Trachea
15. A. Erect
    B. Prone
    C. Supine
16. False (inferiorly and anteriorly)
17. A. Fundus
    B. Greater curvature
    C. Body
    D. Gastric canal
    E. Pyloric portion
    F. Pyloric orifice (or just pylorus)
    G. Angular notch (incisura angularis)
    H. Lesser curvature
    I. Esophagogastric junction (cardiac orifice)
    J. Cardiac antrum
    K. Cardiac notch (incisura cardiaca)
18. A. Fundus (labeled A)
    B. Body or corpus (labeled C)
    C. Pyloric (labeled E)
19. Pyloric antrum and pyloric canal
20. Rugae.
21. A. Pylorus (pyloric sphincter)
    B. Bulb or cap of duodenum
    C. First (superior) portion of duodenum
    D. Second (descending) portion of duodenum
    E. Third (horizontal) portion of duodenum
    F. Fourth (ascending) portion of duodenum
    G. Head of pancreas
    H. Suspensory ligament of duodenum or ligament of Treitz
22. A. Head of pancreas
    B. C loop of duodenum
23. A. Distal esophagus
    B. Area of esophagogastric junction
    C. Lesser curve of stomach
    D. Angular notch-incisura angularis
    E. Pyloric region of stomach
    F. Pyloric valve or sphincter
    G. Duodenal bulb
    H. Second-descending portion of duodenum
    I. Body of stomach
    J. Greater curvature of stomach
    K. Gastric folds or rugae of stomach
    L. Fundus of stomach

Review Exercise B: Mechanical and Chemical Digestion and Body Habitus

1. True
2. A. Pharynx
3. Chyme
4. Rhythmic segmentation
5. A. Carbohydrates
   B. Proteins
   C. Lipids (fats)
6. Enzymes
7. A. Simple sugars
   B. Fatty acids and glycerol
   C. Amino acids
8. Bile
9. A. Small intestine
   B. Stomach
10. Bile
11. Carbohydrates
12. Large intestine
13. Mechanical
14. Chyme
15. A. Hypersthenic

16. C. Hyposthenic/asthenic
17. 1 to 2 in. (2.5 to 5 cm)
18. A. Stomach
    B. Gall bladder
19. Inferior, because of its proximity to the diaphragm
20. 1. A, B
    2. B
    3. B, C
    4. C, D
    5. C, E

Review Exercise C: Contrast Media, Fluoroscopy, and Pathologic Indications and Contraindications for Upper Gastrointestinal Studies

1. True
2. Barium sulfate
3. Radiolucent contrast medium
4. Calcium carbonate
5. Suspension
6. True
7. True
8. One part water to one part barium sulfate (1:1)
9. $BaSO_4$
10. When the mixture may escape into the peritoneal cavity (p. 424)
11. Sensitivity to iodine
12. Better coating and visibility of the mucosa. Polyps, diverticulae, and ulcers are better demonstrated
13. Motility
14. It forces the barium sulfate against the mucosa for better coating
15. A. Output
    B. Input
    C. A. Photospot or cine images are brighter
    D. 1000 to 6000 times
16. C. Bucky slot shield
17. By moving the Bucky all the way to the end of the table
18. C. Reduces exposure to arms and hands of radiologist
19. $1.7 - 3.3 \times 5 = 8.5 - 16.5$ mRad
20. Away from the patient and table and/or behind the radiologist. (Zone F) Would receive less than 2.0 mrad ($0.4 \times 5 = 2.0$ mrad)
21. A. No cassettes are required for filming
    B. Optional post-fluoroscopy overhead images
    C. Multiple frame formatting and multiple original films
    D. Cine loop capability
    E. Image enhancement and manipulation (by computers)
    F. Reduced patient exposure (of 30 to 50%)

22. "Frame hold" capability of specific fluoroscopy images
23. A. 7, B. 5, C. 6, D. 3, E. 2, F. 1, G. 4
24. A. 4, B. 5, C. 8, D. 3, E. 7, F. 1, G. 6, H. 2
25. A. 5, B. 6, C.7, D. 3, E. 2, F. 8, G. 4, H.1

Review Exercise D: Patient Preparation and Positioning for Esophagram and Upper Gastrointestinal Study

1. "Non Per Os," Latin for "nothing by mouth" (pg. 466)
2. False (8 hours NPO for upper GI but not for an esophagram)
3. True
4. Barium soaked cotton balls, barium pills or marshmallows followed by thin barium
5. A. Breathing exercises
   B. Water test
   C. Compression technique
   D. Toe-touch maneuver
6. Valsalva maneuver
7. LPO
8. Esophagogastric junction
9. Oral, water-soluble iodinated contrast media
10. Eight hours
11. Both activities tend to increase gastric secretions
12. D. All of the above
13. Left hand
14. Newborn to 1 year: 2 to 4 ounces
    1 to 3 years: 4 to 6 ounces
    3 to 10 years: 6 to 12 ounces
    Over 10 years: 12 to 16 ounces
15. Christmas tree or tapered adapter
16. C. Sonography
17. B. Radionuclides

18. Places the esophagus between the vertebral column and heart
19. 35 to 40°
20. Optional swimmer's lateral
21. B. Pylorus of stomach and C-loop
22. C. 40 to 70°
23. 100 to 125 kVp
24. Body and pylorus of stomach and duodenal bulb
25. To prevent superimposition of the pylorus over the duodenal bulb, and to better visualize the lesser and greater curvatures of the stomach
26. C. 35 to 45° cephalad
27. B. Lateral
28. Lower
29. A. 10 to 15 mrad
30. Upright (erect)
31. A. RAO
    B. PA
    C. Right lateral
    D. LPO
    E. AP
32. A. RAO
    B. Left lateral
    C. AP
33. Left Upper Quadrant (LUQ)
34. Right
35. False (expiration)

Review Exercise E: Problem Solving for Technical and Positioning Errors

1. When using thin barium, have the patient drink continuously during the exposure. With thick barium, have the patient hold two or three spoonfuls in the mouth and make the exposure immediately after swallowing.
2. When using barium sulfate as a contrast media, 110 to 125 kVp should be used to ensure proper penetration of the contrast filled stomach and visualize the mucosa. 80 to 100 kVp would be adequate for a double contrast study.
3. AP. Since the fundus is more posterior than the body or pylorus, it will fill with barium when the patient is in a supine (AP) position.
4. With a hypersthenic patient, more rotation of up to 70° may be required to better profile the duodenal bulb. (Note: the radiologist under fluoro will frequently oblique the patient as needed for the overhead oblique to best profile the duodenal region.)
5. The LPO position (recumbent) will produce an image where the fundus and body is filled with barium but the duodenal bulb is airfilled.
6. Upper GI series
7. An oral, water-soluble contrast media should be used for an upper GI when ruptured viscus or bowel is suspected (not barium sulfate, which is not water-soluble).
8. With radiolucent foreign bodies in the esophagus, shredded cotton soaked in barium sulfate may be used to help locate it. Marshmallows with barium or a barium capsule may also be used.
9. Would center lower than usual, to the mid L3-4 region or about 1½ to 2 in. (4 to 5 cm) above the level of the iliac crest
10. A mass of undigested material that gets trapped in the stomach-a rare condition, but it can be diagnosed with an upper GI study.
11. Under-obliquity or rotation of the body into the RAO position led to the esophagus being superimposed over the vertebral column
12. Angle the CR 20 to 25° cephalad to open up the body and pylorus of the stomach

SELF-TEST

Directions: This self-test should be taken only after completing **all** of the readings, review exercises, and laboratory activities. The purpose of this test is not only to provide a good learning exercise but also to serve as a good indicator of what your final evaluation grade will be. It is strongly suggested that if you do not get at least a 90% to 95% grade on this self-test, you should review those areas where you missed questions **before** going to your instructor for the final evaluation exam.

1. Which one of the following is **not** a function of the gastrointestinal system?

   A. Intake and digestion of food

   C. Production of hormones

   B. Absorption of nutrients

   D. Elimination of waste products

2. Which one of the following is **not** a salivary gland?

   A. Parotid

   C. Pineal

   B. Sublingual

   D. Submandibular

3. What is another term for an esophagram? _____

4. What is the name of the condition that results from a viral infection of the parotid gland? _____

5. The act of chewing is termed:

   A. Mastication

   C. Aspiration

   B. Deglutition

   D. Peristalsis

6. Which structure in the pharynx prevents aspiration of food and fluid into the larynx:

   A. Uvula

   C. Soft palate

   B. Epiglottis

   D. Laryngopharynx

7. The esophagus extends from C5-6 to:

   A. T9

   C. T10

   B. L1

   D. T11

8. Which one of the following structures does not pass through the diaphragm?

   A. Trachea

   C. Aorta

   B. Esophagus

   D. Inferior vena cava

9. Wavelike involuntary contractions that help propel food down the esophagus are called _____.

10. The Greek term *gaster,* or *gastro,* means_____.

11. Which one of the following aspects of the stomach is defined as an indentation between the body and pylorus?

    A. Cardiac antrum

    C. Incisura cardiaca

    B. Pyloric antrum

    D. Incisura angularis

12. Which aspect of the stomach will fill with air when the patient is prone?

    A. Fundus

    C. Duodenal bulb

    B. Body

    D. Pylorus

13. True/False: The numerous mucosal folds found in the small bowel are called *rugae.*

14. True/False: The lateral margin of the stomach is called the *lesser curvature*.

15. Which aspect of the stomach will barium gravitate to when the patient is in the supine position?

    _____

16. Which two structures create the "romance of the abdomen?"

    _____

17. Match the following aspects of the upper gastrointestinal system with the correct definition.

    ____   1. Pyloric orifice   A. Middle aspect of stomach

    ____   2. Cardiac notch   B. Horizontal portion of duodenum

    ____   3. Fundus   C. Rugae

    ____   4. Fourth portion of duodenum D. Opening between esophagus and stomach

    ____   5. Gastric folds   E. Opening leaving the stomach

    ____   6. Body   F. Found along superior aspect of fundus

    ____   7. Esophagogastric junction   G. Indentation found along lesser curvature

    ____   8. Angular notch   H. Ascending portion of duodenum

    ____   9. Third portion of duodenum I. Most posterior aspect of stomach

18. Identify the structures labeled on Fig. 14-6:

    A. _____

    B. _____

    C. _____

    D. _____

    E. _____

    F. _____

    G. _____

    H. _____

    I. _____

    J. _____

    K. _____

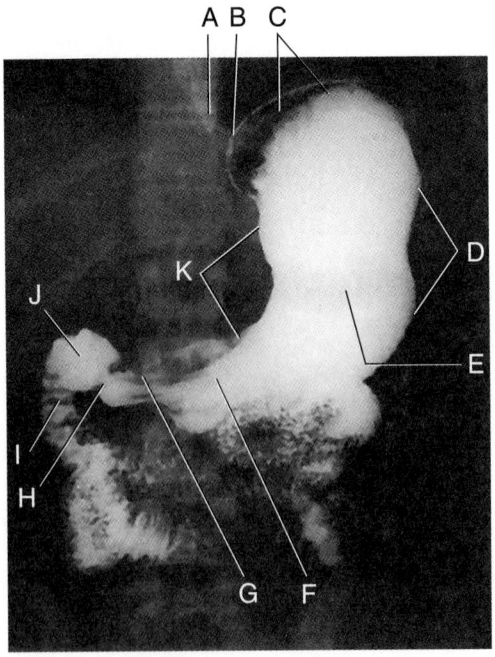

Fig. 14-6 Radiograph of gastrointestinal structures, demonstrating body position.

19. A. Which body position does Fig. 14-6 represent? _____

    B. How could you determine this? _____

20. Which body position does Fig. 14-7 represent? _____

21. A. Which body position does Fig. 14-8 represent? _____

    B. How could you determine this? _____

22. A. Which oblique (anterior or posterior) does Fig. 14-9 represent? _____

    B. How could you determine this _____

    C. Which specific oblique does Fig. 14-10 represent? _____

    D. How could you determine this? _____

23. Which term describes food once it enters the stomach and is mixed with gastric fluids? _____

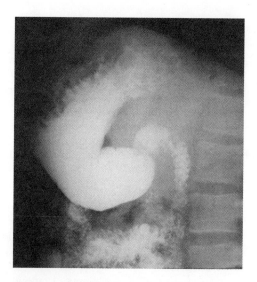

Fig. 14-7 Gastrointestinal radiograph demonstrating body position.

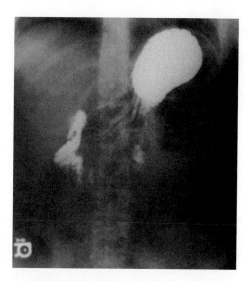

Fig. 14-8 Gastrointestinal radiograph demonstrating body position.

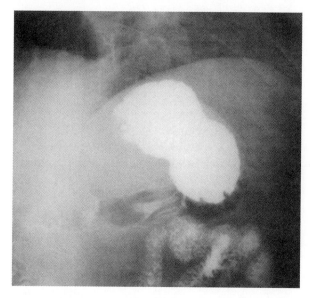

Fig. 14-9 Oblique radiograph of gastrointestinal structures.

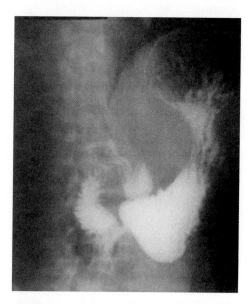

Fig. 14-10 Oblique radiograph of gastrointestinal structures.

24.   Which one of the following nutrients is not digested?

    A.   Vitamins   C.   Carbohydrates

    B.   Lipids   D.   Proteins

25.   The churning or mixing activity of chyme in the small intestine is called:

    A.   Peristalsis   C.   Rhythmic segmentation

    B.   Deglutition   D.   Digestion

26.   A _____ or _____ type of body habitus will usually have a low

    and vertical stomach with the pyloric portion of the stomach at the level of _____.

27.   A high and transverse stomach indicates a _____ body type with the pyloric portion at the

    level of _____.

28.   What is the most common radiopaque contrast media used in the gastrointestinal system?

    _____

29.   What type of radiolucent contrast medium is most commonly used for double-contrast gastrointestinal studies?

    _____

30.   A. What is the ratio of barium to water for a thick mixture of barium sulfate? _____

    B.   What is the ratio for a thin barium mixture? _____

31.   When should a water-soluble contrast media be used during an upper GI rather than barium sulfate?

    _____

32.   Cinefluorography cameras record the image from the _____ (input or output) side of the
    image intensifier?

33.   Image intensified fluoroscopy is _____ brighter than older conventional fluoroscopy with-
    out intensifiers.

    A.   100 times   C.   1000 to 6000 times

    B.   10 times   D.   10,000 to 60,000 times

34.   True/False: Digital fluoroscopy does not require the use of image receptor cassettes.

35.   Digital fluoroscopy leads to 30% to 50% _____ (higher or lower) patient dose as com-
    pared with conventional fluoroscopy.

36.   Protective aprons of _____ mm lead equivalency must be worn during fluoroscopy.

    A.   1.0   C.   0.25

    B.   0.50   D.   0.15

37.   A large, outpouching of the upper esophagus is:

    A.   Zenker's diverticulum   C.   Barrett's esophagus

    B.   Achalasia   D.   Esophageal varices

38. Other than the esophagram, what other imaging modality is used to diagnose Barrett's esophagus?

   A.   Computed tomography   C. Magnetic resonance

   B.   Nuclear medicine   D. Sonography

39. A phytobezoar is:

   A.   Outpouching of the mucosal wall   C.   Rare tumor

   B.   Trapped mass of hair in the stomach   D.   Trapped vegetable fiber in the stomach

40. What is the reason that the patient may be asked to swallow a mouthful of water drawn through a straw during an esophagram?

   _____

41. How much obliquity should be used for the RAO esophagram projection? _____

42. Why is an RAO rather than an LAO preferred for an esophagram?

   _____

43. Why is the AP projection of the esophagus not a preferred projection for the esophagram series?

   _____

44. What can be added to the barium sulfate and swallowed to detect a radiolucent foreign body lodged in the esopha-

   gus? _____

45. Which upper GI position will best demonstrate the retrogastric space? _____

46. An upper GI series is performed on an asthenic patient. A radiograph of the RAO position reveals that the duodenal bulb and C-loop are not in profile. The technologist obliqued the patient 50 degrees. What modification of the position is required during the repeat exposure?

   _____

47. A radiograph taken during a double-contrast, upper GI demonstrates that the fundus is barium-filled, and the duodenal bulb is air-filled. This was either an AP or a PA radiograph, which needs to be repeated. Which specific position does this radiograph represent?

   _____

48. **Situation:** A patient with a clinical history of cirrhosis of the liver with GI bleeding comes to the radiology department. What may be the most likely reason that an esophagram was ordered for this patient?

   _____

49. During an esophagram, the radiologist asks the patient to try to bear down as if having a bowel movement. What is the maneuver called and why did the radiologist make such a request?

   _____

50. During an upper GI, the radiologist reports that she sees a "halo" sign in the duodenum. What form of pathology did the radiologist observe?

   _____

15

Lower Gastrointestinal System

CHAPTER OBJECTIVES

After you have completed **all** the activities of this chapter, you will be able to:

_____ 1. List three divisions of the small intestine and the major parts of the large intestine.

_____ 2. Identify the function, location, and pertinent anatomy of the small and large bowel.

_____ 3. Differentiate between the terms _colon_ and _large intestine._

_____ 4. Identify on drawings and radiographs, specific anatomy of the lower gastrointestinal canal from the duodenum through the anus.

_____ 5. Identify the sectional differences that differentiate the large intestine from the small intestine.

_____ 6. List specific pathologic indications and contraindications for a small bowel series and for a barium enema examination.

_____ 7. Match specific types of pathology to the correct radiographic appearances and signs.

_____ 8. Identify patient preparation for a small bowel series and for a barium enema.

_____ 9. List five safety concerns that must be followed during a barium enema procedure.

_____ 10. Identify the radiographic procedure and sequence for a small bowel series.

_____ 11. Identify the purpose, pathologic indications, and the methodology for the enteroclysis and the intubation method procedures.

_____ 12. Identify the patient preparation, room preparation, and the fluoroscopic procedure for a barium enema.

_____ 13. Identify the purpose, clinical indications, and methodology for an evacuative proctogram.

_____ 14. Identify the correct procedure for inserting a rectal tube.

_____ 15. List specific information related to the basic positions or projections of a small bowel series and barium enema examination to include size and type of, image receptor, central ray location, direction and angulation of the central ray, and the anatomy best demonstrated.

_____ 16. Identify the advantages, procedure, and positioning for an air contrast barium enema.

_____ 17. Identify patient dose ranges for skin, midline, and gonads for each small bowel and barium enema projection.

_____ 18. Given various hypothetical situations, identify the correct modification of a position and/or exposure factors to improve the radiographic image.

POSITIONING AND FILM CRITIQUE

_____ 1. Using a peer, position for basic and special projections for the small bowel and barium enema series.

_____ 2. Critique and evaluate small bowel and barium enema series radiographs based on the four divisions of radiographic criteria: (1) structures shown, (2) position, (3) collimation and CR, and (4) exposure criteria.

_____ 3. Distinguish between acceptable and unacceptable small bowel and barium enema series radiographs resulting from exposure factors, motion, collimation, positioning, or other errors.

Learning Exercises

Complete the following review exercises after reading the associated pages in the textbook as indicated by each exercise. Answers to each review exercise are given at the end of the review exercises.

PART I: Radiographic Anatomy

Review Exercise A: Radiographic Anatomy and Function of the Lower Gastrointestinal System (see textbook pp. 480-485)

1. List the three divisions of the small bowel in descending order starting with the widest division:

    A. _____   B. _____   C. _____

2. Which division of the small bowel is the shortest? _____

3. Which division of the small bowel is the longest? _____

4. Which division of the small bowel has a feathery or coiled-spring appearance during a small bowel series?

    _____

5. A. If removed and stretched out during autopsy, how long is the average small bowel? _____

    B. In a person with good muscle tone, the length of the entire small bowel is _____

    C. The average length of the large intestine is _____

6. In which two abdominal quadrants would the majority of the jejunum be found?

    _____

7. Which muscular band marks the junction between the duodenum and jejunum?

    _____

8. Which two aspects of the large intestine are **not** considered part of the colon?

    _____

9. The colon consists of _____ sections and _____ flexures.

10. List the two functions of the ileocecal valve: A. _____

    B. _____

11. What is another term for the appendix? _____

12. Match the following aspects of the small and large intestine to the following characteristics:

    _____ 1. Jejunum   A. Longest aspect of the colon

    _____ 2. Duodenum   B. Widest portion of the colon

    _____ 3. Ileum   C. A blind pouch inferior to the ileocecal valve

    _____ 4. Cecum   D. Aspect of small intestine that is the smallest in diameter but longest in length

    _____ 5. Appendix   E. Distal part; also called the *iliac colon*

    _____ 6. Ascending colon   F. Shortest aspect of small intestine

    _____ 7. Descending colon   G. Lies in pelvis but possesses a wide freedom of motion

    _____ 8. Transverse colon   H. Makes up 40% of the small intestine

    _____ 9. Sigmoid colon   I. Found between the cecum and transverse colon

13. A. What is the term for the three bands of muscle that pull the large intestine into

      pouches?_____

     B. These pouches or sacculations, seen along the large intestine wall, are called _____.

14. The part of the large intestine directly anterior to the coccyx is the _____

15. Identify the labeled structures demonstrated on Fig. 15-1 and Fig. 15-2. Include secondary names where indicated.

     Fig. 15-1

     A. _____ (_____)

     B. _____

     C. _____

     D. _____

     E. _____ (_____) _____

     F. _____

     G. _____ (_____) _____

     H. _____

     I. _____

     J. _____

     K. _____

     L. _____

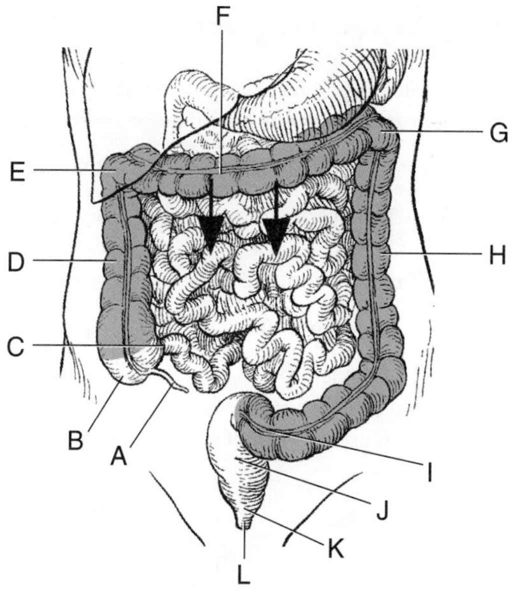

Fig. 15-1 Structures of the lower gastrointestinal tract, anterior view.

Fig.   15-2

M. _____

N. _____

O. _____

P. _____

Q. _____

R. _____

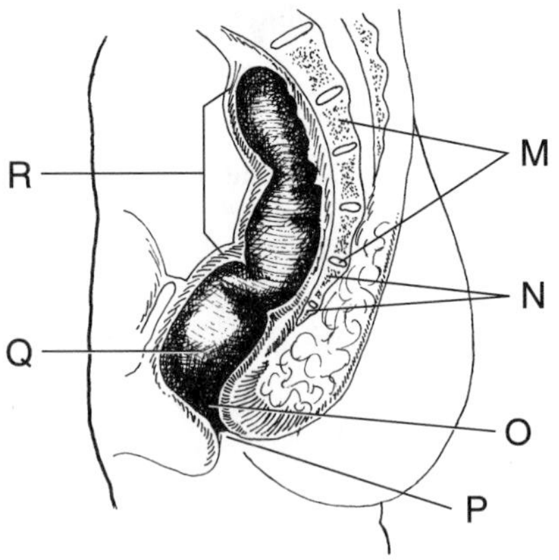

Fig. 15-2 Structures of the lower gastrointestinal tract, lateral view.

16. Which portion of the small intestine is located **primarily** to the left of the midline? _____

17. Which portion of the small intestine is located **primarily** in the RLQ? _____

18. Which portion of the small intestine has the smoothest internal lining and does **not** present a feathery appearance when barium filled? _____

19. Which aspect of the small intestine is **most fixed** in position? _____

20. In which quadrant does the terminal ileum connect with the large intestine? _____

21. The widest portion of the large bowel is the _____.

22. Which flexure of the large bowel usually extends more superiorly? _____

23. Inflammation of the appendix is called _____.

24. Which of the following structures will fill with air during a barium enema with the patient supine? (More than one answer may be correct.)

A. Ascending colon   C. Rectum   E. Descending colon

B. Transverse colon   D. Sigmoid colon

25. Which aspect of the GI tract is primarily responsible for digestion, absorption, and reabsorption?

A. Small intestine   C. Large intestine

B. Stomach   D. Colon

26. Which aspect of the GI tract is responsible for the synthesizing and absorption of vitamins B and K, and amino acids?

A. Duodenum   C. Large intestine

B. Jejunum   D. Stomach

27. Four types of digestive movements occurring in the large intestine are listed below as A through D. Which one of these movement types also occur in the small intestine? _____

A. Peristalsis   C. Mass peristalsis

B. Haustral churning   D. Defecation

CHAPTER 15   REVIEW EXERCISE B: Pathologic Indications and Radiographic Procedures for the Small Bowel Series and
Barium Enema

27

28. Identify the gastrointestinal structures labeled on Fig. 15-3.

A. _____

B. _____

C. _____

D. _____

E. _____

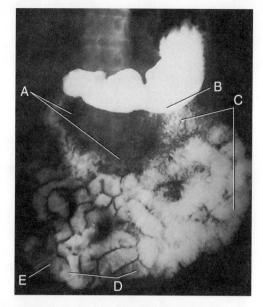

Fig. 15-3 Structure identification on a PA, 30-minute small bowel radiograph.

29. Identify the gastrointestinal structures labeled on Fig. 15-4.

A. _____

B. _____

C. _____

D. _____

E. _____

F. _____

G. _____

H. _____

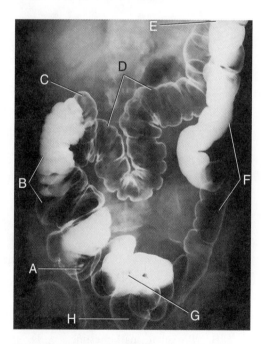

Fig. 15-4 Structure identification on an AP, barium enema radiograph.

PART II: Radiographic Positioning

Review Exercise B: Pathologic Indications and Radiographic Procedures for the Small Bowel Series and Barium Enema (see textbook pp. 486-504)

1. Which of the following conditions relate to a radiographic study of the small bowel?

    A. May perform as a double-contrast media study

    B. An enteroclysis procedure

    C. Timing of the procedure is necessary

    D. All of the above

2. Match the following definitions or statements to the correct pathologic indication for the small bowel series:

    _____ A. Common birth defect found in the ileum   1. Ileus

    _____ B. Common parasitic infection of the small intestine 2. Neoplasm

    _____ C. Obstruction of the small intestine   3. Meckel's diverticulum

    _____ D. Patient with lactose or sucrose sensitivities   4. Malabsorption syndrome

    _____ E. New growth   5. Enteritis

    _____ F. A form of sprue   6. Celiac disease

    _____ G. Inflammation of the intestine   7. Regional enteritis

    _____ H. Chronic inflammatory disease of the GI tract   8. Giardiasis

3. Match the following pathologic conditions or diseases to the correct radiographic appearance:

    _____ A. Circular staircase or herringbone sign   1. Adenocarcinoma

    _____ B. Cobblestone appearance   2. Meckel's diverticulum

    _____ C. Napkin ring sign   3. Ileus

    _____ D. Dilatation of the intestine with thickening   4. Giardiasis of circular folds

    _____ E. Large diverticulum of the ileum   5. Regional enteritis

4. Giardiasis is a condition acquired through:
    A. Contaminated food   C. Person-to-person contact
    B. Contaminated water   D. All of the above

5. Meckel's diverticulum is best diagnosed with which imaging modality
    A. Small bowel series   C. Magnetic resonance imaging
    B. Enteroclysis   D. Nuclear medicine

6. Whipple's disease is a disorder of the:
    A. Distal small intestine   C. Proximal large intestine
    B. Proximal small intestine D. Distal large intestine

7. List the two conditions that may prevent the use of barium sulfate during a small bowel series?
    A. _____   B. _____

8. What type of patients should be given extra care when using a water-soluble contrast media?

    _____

9. How much barium sulfate is generally given to an adult patient for a small-bowel-only series? _____

10. When is a small bowel series deemed completed?

    _____

CHAPTER 15   REVIEW EXERCISE B: Pathologic Indications and Radiographic Procedures for the Small Bowel Series and Barium Enema

29

11. How long does it usually take to complete a small bowel series? _____

12. When is the first radiograph generally taken during a small bowel series? _____

13. True/False: Fluoroscopy is sometimes used during a small bowel series to visualize the ileocecal valve.

14. True/False: It takes approximately 12 hours for barium sulfate, given orally, to reach the rectum.

15. The term *enteroclysis* describes what type of a small bowel study? _____

16. Which two clinical conditions are best evaluated through an enteroclysis procedure?

    _____

17. What type of contrast media is used for an enteroclysis?

    _____

18. The tip of the catheter is advanced to the _____ during an enteroclysis.

    A. Duodenojejunal flexure (suspensory ligament)   C. Pyloric sphincter

    B. C-loop of duodenum   D. Ileocecal sphincter

19. A procedure to alleviate postoperative distention of a small intestine obstruction is called:

    A. Diagnostic intubation   C. Therapeutic intubation

    B. Enteroclysis   D. Small bowel series

20. What is the recommended patient preparation before a small bowel series?

    _____

21. Which position is recommended for small bowel radiographs? Why?

    _____

22. Match the following definitions or statements to the correct pathologic indication for the barium enema:

    _____ A. A twisting of a portion of the intestine on its own mesentery   1. Polyp

    _____ B. Outpouching of the mucosal wall   2. Diverticulum

    _____ C. Inflammatory condition of the large intestine   3. Intussusception

    _____ D. Severe form of colitis   4. Volvulus

    _____ E. Telescoping of one part of the intestine into another   5. Ulcerative colitis

    _____ F. Inward growth extending from the lumen of the intestinal wall   6. Colitis

23. Which type of patient usually experiences intussusception? _____

24. A condition of numerous herniations of the inner wall of the colon is called _____

25. Which one of the following pathologic indications may produce a "tapered or corkscrew" radiographic sign during a barium enema?

    A. Diverticulosis   C. Volvulus

    B. Ulcerative colitis   D. Diverticulitis

26. Which one of the following conditions may produce the "stove pipe" radiographic sign during a barium enema?

    A.   Ulcerative colitis   C.   Diverticulosis

    B.   Appendicitis   D.   Adenocarcinoma

27. True/False: The barium enema is a commonly recommended procedure for diagnosing possible acute appendicitis.

28. Which four conditions would prevent the use of a laxative cathartic before a barium enema procedure?

    A. _____   C. _____

    B. _____   D. _____

29. True/False: Any stool retained in the large intestine may require cancellation of a barium enema.

30. True/False: An example of an irritant cathartic is magnesium citrate.

31. True/False: Synthetic latex enema tips or gloves do not cause problems for latex-sensitive patients.

32. List the three types of enema tips commonly used (all are considered single-use and disposable):

    A. _____   B. _____   C. _____

33. What water temperature is recommended for barium enema mixtures? _____

34. To minimize spasm during a barium enema, _____ can be added to the contrast media mixture.

    A.   Glucagon   C.   Saline

    B.   Lidocaine   D.   Valium

35. What is the name of the patient position recommended for insertion of the rectal enema tip?

    _____

36. The initial insertion of the rectal enema tip should be pointed toward the:

    A.   Symphysis pubis   C.   Umbilicus

    B.   Bladder   D.   Tip of coccyx

37. Which one of the following procedures is most effective to demonstrate small polyps in the colon?

    A.   Single-contrast barium enema   C.   Enteroclysis

    B.   Double-contrast barium enema   D.   Evacuative proctogram

38. Which one of the following procedures uses the thickest mixture of barium sulfate?

    A.   Single-contrast barium enema   C.   Evacuative proctogram

    B.   Double-contrast barium enema   D.   Enteroclysis

39. Which one of the following clinical conditions is best demonstrated with evacuative proctography?

    A.   Intussusception   C.   Rectal prolapse

    B.   Volvulus   D.   Diverticulosis

40. Which aspect of the large intestine must be demonstrated during evacuative proctography?

    A.   Sigmoid colon   C.   Anorectal angle

    B.   Haustra   D.   Rectal ligament

41. Into which position is the patient placed for imaging during the evacuative proctogram?

    A.   AP spine   C.   Ventral decubitus

    B.   Left or right lateral decubitus   D.   Lateral

42. True/False: A special tapered enema tip is inserted into the stoma before a colostomy barium enema.

43. True/False: The enema bag should not be more than 36 in. (90 cm) above the table-top before the beginning of the procedure.

44. True/False: The technologist should review the patient's chart before a barium enema to determine if a sigmoidoscopy or colonoscopy was performed recently.

45. True/False: Both computed tomography and sonography may be performed to aid in diagnosing appendicitis.

REVIEW EXERCISE C: Positioning of the Lower Gastrointestinal System (see textbook pp. 505-517)

1. Why is the Chassard-Lapine position not commonly performed as part of a barium enema routine?

    A.   Produces a poor image of the rectosigmoid colon   C.   Requires the use of a 14 × 17 in.   cassette

    B.   High gonadal dose and difficult position for patients   D.   Must use a long SID (>72 in)

2. Which two alternate special projections, other than the Chassard-Lapine position, demonstrate the rectosigmoid region as commonly performed by 40% or more of clinical institutions.

    _____

3. The _____ projection is a recommended alternate projection for the lateral rectum with a double-contrast BE exam.

4. Where is the CR centered for the 15-minute radiograph during a small bowel series?

    A.   Iliac crest   C.   2 inches (5 cm) above iliac crest

    B.   Xiphoid process   D.   ASIS

5. What kVp is recommended for a small bowel series (with barium)? _____

6. What are the breathing instructions for a PA projection during a small bowel series?

    _____

7. Once the small bowel procedure has gone beyond 2 hours, radiographs are taken generally every

    _____.

8. Which ionization chambers should be activated for both PA small bowel and AP and oblique barium enema projections?

    A.   All three chambers   C.   Left and right upper chambers

    B.   Center chamber only   D.   AEC should not be used for barium procedures

9. How much midline dose (also female gonadal dose) is acquired for a PA small bowel or barium enema projection of a small to average-size patient?

    A.   5 to 10 mrad   C.   100 to 200 mrad

    B.   30 to 50 mrad   D.   400 to 500 mrad

10. Which type of patient may require two 35 x 43 cm (14 x 17 in.) crosswise cassettes for an AP barium enema projection?

    A. Hypersthenic   C. Hyposthenic

    B. Sthenic   D. Asthenic

11. Which position(s) taken during a barium enema will best demonstrate the right colic flexure?

    _____

12. How much rotation is required for oblique barium enema projections? _____

13. Which position should be taken if the patient cannot lie prone on the table for the anterior oblique to visualize the

    left colic flexure? _____

14. Which of the following barium enema positions provides the greatest amount of skin dose?

    A. Decubitus position (AP)   C. Obliques

    B. Lateral   D. AP axial

15. Which projection, taken during a double-contrast barium enema, will produce an air-filled image of the right colic

    flexure, ascending colon, and cecum? _____

16. Where is the CR centered for a lateral projection of the rectum? _____

17. True/False: If a retention-type enema tip is used, it should be removed after fluoroscopy is completed before overhead filming to better visualize the rectal region.

18. Which aspect of the large intestine is best demonstrated with an AP axial projection? _____

19. What is the advantage of performing an AP axial oblique projection rather than an AP axial?

    _____

20. A. What is another term describing the AP and PA axial projections? _____

    B. What CR angle is required for the AP axial? _____

    C. What CR angle is required for the PA axial? _____

21. Which projection for a double-contrast barium enema series best demonstrates the descending colon for possible

    polyps? _____

22. Which one of the following substances can be given to the patient to help stimulate evacuation following a barium enema?

    A. Milk   C. Wine or beer

    B. Coffee or hot tea D. Garlic bread

23. What kVp range is recommended for a postevacuation projection following a barium enema? _____

24. A. What is the recommended kVp for a single-contrast barium enema study? _____

    B. What is the recommended kVp for a double-contrast study? _____

REVIEW EXERCISE D: Problem Solving for Technical and Positioning Errors (see textbook pp. 486-517)

1. **Situation:** A radiograph of a double-contrast barium enema projection reveals an obscured anatomical side marker. The technologist is unsure whether it is an AP or PA recumbent projection. The transverse colon is primarily filled with barium, with the ascending and descending colon containing a lesser amount. Which position does this radiograph represent?

   _____

   _____

2. **Situation:** A radiograph of a lateral decubitus projection taken during an air-contrast barium enema reveals that the upside aspect of the colon is overpenetrated. The following factors were used during this exposure: 120 kVp, 30 mAs, 40 in. (102 cm) SID, high-speed screens, and compensating filter for the air-filled aspect of the large intestine. Which one of these factors must be modified during the repeat exposure?

   _____

   _____

3. **Situation:** A radiograph of an AP axial barium enema projection of the rectosigmoid segment reveals that there is considerable superimposition of the sigmoid colon and rectum. The following factors were used during this exposure: 120 kVp, 20 mAs, 40 in. (102 cm) SID, 35° caudad CR angle, and collimation. Which one of these factors must be modified or corrected for the repeat exposure?

   _____

   _____

4. **Situation:** A barium enema study performed on a hypersthenic patient reveals that the majority of the radiographs demonstrate that the left colic flexure was cut off. What can be done during the repeat exposures to avoid this problem?

   _____

   _____

   _____

5. **Situation:** A technologist has inserted an air-contrast retention tip for a double-contrast BE study. He is not sure how much to inflate the retention balloon. Should he inflate it as much as the patient can tolerate, or is there a better alternative?

   _____

   _____

   _____

6. **Situation:** A student technologist is told to place the patient onto the x-ray table in a Sims position in preparation for the tip insertion for a barium enema. Describe how the patient should be positioned.

   _____

   _____

   _____

7. **Situation:** A patient with a clinical history of regional enteritis comes to the radiology department. What type of procedure would be most diagnostic for this condition?

   _____

   _____

8. **Situation:** A patient is referred to the radiology department for a presurgical, small bowel series. What modification to the standard study needs to be made for this particular patient?

   _____

   _____

9. **Situation:** A patient comes to the radiology department for a small bowel series. However, due to a stroke, the patient is unable to swallow the contrast media. What type of study should be performed for this patient?

   _____

   _____

10. **Situation:** A young infant with a possible intussusception is brought to the emergency room. Which radiographic procedure may serve a therapeutic role for correcting this condition?

   _____

   _____

11. **Situation:** Before a barium enema, the technologist experienced difficulty in inserting the enema rectal tip (without causing significant pain for the patient). What should the technologist do to complete this task?

   _____

12. **Situation:** During the fluoroscopy aspect of a barium enema, the radiologist detects an unusual defect within the right colic flexure. She asks that the technologist provide the best images possible of this region. Which two projections will best demonstrate the right colic flexure?

   _____

13. **Situation:** A patient with a clinical history of possible enteritis comes to the radiology department. Which type of radiographic GI study would most likely be indicated for this condition. (Of course, this would have to be requested by the referring physician.)

   _____

14. **Situation:** A patient's clinical history includes possible giardiasis. What radiographic procedures would likely be indicated for this condition?

   _____

15. **Situation:** A patient came to the radiology with a request for a small bowel series. The patient's chart indicates a possible large bowel obstruction.

   _____

   What radiographic exams and/or projections should be performed first before giving the patient barium to ingest for a small bowel series?

   _____

PART III: Laboratory Activities (see textbook pp. 505-517)

You must gain experience in positioning each part of the lower GI procedures before performing the following exams on actual patients. You can get experience in positioning and radiographic evaluation of these projections by performing exercises using radiographic phantoms and practicing on other students (although you will not be taking actual exposures).

LABORATORY EXERCISE A: Radiographic Evaluation

1. Evaluate and critique the radiographs produced during the previous experiments, additional radiographs of esophagrams, and lower GI procedures provided by your instructor.   Evaluate each position for the following points. (Check off when completed.):

    _____ Evaluate the completeness of the study.   (Are all of the pertinent anatomic structures included on the radiograph?)

    _____ Evaluate for positioning or centering errors (e.g., rotation, off centering)

    _____ Evaluate for correct exposure factors and possible motion.
    (Are the density and contrast of the images acceptable?)

    _____ Determine whether markers and an acceptable degree of collimation and/or area shielding are visible on the images.

LABORATORY EXERCISE B: Physical Positioning

On another person, simulate performing all basic and special projections of the lower GI as follows.   (Check off each when completed satisfactorily.) Include the following six steps as described in the textbook.

Step 1. Appropriate size and type of film holder with correct markers
Step 2. Correct CR placement and centering of part to CR and/or film
Step 3. Accurate collimation
Step 4. Area shielding of patient where advisable
Step 5. Use of proper immobilizing devices when needed
Step 6. Approximate correct exposure factors, breathing instructions where applicable, and "making" exposure

	Step 1	Step 2	Step 3	Step 4	Step 5	Step 6
• PA 15- or 30-minute small bowel	_____	_____	_____	_____	_____	_____
• PA 1- or 2-hour small bowel	_____	_____	_____	_____	_____	_____
• PA or AP barium enema	_____	_____	_____	_____	_____	_____
• RAO and LAO barium enema	_____	_____	_____	_____	_____	_____
• LPO and RPO barium enema	_____	_____	_____	_____	_____	_____
• Right and left lateral decubitus	_____	_____	_____	_____	_____	_____
• AP and LPO axial	_____	_____	_____	_____	_____	_____
• PA and RAO axial	_____	_____	_____	_____	_____	_____
• Lateral rectum	_____	_____	_____	_____	_____	_____
• Ventral decubitus lateral rectum	_____	_____	_____	_____	_____	_____

Answers to Review Exercises

Review Exercise A: Radiographic Anatomy and Function of the Lower Gastrointestinal System

1. A. Duodenum
   B. Jejunum
   C. Ileum
2. Duodenum
3. Ileum
4. Jejunum
5. A. 23 feet or 7 meters
   B. 15 to 18 feet or 4.5 to 5.5 meters
   C. 5 feet or 1.5 meters
6. LUQ and LLQ
7. Suspensory ligament of the duodenum or ligament of Treitz (this site is a reference point for certain small bowel exams because it remains in a relatively fixed position).
8. Cecum and rectum
9. 4 sections, 2 flexures
10. A. Prevents contents from the ileum to pass too quickly into cecum
    B. Prevents reflux back into the ileum
11. Vermiform appendix
12. 1. H, 2. F, 3. D, 4. B, 5. C,
    6. I, 7. E, 8. A, 9. G
13. A. Taeniae coli
    B. Haustra
14. Rectal ampulla
15. A. Appendix (vermiform process)
    B. Cecum
    C. Ileocecal valve
    D. Ascending colon
    E. Right colic (hepatic) flexure
    F. Transverse colon
    G. Left colic (splenic) flexure
    H. Descending colon
    I. Sigmoid colon
    J. Rectum
    K. Anal canal
    L. Anus
    M. Sacrum
    N. Coccyx
    O. Anal canal
    P. Anus
    Q. Rectal ampulla
    R. Rectum
16. Jejunum
17. Ileum
18. Ileum
19. Duodenojejunal junction
20. Right lower quadrant (RLQ)
21. Cecum
22. Left colic (splenic)
23. Appendicitis
24. B. Transverse colon
    D. Sigmoid colon
25. A. Small intestine
26. C. Large intestine
27. A. Peristalsis
28. A. Duodenum
    B. Area of suspensory ligament/duodenojejunal junction
    C. Jejunum
    D. Ileum
    E. Area of ileocecal valve
29. A. Cecum
    B. Ascending colon
    C. Right colic (hepatic) flexure
    D. Transverse colon
    E. Left colic (splenic) flexure
    F. Descending colon
    G. Sigmoid colon
    H. Rectum

Review Exercise B: Pathologic Indications and Radiographic Procedures for the Small Bowel Series and Barium Enema

1. D. All of the above
2. A. 3
   B. 8
   C. 1
   D. 4
   E. 2
   F. 6
   G. 5
   H. 7
3. A. 3
   B. 5
   C. 1
   D. 4
   E. 2
4. D. All of the above
5. D. Nuclear medicine
6. B. Proximal small intestine
7. A. Possible perforated hollow viscus
   B. Large bowel obstruction
8. Young and dehydrated
9. 2 cups or 16 ounces
10. When the contrast medium passes through the ileocecal valve
11. 2 hours
12. 15 to 30 minutes after ingesting the contrast medium
13. True
14. False (24 hours)
15. Double-contrast method
16. Regional enteritis (Crohn's disease) and malabsorption syndromes
17. High-density barium sulfate and air or methylcellulose
18. A. Duodenojejunal flexure (suspensory ligament)
19. C. Therapeutic intubation
20. NPO for at least 8 hours before procedure; no smoking or gum chewing
21. Prone. To separate the loops of bowel
22. A. 4
    B. 2
    C. 6
    D. 5
    E. 3
    F. 1
23. Infants
24. Diverticulosis
25. C. Volvulus
26. A. Ulcerative colitis
27. False
28. A. Gross bleeding
    B. Severe diarrhea
    C. Obstruction
    D. Inflammatory lesions
29. True
30. False (castor oil is an irritant cathartic)
31. True
32. A. Plastic disposable
    B. Rectal retention
    C. Air-contrast retention
33. Room temperature (85 to 90 degrees)
34. B. Lidocaine
35. Sims position
36. C. Umbilicus
37. B. Double contrast barium enema
38. C. Evacuative proctogram
39. C. Rectal prolapse
40. C. Anorectal angle
41. D. Lateral
42. True
43. False (not more than 24 in. (60 cm) above tabletop when beginning the procedure)
44. True
45. True

Review Exercise C: Postioning of the Lower Gastrointestinal System

1. B. High gonadal dose and difficult position for patients
2. AP or PA axial (butterfly)
3. Ventral decubitus
4. C. 2 inches (5 cm) above iliac crest
5. 100 to 125 kVp
6. Make exposure on expiration
7. Hour
8. A. All three chambers
9. B. 30 to 50 mrad
10. A. Hypersthenic
11. RAO or LPO

12. 35 to 45°
13. RPO
14. B. Lateral
15. Left lateral decubitus
16. Level of ASIS at the midcoronal plane
17. False (generally should not be removed until after overhead filming is completed unless directed to do so by the radiologist)
18. Rectosigmoid segment
19. Creates less superimposition of the rectosigmoid segments
20. A. Butterfly projections
    B. AP: CR angled 30 to 40° cephalad C. PA: CR 30 to 40° caudad
21. Right lateral decubitus (left side up)
22. B. Coffee or hot tea
23. 80 to 90 kVp
24. A. 100 to 125 kVp
    B. 80 to 90 kVp

Review Exercise D: Problem Solving for Technical and Positioning Errors

1. PA prone. Since the transverse colon is an intraperitoneal aspect of the large intestine located more anteriorly, it will fill with barium in the PA prone position.

2. Even with the use of a compensating filter, a reduction in kVp is required. Since less barium sulfate is used during an air-contrast procedure, the kVp range should be 80 to 90.
3. The CR was angled in the wrong direction. The AP axial projection requires a 30 to 40° cephalad angle.
4. Use two 14 x 17 in. (35 x 43 cm) crosswise cassettes for the AP/PA and oblique projections, one centered higher and one lower. Since hypersthenic patients have a wider distribution of the large intestine, two crosswise-placed cassettes will ensure that all of the pertinent anatomy is demonstrated.
5. Retention catheters should only be fully inflated by the radiologist under fluoroscopic control.
6. Lay on left side and flex head and upper body forward, drawing the right leg up above the partially flexed left leg.
7. Enteroclysis, a double-contrast small bowel procedure. A basic small bowel series may also demonstrate this condition, but the enteroclysis with double contrast is more effective in demonstrating mucosal changes.

8. Since the patient is having surgery soon after the small bowel series, a water-soluble, iodinated contrast media should be used. Barium sulfate should not be given to presurgical patients.
9. A diagnostic, intubation small bowel series would be preferred. A nasogastric tube would be passed into the small intestine, allowing the contrast media to be instilled. This procedure is effective for patients who can't swallow.
10. A barium enema or air enema often leads to re-expansion of the telescoped aspect of the large intestine (see textbook, p. 659).
11. Inform the radiologist and have him or her insert it under fluoroscopy guidance
12. RAO or LPO projections
13. A small bowel series (enteritis is an inflammation or infection of the small intestine)
14. An upper GI, small bowel combination series (gastroenteritis is an inflammation or infection of both the stomach and small intestine)
15. An acute abdominal series and a barium enema to rule out a possible large bowel obstruction. (Barium by mouth is contraindicated with a possible large bowel obstruction.)

SELF-TEST

My Score = _____%

Directions: This self-test should be taken only after completing all of the readings, review exercises, and laboratory activities for a particular section.   The purpose of this test is not only to provide a good learning exercise but also to serve as a good indicator of what your final evaluation grade will be. It is strongly suggested that if you do not get at least a 90% to 95% grade on each self-test, you should review those areas in which you missed questions before going to your instructor for the final evaluation exam for this chapter. (There are 78 questions or blanks—each is worth 1.3 points.)

1.   During life, how long is the entire small intestine?

A. 15 to 18 feet (4.5 to 5.5 meters)   C.   5 to 10 feet (1.5 to 3 meters)

B.   20 to 25 feet (6 to 7.5 meters)   D.   30 to 40 feet (9 to 12 meters)

2.   Which aspect of the small intestine is considered the longest?

A.   Duodenum   C.   Ileum

B.   Jejunum   D.   Cecum

3.   What is the name for the band of muscular tissue found at the junction of the duodenum and jejunum?

A.   Valvulae conniventes   C.   Duodenal flexure

B.   Haustra   D.   Suspensory ligament of the duodenum

4.   Which aspect of the small intestine possesses the smallest diameter?

A.   Ileum   C.   Cecum

B.   Duodenum   D.   Jejunum

5.   The part of the intestine with a "feathery" and "coiled spring" appearance when filled with barium is the:

A.   Ileum   C.   Jejunum

B.   Duodenum   D.   Cecum

6.   List the two aspects of the large intestine not considered part of the colon.

A.   _____   B.   _____

7.   What is another term for the appendix ? _____

8.   True/False: The rectum possesses two anteroposterior curves that have a direct impact on rectal enema tip insertions.

9.   True/False: The small sacculations found within the jejunum are called *haustra*.

10.   Which colic flexure (right or left) is located 1 to 2 inches (2.5 to 5 cm) higher or more superior in the abdomen?

_____

11. Identify the labeled structures on the following radiographs (Fig. 15-5 and Fig. 15-6). Include secondary names where indicated by parentheses.

Fig.15-5:

A. _____

B. _____

C. _____

D. _____

E. _____

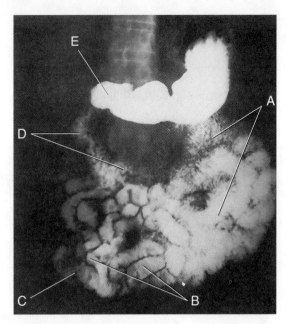

Fig. 15-5 Structure identification on a gastrointestinal radiograph.

Fig.15-6:

F. _____ (_____) _____

G. _____

H. _____

I. _____

J. _____

K. _____

L. _____ (_____) _____

M. _____

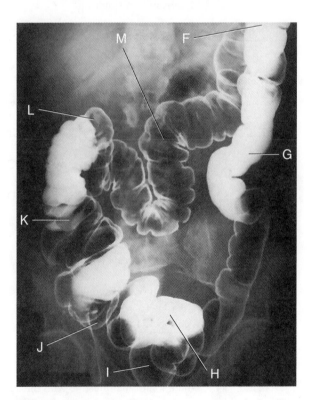

Fig. 15-6 Structure identification on a gastrointestinal radiograph.

12. Which one of the following structures is considered to be most anterior?

A. Cecum   C. Transverse colon

B. Rectum   D. Ascending colon

13. Where does the reabsorption of inorganic salts occur in the gastrointestinal tract?

    A. Duodenum   C. Stomach

    B. Large intestine   D. Jejunum

14. Which one of the following digestive movements occurs in the small intestine?

    A. Haustral churning   C. Mass peristalsis

    B. Rhythmic segmentation   D. Mastication

15. Match the following pathologic indications to their correct definition:

    _____ 1. Meckel's diverticulum   A. Telescoping of the bowel into another

    _____ 2. Diverticulosis   B. A new growth extending from mucosal wall

    _____ 3. Enteritis   C. A twisting of the intestine on its own mesentery

    _____ 4. Whipple's Disease   D. Caused by an outpouching of the intestinal wall

    _____ 5. Polyp   E. Chronic inflammatory condition of small intestine

    _____ 6. Malabsorption syndrome   F. Outpouching located in distal ileum

    _____ 7. Diverticulitis   G. Unable to process certain nutrients

    _____ 8. Volvulus   H. May be caused by cutting off blood supply to it or infection

    _____ 9. Intussusception   I. Inflammation of the small intestine

    _____ 10. Regional enteritis   J. Inflammation of small herniations in the intestinal wall

    _____ 11. Ulcerative colitis   K. Caused by a flagellate protozoan

    _____ 12. Giardiasis   L. Disorder of proximal small intestine

    _____ 13. Appendicitis   M. Chronic inflammatory condition of the large intestine

16. Match the following radiographic appearances to the correct pathologic indication:

    _____ 1. A tapered or corkscrew appearance seen during a barium enema   A. Ulcerative colitis

    _____ 2. Apple-core lesion   B. Diverticulosis

    _____ 3. String sign   C. Intussusception

    _____ 4. Dilatation of the intestine with thickening of the circular folds   D. Volvulus

    _____ 5. Stovepipe appearance of colon   E. Regional enteritis

    _____ 6. Mushroom-shaped dilatation with a small amount of barium
             passing beyond it   F. Polyp

                                                                                  G. Neoplasm
    _____ 7. Jagged or sawtooth appearance of the intestinal mucosa

                                                                                  H. Giardiasis
    _____ 8. Inward growth from intestinal wall

17. Which of the following imaging modalities/procedures is performed to diagnose an intussusception?

    A. Barium enema   C. Nuclear medicine scan

    B. Enteroclysis   D. CT

18. True/False: The barium enema is recommended to diagnose appendicitis.

19. What breathing instructions should be given to the patient during insertion of the enema tip?

    _____

20. Why is the PA rather than an AP position recommended for a small bowel series?

    _____

21. What is the minimum amount of time a patient needs to remain NPO before a small bowel series?

    _____

22. What is another term for a laxative? _____

23. Which type of rectal enema tip is ideal for the patient with a relaxed anal sphincter? _____

24. What is the name of the drug that can be given to help control spasm during a barium enema?

    _____

25. What drug can be added to the barium sulfate mixture to minimize spasm during a barium enema?

    _____

26. Which one of the following pathologic indications is best diagnosed during an evacuative proctogram?

    A. Regional enteritis   C. Volvulus

    C. Diverticulosis   D. Prolapse of rectum

27. Which region of the large intestine must be visualized during an evacuative proctogram study?

    A. Cecum   C. Ileocecal valve

    B. Anorectal angle   D. Left colic flexure

28. True/False: A small balloon retention catheter may be placed within the stoma of the colostomy to deliver contrast media during a barium enema.

29. Which oblique position, the LAO or RAO, best demonstrates the ascending colon and cecum? _____

30. What is the average length of time in a routine small bowel series for the barium to reach the large intestine?

    _____

31. Which one of the following commercial contrast media would be used during an evaluative proctogram?

    A. Hypaque   C. Gastroview

    B. Gastrographin   D. Anatrast

32. Which ionization chambers should be activated for a lateral barium enema projection of the rectum?

    A. All three chambers   C. Center chamber only

    B. Right and left upper chambers   D. Right upper chamber only

33. How much obliquity of the body is required for the LAO barium enema projection? _____

34. The CR and film should be centered about _____ higher for the 15- or 30-minute small bowel image than for the later images.

35. The term *evacuative proctography* is sometimes used for a lower GI tract procedure may also be commonly called

    _____ .

36. A patient is unable to lie prone on the radiographic table during a barium enema. Which specific position will best

    demonstrate the right colic flexure? _____

37. **Situation:** A patient is scheduled for an air-contrast barium enema. During the fluoroscopy phase of the study, the radiologist detects a possible polyp in the lower descending colon. Which specific position will best demonstrate this region of the colon?

    _____

    _____

38. **Situation:** A patient with a clinical history of a rectocele comes to the radiology department. Which radiographic procedure will best diagnose this condition?

    _____

39. True/False: A PA axial oblique (RAO) barium enema projection is an optional projection to demonstrate the right colic flexure.

40. True/False: On a hypersthenic-type patient, a 35 x 43 cm (14 x 17 inches) film placed lengthwise centered correctly will generally include the entire barium-filled large intestine on one film.

41. True/False: The female gonadal dose for a lateral barium enema projection is approximately 15 to 20 times greater than for a lateral decubitus (AP) projection.

42. The skin dose range for a lateral rectum position on an average size patient is:

    A. 50 to 100 mrad   C. 500 to 1000 mrad

    B. 200 to 400 mrad   D. 2000 to 3000 mrad

43. A. The RAO position best demonstrates the _____ (right or left) colic flexure with the

       CR and image receptor centered to the level of _____ .

    B. The LAO position best demonstrates the _____ (right or left) colic flexure with the CR

       and image receptor centered to the level of _____ .

CHAPTER 16

Gallbladder and Biliary Ducts

CHAPTER OBJECTIVES

After you have completed **all** the activities of this chapter, you will be able to:

_____ 1. Identify specific anatomy and functions of the liver, gallbladder, and biliary ductal system.

_____ 2. Describe the production, storage, and purpose of bile.

_____ 3. On drawings and radiographs, identify specific anatomy of the biliary system.

_____ 4. Describe the impact of body habitus on the position of the gallbladder.

_____ 5. Define specific terms related to conditions and procedures of the biliary system.

_____ 6. Define specific pathologies of the biliary system.

_____ 7. Match specific biliary pathologies to the correct radiographic appearances and signs.

_____ 8. Identify special and alternative radiographic procedures of the biliary system.

_____ 9. List the advantages of ultrasound of the gallbladder as compared to the oral cholecystogram.

_____ 10. List information related to the operative, percutaneous transhepatic, T-tube, and laproscopic cholangiogram and endoscopic retrograde cholangiopancreatogram procedures, including purpose of study, contraindications, imaging, and post-procedure care.

_____ 11. List information related to the basic and special projections for an oral cholecystogram, including size and type of image receptor, central ray location, direction and angulation of the central ray, and anatomy best visualized.

_____ 12. Identify the patient dose ranges for skin, midline, and gonads for various oral cholecystogram projections.

_____ 13. Given various hypothetical situations, identify the correct modification of a position and/or exposure factors to improve the radiographic image.

POSITIONING AND FILM CRITIQUE

_____ 1. Using a peer, position for basic and special projections for an oral cholecystogram procedure.

_____ 2. Critique and evaluate oral cholecystogram and cholangiogram radiographs based on the four divisions of radiographic criteria: (1) structures shown, (2) position, (3) collimation and CR, and (4) exposure criteria.

_____ 3. Distinguish between acceptable and unacceptable biliary study radiographs resulting from exposure factors, motion, collimation, positioning, or other errors.

Learning Exercises

Complete the following review exercises after reading the associated pages in the textbook as indicated by each exercise. Answers to each review exercise are given at the end of the review exercises.

PART I: Radiographic Anatomy

Review Exercise A: Radiographic Anatomy of the Gallbladder and Biliary System (see textbook pp. 520-522)

1. What is the average weight of the adult human liver? _____

2. Which abdominal quadrant contains the gallbladder? _____

3. What is the name of the soft tissue structure that separates the right from the left lobe of the liver?

   _____

4. Which lobe of the liver is larger, the right or left? _____

5. List the other two lobes of the liver (in addition to right and left lobes):

   A. _____   B. _____

6. True/False: The liver performs over 100 functions.

7. True/False: The average healthy adult liver produces 1 gallon, or 3000 to 4000 ml, of bile per day.

8. List the three primary functions of the gallbladder:

   A. _____

   B. _____

   C. _____

9. What is the name of the hormone that causes the gallbladder to contract? _____

10. True/False: The hormone identified in question 9 is secreted by the liver.

11. True/False: Concentrated levels of cholesterol in bile may lead to gallstones.

12. What is a common site for impaction, or lodging, of gallstones? _____

13. True/False: In about 40% of individuals, the hepatopancreatic ampulla is totally separated into two ducts rather than the one enlarged ampulla.

14. True/False: An older term for the main pancreatic duct is *the duct of Vater.*

15. The gallbladder is located more (posteriorly or anteriorly) within the abdomen? _____

16. Match the following structures to their primary location within the abdomen.

    _____ 1. Liver   A. Near midsagittal plane

    _____ 2. Gallbladder on asthenic patient   B. To left of midsagittal plane

    _____ 3. Gallbladder on hypersthenic patient   C. To right of midsagittal plane

    _____ 4. Gallbladder on hyposthenic patient

17. Identify the major components of the gallbladder and the biliary system on Fig. 16-1:

    A. _____

    B. _____

    C. _____

    D. _____

    E. _____

    F. _____

    G. _____

    H. _____

    I. _____

    J. _____

    K. _____

    L. _____

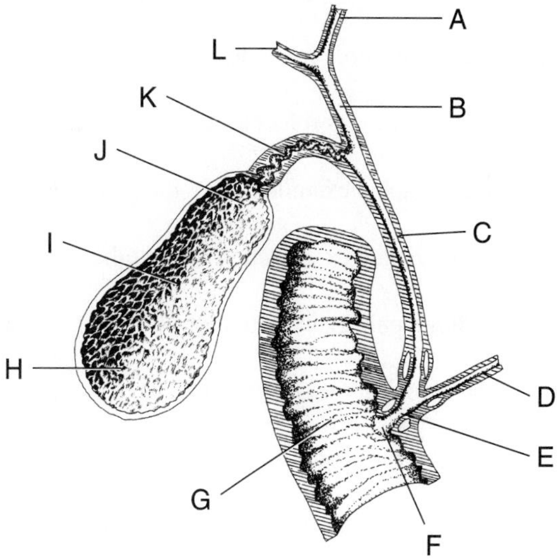

Fig. 16-1 Components of the gallbladder and biliary system.

18. Identify the labeled structures on this sagittal view of the abdomen (Fig. 16-2):

    A. _____

    B. _____

    C. _____

    D. _____

    E. _____

    F. _____

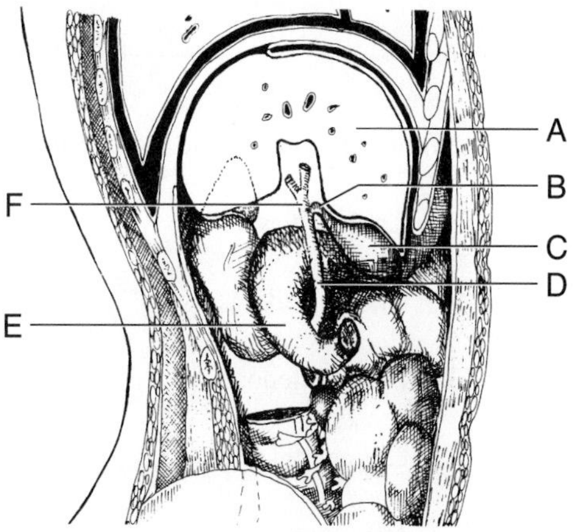

Fig. 16-2 Lateral, cut-away view of components of the gallbladder and biliary system.

19. What position should the patient be placed in if the primary purpose is to drain the gallbladder into the duct system?

_____

20. Which projection (AP or PA) would place the gallbladder closest to the image receptor for the best visualization?

_____

21. Which radiographic oblique position will project the gallbladder away from the spine? _____

PART II: Radiographic Positioning

REVIEW EXERCISE B: Radiographic Procedures and Positioning of the Gallbladder and Biliary Ducts (see textbook pp. 523-538)

1. The prefix *chole* refers to _____ .

2. The prefix *cysto* refers to _____ .

3. Radiographic examination of the gallbladder is called _____ .

4. Radiographic examination of the biliary ducts is called _____ .

5. Radiographic examination of both the gallbladder and biliary ducts is called _____ .

6. The acronym *OCG* refers to _____ .

7. Oral types of contrast media designed to visualize the gallbladder are called _____ .

8. List the three biliary functions measured during an OCG

   A. _____

   B. _____

   C. _____

9. In addition to hypersensitivity to iodinated compounds, what are the three other contraindications for an OCG?

   A. _____   C. _____

   B. _____

10. Match the following pathologic indications with their correct definition:

   _____ 1. Cholelithiasis   A. Defects present at birth

   _____ 2. Cholecystitis   B. Emulsion of biliary stones

   _____ 3. Biliary stenosis   C. Condition of having gallstones

   _____ 4. Congenital anomalies   D. Inflammation of the gallbladder

   _____ 5. Neoplasm   E. Benign or malignant tumors

   _____ 6. Milk calcium bile   F. Narrowing of the biliary ducts

11. True/False: Most gallstones contain enough calcium to be at least minimally visualized on a plain abdomen radiograph.

12. True/False: Chronic cholecystitis is usually associated with gallstones.

13. True/False: Acute cholecystitis may produce a thickened gallbladder wall.

14. True/False: A nonvisualized gallbladder is always the result of a pathologic condition.

15. True/False: The patient must take laxatives 8 hours before an OCG to ensure that the colon is free of feces, which may obscure the gallbladder.

16. True/False: The evening meal before an OCG should contain a slight amount of fat.

17. True/False: Most disorders of the gallbladder and biliary duct are caused by gallstones.

18. How many hours before an OCG should the cholecystopaques be taken? _____

19. What is the optimal kVp range for an OCG? _____

20. What five questions should a patient be asked before taking the cholecystogram scout?

    A. _____

    B. _____

    C. _____

    D. _____

    E. (Female) _____

21. What is the purpose of the fatty meal or CCK study? _____

22. List four advantages of a gallbladder ultrasound instead of the conventional OCG:

    A. _____

    B. _____

    C. _____

    D. _____

23. What special imaging equipment is required if the surgeon desires a real-time image during an operative cholangiogram?

    _____

24. Why will the surgeon sometimes dilute the contrast media with saline before an operative cholangiogram?

    _____

25. List the three advantages to a laparoscopic cholangiogram as compared to the conventional operative cholangiogram:

    A. _____

    B. _____

    C. _____

26. Postoperative (T-tube) cholangiograms are generally performed in (surgery or in the radiology department)

    _____.

27. Which one of the following procedures may be performed during a postoperative (T-tube) cholangiogram?

    A. Remove the gallbladder   C. Remove a biliary stone

    B. Remove a liver cyst   D. Catheterize the hepatic portal vein

28. Which one of the following clinical conditions is best suited for a percutaneous cholangiogram (PTC)?

    A. Obstructive jaundice   C. Liver hemorrhage

    B. Ascites   D. Cholelithiasis

29. Why is a chest radiograph commonly ordered following a PTC? _____

30. Which one of the following is not an expected risk associated with a PTC?

    A. Liver hemorrhage   C. Escape of bile

    B. Pneumothorax   D. Cholecystitis

31. A radiographic procedure of examining the biliary and main pancreatic ducts is called a(n):

    A. (write out full term) _____

    B. What initials are commonly used for this procedure? _____

    C. What type of special endoscope is commonly used for this procedure? _____

    D. Which member of the health care team usually performs this procedure? _____

    E. Why should a patient remain NPO at least 1 hour following this procedure? _____

32. Match the following biliary procedures with the means of introducing the contrast media during these procedures:

    _____ 1. ERCP   A. Direct injection through a catheter placed during an endoscopic process

    _____ 2. PTC   B. No contrast media required

    _____ 3. T-tube cholangiogram   C. Oral ingestion

    _____ 4. Immediate cholangiogram   D. Direct injection by a needle

    _____ 5. OCG   E. Direct injection through indwelling drainage tube puncture

    _____ 6. Cholecystosonography   F. Direct injection through catheter during surgery

33. True/False: Conditions such as sickle cell anemia may produce gallstones in pediatric patients

34. True/False: A HIDA nuclear medicine scan is intended to diagnose cirrhosis of the liver.

35. Which imaging modality/procedure is recommended for a gallbladder study on a pediatric patient?

    A. OCG   C. MRI

    B. Sonography   D. CT

36. True/False: Gallbladder projections result in approximately equal amounts of gonadal dose for males and females.

37. True/False: The right upper AEC pickup cell is recommended for gallbladder projections.

38. The gallbladder is usually found on the sthenic patient at the level of _____ .

    A. T12   B. L4   C. T10   D. L2

39. Centering for a PA scout projection on a hypersthenic patient is usually _____ as compared with a sthenic patient.

    A. Lower and more midline   C. Higher and midline

    B. About the same location   D. Higher and more lateral

40. Which oblique position will project the gallbladder away from the spine? _____

41. How much obliquity is required for this projection taken on (A) an asthenic patient? _____

    (B) a hypersthenic patient? _____

42. Which two possible positions during an OCG will stratify any possible gallstones? _____

43. Which specific decubitus position should be performed to demonstrate possible stratification (layering out) of gall-

    stones? _____

44. What is the gonadal dose given to a female patient with a decubitus projection during an OCG?

    A. Not measurable   C. 50 to 100 mrad

    B. 5 to 10 mrad   D. 200 to 400 mrad

45. How much lower should centering be for an erect gallbladder projection as compared with a recumbent projection?

    _____

REVIEW EXERCISE C: Problem Solving for Technical and Positioning Errors (see textbook pp. 523-538)

1. **Situation:** An asthenic-type patient comes to the radiology department for an oral cholecystogram. The PA scout film fails to reveal the location of the gallbladder. The following factors were used during the initial exposure: 10 x 12 lengthwise cassette, 70 kVp, 30 mAs, 40 in. (102 cm) SID, Bucky, CR centered to the level of L2. Which of these factors can be modified to increase the chances of locating the gallbladder?

    _____

    _____

2. **Situation:** A radiograph of a PA scout projection for the gallbladder reveals that the gallbladder is only faintly visible. The patient assures the technologist that she had taken all the required tablets. The following factors were used during the exposure: 85 kVp, AEC with center cell, Bucky, CR centered to the level of L2. Which of these factors can be modified to improve the visibility of the gallbladder?

    _____

3. **Situation:** A radiograph of an LAO projection reveals that the gallbladder is superimposed over the spine. What type of positioning modification is needed to prevent this superimposition during the repeat exposure?

    _____

    _____

4. **Situation:** During an operative cholangiogram, the resultant radiograph reveals that the biliary ducts are superimposed over the spine. As requested by the surgeon, the initial projection was taken AP in the supine position. What can be done to shift the biliary ducts away from the spine during the repeat exposure?

    _____

    _____

5. **Situation:** A patient with right upper quadrant pain enters the emergency room. The physician is concerned about gallstones, but the patient states that he is hypersensitive to iodine. Which procedure of the biliary system would be ideal for this patient?

    _____

    _____

6. **Situation:** A patient with signs of obstructive jaundice enters the emergency room. The patient's skin has a yellow tinge to it. Which radiographic study of the biliary system would be recommended for this patient?

    _____

    _____

7. **Situation:** During an OCG, the patient's gallbladder is well-visualized with contrast media. But the radiologist is concerned about the function of the gallbladder. Which particular study would evaluate the function of the gallbladder?

    _____

    _____

8. **Situation:** A patient who may have a stone in the main pancreatic duct enters the emergency room. Which procedure would be ideal to demonstrate this duct and determine if a stone is present?

    _____

    _____

9. **Situation:** A patient with a history of acute cholecystitis comes to the radiology department for an OCG. The scout image does not demonstrate an opacified gallbladder. What other procedure (s) can be ordered to visualize the gallbladder and biliary ducts?

    _____

    _____

10. **Situation:** A patient who may have a neoplasm of the gallbladder comes to the radiology department. Which imaging modalities or procedures would best diagnose this condition?

    _____

    _____

PART III: Laboratory Exercises (see textbook pp. 533-538)

Although it is impossible to duplicate many aspects of biliary studies on a phantom in the lab, evaluation of actual radiographs and physical positioning is possible. You can get experience in positioning and radiographic evaluation of these projections by performing exercises using radiographic phantoms and practicing on other students (although you will not be taking actual exposures). Technologists must learn the positioning routine, room setup, and fluoroscopy procedure for their particular facility.

LABORATORY EXERCISE A: Radiographic Evaluation

Using actual radiographs of OCG and cholangiogram procedures provided by your instructor, evaluate and critique each position for the following points.   (Check off when completed.):

_____   Evaluate the completeness of the study. (Are all of the pertinent anatomic structures included on the radiograph?)

_____   Evaluate for positioning or centering errors (e.g., rotation, off centering)

_____   Evaluate for correct exposure factors and possible motion. (Is the contrast media properly penetrated?)

_____   Determine whether patient obliquity is correct for specific positions.

_____   Determine whether markers and an acceptable degree of collimation and/or area shielding are visible on the images.

LABORATORY EXERCISE B: Physical Positioning

On another person, simulate performing all basic and special projections of an OCG as follows.   (Check off each when completed satisfactorily.) Include the following six steps as described in the textbook.

Step 1.   Appropriate size and type of image receptor with correct markers
Step 2.   Correct CR placement and centering of part to CR and/or image receptor
Step 3.   Accurate collimation
Step 4.   Area shielding of patient where advisable
Step 5.   Use of proper immobilizing devices when needed
Step 6.   Approximate correct exposure factors, breathing instructions where applicable, and "making" exposure

Projections	Step 1	Step 2	Step 3	Step 4	Step 5	Step 6
• PA scout	_____	_____	_____	_____	_____	_____
• LAO	_____	_____	_____	_____	_____	_____
• Right lateral decubitus	_____	_____	_____	_____	_____	_____
• PA erect	_____	_____	_____	_____	_____	_____

Optional:

• RPO for biliary ducts	_____	_____	_____	_____	_____	_____

Answers to Review Exercises

Review Exercise A: Radiographic Anatomy of the Gallbladder and Biliary System

1. 3 to 4 pounds (1.5 kg) or $\frac{1}{60}$ of total body weight
2. Right upper quadrant
3. Falciform ligament
4. Right
5. A. Quadrate
   B. Caudate
6. True
7. False (1 qt or 800 to 1000 ml)
8. A. Store bile
   B. Concentrate bile
   C. Contract to release bile into duodenum
9. Cholecystokinin (CCK)
10. False (by the duodenal mucosa)
11. True
12. Duodenal papilla
13. True
14. False (duct of Wirsung)
15. Anteriorly
16. 1. C, 2. A, 3. C, 4. C
17. A. Left hepatic duct
    B. Common hepatic duct
    C. Common bile duct
    D. Pancreatic duct
    E. Hepatopancreatic ampulla (ampulla of Vater)
    F. Duodenal papilla
    G. Duodenum
    H. Fundus of gallbladder
    I. Body of gallbladder
    J. Neck of gallbladder
    K. Cystic duct
    L. Right hepatic duct
18. A. Liver
    B. Cystic duct
    C. Gallbladder
    D. Common bile duct
    E. Duodenum
    F. Common hepatic duct
19. Supine
20. PA
21. LAO

Review Exercise B: Radiographic Procedures and Positioning of the Gallbladder and Biliary Ducts

1. Bile
2. Bladder or sac
3. Cholecystography
4. Cholangiography
5. Cholecystocholangiography
6. Oral cholecystogram
7. Cholecystopaques
8. A. Functional ability of the liver to remove contrast media
   B. Patency and condition of the biliary ducts
   C. Concentrating and contracting ability of the gallbladder
9. A. Advanced hepatorenal disease
   B. Active gastrointestinal disease
   C. Pregnancy
10. 1. C, 2. D, 3. F, 4. A, 5. E, 6. B
11. False (only about 15 % are visualized)
12. True
13. True
14. False (may be other reasons)
15. False (only NPO 8 hrs)
16. True
17. True
18. 10 to 12 hours before the procedure
19. 70 to 80 kVp
20. A. How many pills were taken and at what time?
    B. Any reaction from the pills?
    C. Did you have breakfast?
    D. Do you still have your gallbladder?
    E. Is there a possibility of pregnancy?
21. Measure the function of the gallbladder
22. A. No ionizing radiation
    B. Better detection of small calculi
    C. No contrast media is required
    D. Is a less time-consuming procedure
23. Mobile digital C-arm fluoroscopy
24. Reduce the risk of spasm of the biliary ducts
25. A. It can be performed as an outpatient procedure
    B. It is a less invasive procedure
    C. Reduced hospital time and cost
26. In the radiology department
27. C. Remove a biliary stone
28. A. Obstructive jaundice
29. Rule out a possible pneumothorax
30. D. Cholecystitis
31. A. Endoscopic retrograde cholangiopancreatogram
    B. ERCP
    C. Duodenoscope or video endoscope
    D. Gastroenterologist
    E. Prevent aspiration of food or liquid into the lungs
32. 1. A, 2. D, 3. E, 4. F, 5. C, 6. B
33. True
34. False (HIDA scans are a study of the gallbladder and biliary ducts)
35. B. Sonography
36. False (female ≈6 mrad; males 0.1 mrad)
37. False (the center cell should be used)
38. D. L2
39. D. Higher and more lateral
40. LAO (or RPO if the patient cannot lie supine)
41. A. 40°
    B. 15°
42. Erect or right lateral decubitus
43. Right lateral decubitus (PA)
44. B. 5 to 10 mrad
45. 1 to 2 in (2.5 to 5 cm)

Review Exercise C: Problem Solving for Technical and Positioning Errors

1. Center the CR lower and more midline for an asthenic patient. Also, using a 14 x 17 in. (35 x 43 cm) cassette for the scout, instead of a 10 x 12 in. (24 x 30 cm), will provide greater coverage of the abdomen.
2. Lower the kVp to the 70 to 76 range
3. Increase obliquity to project the gallbladder away from the spine
4. Request that the patient be rotated into a 15 to 25° RPO position
5. Ultrasound of the gallbladder. It does not require any contrast media
6. Percutaneous transhepatic cholangiogram (PTC) (The PTC may also be preceded by an ultrasound study.)
7. Fatty meal or CCK study
8. ERCP
9. Sonography or nuclear medicine-HIDA scan
10. Sonography or computed tomography

SELF-TEST

Directions: This self-test should be taken only after completing **all** of the readings, review exercises, and laboratory activities for a particular section. The purpose of this test is not only to provide a good learning exercise but also to serve as a good indicator of what your final evaluation grade will be. It is strongly suggested that if you do not get at least a 90% to 95% grade on each self-test, you should review those areas in which you missed questions **before** going to your instructor for the final evaluation exam for this chapter. (There are 70 questions or blanks—each is worth 1.4 points.)

1. The gallbladder is located in the _____ margin of the liver.

    A. Anterior inferior   C. Mid aspect

    B. Posterior superior   D. Anterior superior

2. Which one of the following is **not** a major lobe of the liver?

    A. Caudate   C. Inferior

    B. Quadrate   D. Left

4. What is the name of the soft-tissue structure that divides the liver into left and right lobes?

    _____

5. What is the primary function of bile? _____

6. Which duct is formed by the union of the left and right hepatic ducts? _____

7. What is the average capacity of the gallbladder? _____

8. Which chemical process leads to concentration of bile within the gallbladder? _____

9. Which hormone leads to contraction of the gallbladder to release bile? _____

10. Which duct carries bile from the cystic duct to the duodenum? _____

11. Match the following biliary structures to their correct description or definition:

    _____ 1. Pancreatic duct   A. Series of mucosal folds in cystic duct

    _____ 2. Fundus   B. A protrusion into the duodenum

    _____ 3. Hepatopancreatic ampulla   C. Middle aspect of gallbladder

    _____ 4. Spiral valve   D. Duct connected directly to gallbladder

    _____ 5. Hepatopancreatic sphincter   E. Narrowest portion of gallbladder

    _____ 6. Duodenal papilla   F. Broadest portion of gallbladder

    _____ 7. Cystic duct   G. Enlarged chamber in distal aspect of common bile duct

    _____ 8. Neck   H. Duct of Wirsung

    _____ 9. Body   I. Circular muscle

12. Which general body position will encourage drainage of bile/contrast media from the gallbladder?

   _____

   Why? _____

13. Identify the labeled parts and/or structures on the radiograph of an OCG (Fig. 16-3) and of biliary ducts from two different operative cholangiogram procedures (Fig. 16-4).

   Fig.   16-3

   A. _____

   B. _____

   C. _____

   D. _____

   Fig. 16-4

   E. _____

   F. _____

   G. _____

   H. _____

   I. _____

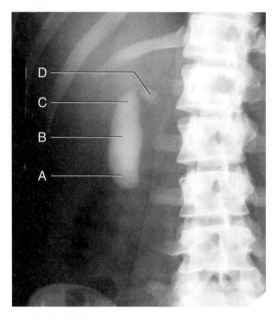

Fig. 16-3 Radiograph of an OCG and of biliary ducts.

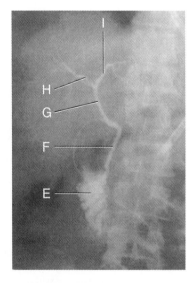

Fig. 16-4 Radiograph of an operative cholangiogram procedure.

14. Match the prefixes and terms on the left with the correct description on the right.

     _____ 1. Cysto-

     A. Radiographic study of gallbladder and biliary ducts

     _____ 2. Chole-

     B. Radiographic study of gallbladder

     _____ 3. Cholecystocholangiogram

     C. Radiographic study of biliary ducts

     _____ 4. Cholecystogram

     D. Condition of having gallstones

     _____ 5. Cholangiogram

     E. Inflammation of gallbladder

     _____ 6. Cholecystopaque

     F. Oral contrast media for gallbladder

     _____ 7. Cholecystitis

     G. OCG

     _____ 8. Oral cholecystogram

     H. Denotes sac or bladder

     _____ 9. Cholelithiasis

     I. Denotes bile

15. True/False: Drugs have been developed that will dissolve gallstones and may avoid the need to have surgery in select cases.

16. True/False: Gallbladders with acute cholecystitis rarely become radiopaque during an OCG.

17. Match the following pathologic indications with the correct definition and/or statement:

     _____ 1. Biliary stenosis

     A. Emulsion of biliary stones

     _____ 2. Congenital anomalies

     B. May be caused by bacterial infection or ischemia of the gallbladder

     _____ 3. Chronic cholecystitis

     C. Narrowing of one of the biliary ducts

     _____ 4. Choledocholithiasis

     D. Although benign, they may affect production, storage, or release of bile

     _____ 5. Acute cholecystitis

     E. Signs may include calcification of the gallbladder wall

     _____ 6. Milk calcium bile

     F. Approximately 80% of the patients with this condition have gallstones

     _____ 7. Carcinoma of gallbladder

     G. Stones in the biliary ducts

18. How long should a patient remain NPO before an OCG? _____

19. How far in advance should the oral contrast media be taken for an OCG? _____

20. Which kVp range is ideal for an OCG? _____

21. Why is a patient placed into the RPO position during a fatty meal or CCK procedure?

_____

22. How long does it take the gallbladder to begin to contract after an injection of CCK? _____

23. True/False: Ultrasound of the gallbladder requires that the patient be NPO for at least 8 hours before the study.

24. True/False: Ultrasound of the gallbladder is considered a noninvasive procedure.

25. How is the contrast media instilled into the biliary ducts during an operative cholangiogram?

    _____

26. On average, how much contrast media is injected during an operative cholangiogram?

    _____

27. What must the technologist do with respect to the grid-image receptor if the OR table is tilted during an operative

    cholangiogram? _____

    _____

28. Why is a laparoscopic cholecystectomy considered less invasive as compared with traditional cholecystectomy?

    _____

29. What is the most common clinical reason for performing a T-tube cholangiogram?

    _____

30. Which one of the following conditions is a pathologic indication for a percutaneous transhepatic cholangiogram
    (PTC)?
    A. Chronic cholecystitis   C. Neoplasm of the gallbladder
    B. Obstructive jaundice   D. Cholelithiasis

31. What type of needle is most often used for a PTC?
    A. 6-inch spinal needle   C. 18-gauge angiocath
    B. 18-gauge butterfly   D. Skinny needle

32. Match the following by indicating which procedure is performed in the operating room by a surgeon and which is per-
    formed in the radiology department by a radiologist.

    _____ A. T-tube cholangiogram   S. In operating room by a surgeon

    _____ B. Operative cholangiogram   R. In radiology department by a radiologist

    _____ C. Percutaneous transhepatic cholangiogram

33. True/False: An ERCP can be considered both a diagnostic and therapeutic procedure.

34. True/False: A percutaneous transhepatic cholangiogram (PTC) is generally performed in the radiology department
    and involves placing a needle through the liver directly into a biliary duct.

35. True/False: A pediatric patient with hemolytic anemia may develop gallstones.

36. True/False: A HIDA scan is a special MRI study of the liver using a contrast agent.

37. True/False: CT is an excellent imaging modality for demonstrating tumors of the liver, gallbladder, or pancreas.

38. Which ionization chamber needs to be activated for an LAO projection of the gallbladder?

    _____

39. What is the primary difference between the operative cholangiogram and the T-tube cholangiogram? (Both are performed to visualize possible choleliths.)

_____

_____

40. **Situation:** A radiograph of an LAO projection reveals that the gallbladder is superimposed over the spine. What modification is needed during the repeat exposure to avoid this problem?

_____

41. Why is the erect gallbladder projection preferred as a PA rather than an AP projection?

_____

42. **Situation:** During an OCG, the radiologist believes that stones may be present in the gallbladder. She requests that the technologist provide a projection to stratify any possible stones. Which two projections may accomplish this goal?

_____

43. **Situation:** A patient scheduled for an OCG complains that she can't lie prone or on her right side due to recent surgery. Which position could be performed to ensure that the gallbladder will not be superimposed over the spine?

_____

44. **Situation:** A patient with a history of possible gallstones is scheduled for an OCG. During the patient interview, she states that she had a piece of bacon before coming into the hospital. When the scout image is taken, the gallbladder is not visualized. What other imaging options can the radiologist order to determine if there are gallbladder stones?

_____

45. Which one of the following studies is considered an invasive procedure?

    A. OCG   C. Sonography of the gallbladder
    B. CT of the gallbladder   D. PTC

CHAPTER 17

Urinary System

CHAPTER OBJECTIVES

After you have completed **all** the activities of this chapter, you will be able to:

_____ 1. Identify the location and pertinent anatomy of the urinary system to include the adrenal glands.

_____ 2. Identify specific structures of the macroscopic and microscopic anatomy and physiology of the kidney.

_____ 3. Identify the orientation of the kidneys, ureters and urinary bladder with respect to the peritoneum and other structures of the abdomen.

_____ 4. List the primary functions of the urinary system.

_____ 5. Describe the spatial relationship between the male and female reproductive system and the urinary system.

_____ 6. On drawings and radiographs, identify specific anatomy of the urinary system

_____ 7. Identify key lab values and drug concerns that must be verified prior to intravenous injections of contrast media.

_____ 8. Identify characteristics specific to either ionic or nonionic contrast media.

_____ 9. Differentiate between mild, moderate, and severe reactions and from side effects to injected contrast media. List several examples of each.

_____ 10. Identify the steps and safety measures to be observed during a venipuncture procedure.

_____ 11. List safety measures to be followed before and during the injection of an iodinated contrast media.

_____ 12. Define specific urinary pathologic terminology and indications.

_____ 13. Match specific types of urinary pathology to the correct radiographic appearances and signs.

_____ 14. List the purpose, contraindications, and six high-risk patient conditions for intravenous urography.

_____ 15. Identify two methods utilized to enhance pelvicalyceal filling during intravenous urography and contraindications for their use.

_____ 16. Identify the purpose of the nephrogram and nephrotomogram.

_____ 17. Identify specific aspects related to the retrograde urogram and how this procedure differs from an intravenous urogram.

_____ 18. Identify specific aspects related to the retrograde cystogram.

_____ 19. Identify specific aspects related to the retrograde urethrogram.

_____ 20. List specific information related to the basic and special projections for excretory urography, retrograde urography, cystography, urethrography, and voiding cystourethrography to include size and type of image receptor, central ray location, direction and angulation of central ray, and anatomy best visualized.

_____ 21. Identify the patient dose ranges for skin, midline, and gonads for specific urinary system projections.

_____ 22 Given various hypothetical situations, identify the correct modification of a position and/or exposure factors to improve the radiographic image.

POSITIONING AND FILM CRITIQUE

_____ 1. Using a peer, position for basic and special projections for an intravenous urogram procedure.

_____ 2. Critique and evaluate urinary study radiographs based on the four divisions of radiographic criteria: (1) structures shown, (2) position, (3) collimation and CR, and (4) exposure criteria.

_____ 3. Distinguish between acceptable and unacceptable urinary study radiographs due to exposure factors, motion, collimation, positioning, or other errors.

Learning Exercises

Complete the following review exercises after reading the associated pages in the textbook as indicated by each exercise. Answers to each review exercise are given at the end of the review exercises.

PART I: Radiographic Anatomy

REVIEW EXERCISE A: Radiographic Anatomy of the Urinary System (see textbook pp. 540-546)

1. The kidneys and ureters are located in the _____ space.

   A. Intraperitoneal   C. Extraperitoneal

   B. Infraperitoneal   D. Retroperitoneal

2. The _____ glands are located directly superior to the kidneys.

3. Which structures create a 20° angle of the upper pole of the kidney in relation to the lower pole?

   _____

4. What is the specific name for the mass of fat that surrounds each kidney? _____

5. What degree of rotation from supine is needed to place the kidneys parallel to the film?

   _____

6. Which two bony landmarks can be palpated to locate the kidneys? _____

7. Which term describes an abnormal drop of the kidneys when the patient is placed erect?

   _____

8. List the three functions of the urinary system.

   A. _____

   B. _____

   C. _____

9. A buildup of nitrogenous waste in the blood is called:

   A. Hemotoxicity   C. Sepsis

   B. Uremia   D. Renotoxicity

10. The longitudinal fissure, found along the central medial border of the kidney, is called the _____ .

11. The peripheral or outer portion of the kidney is called the _____ .

12. The term that describes the total functioning portion of the kidney is _____ .

13. The microscopic function and structural unit of the kidney is the _____ .

14. Which structure of the medulla is made up of a collection of tubules that drain into the minor calyx?

    _____

15. What is another name for the glomerular capsule? _____

16. True/False: The glomerular capsule and proximal and distal convoluted tubules are located in the medulla of the kidney.

17. True/False: The efferent arterioles carry blood to the glomeruli.

18. Identify the renal structures labeled on Fig. 17-1:

    A. _____

    B. _____

    C. _____

    D. _____

    E. _____

    F. _____

    G. _____

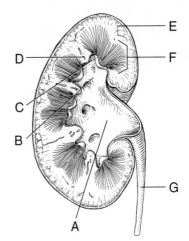

Fig. 17-1 Cross-section of a kidney.

19. Identify the structures making up a nephron and collecting duct (Fig. 17-2). With each structure, check whether it is located in the cortex or medulla portion of the kidney.

STRUCTURE	CORTEX	MEDULLA
A. _____	_____	_____
B. _____	_____	_____
C. _____	_____	_____
D. _____	_____	_____
E. _____	_____	_____
F. _____	_____	_____
G. _____	_____	_____
H. _____	_____	_____
I. _____	_____	_____

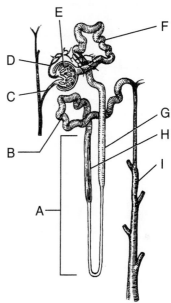

Fig. 17-2 Structures of a nephron and collecting duct.

20. Which two processes move urine through the ureters to the bladder?

    A. _____   B. _____

21. Which one of the following structures is located most anterior?

    A. Proximal ureters   C. Urinary bladder

    B. Kidneys   D. Suprarenal glands

22. What is the name of the junction found between the distal ureters and urinary bladder? _____

23. What is the name of the inner posterior region of the bladder formed by the two ureters entering and the urethra exiting?

    _____

24. What is the name of the small gland found just inferior to the male bladder? _____

25. The total capacity for the average adult bladder is:

    A. 100 to 200 milliliters   C. 350 to 500 milliliters

    B. 200 to 300 milliliters   D. 500 to 700 milliliters

26. Which one of the following structures is considered to be most posterior?

    A. Ovaries   C. Vagina

    B. Urethra   D. Kidneys

27. Identify the urinary structures labeled on Fig.17-3.

    A. _____

    B. _____

    C. _____

    D. _____

    E. _____

    F. _____

    G. _____

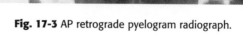

Fig. 17-3 AP retrograde pyelogram radiograph.

PART II: Radiographic Positioning, Contrast Media, and Pathology

REVIEW EXERCISE B: Contrast Media, Contrast Media Reactions, and Venipuncture (see textbook pp. 547-554)

1. List the two ways contrast media are administered in urography.

   A. _____   B. _____

2. The two major types of iodinated contrast media used for urography are ionic and nonionic. For each of the following characteristics, indicate which apply to ionic (I) and which to nonionic (N) contrast media:

   _____ 1. Uses a parent compound of a benzoic acid

   _____ 2. Will not significantly increase the osmolality of the blood plasma

   _____ 3. Incorporates sodium or meglumine to increase solubility of the contrast media

   _____ 4. Creates a hypertonic condition in the blood plasma

   _____ 5. Is more expensive

   _____ 6. Produces less severe reactions

   _____ 7. Is a near-isotonic solution

   _____ 8. Greater risk of disrupting homeostasis

   _____ 9. Uses a parent compound of an amide or glucose group

   _____ 10. May increase the severity of side effects

3. Which one of the following compounds is a common **anion** found in ionic contrast media?

   A. Diatrizoate or iothalamate   C. Benzoic acid

   B. Sodium or meglumine   D. None of the above

4. Any disruption in the physiological functions of the body that may lead to a contrast media reaction is

   called _____ .

   A. Homeostasis   C. Vasovagal

   B. Anaphylactoid   D. Chemotoxic

5. The normal creatinine level for an adult should range between: _____

6. Normal BUN levels for an adult should range between: _____

7. A. Glucophage is a drug that is taken for the management of _____

   B. The American College of Radiology recommends that Glucophage be withheld _____

   hours before a contrast media procedure and not taken for _____ hours following a

   contrast media procedure.

8. List the six conditions that may place a patient at greater risk of a contrast media reaction:

   A. _____

   B. _____

   C. _____

   D. _____

   E. _____

   F. _____

9. True/False: Mild contrast media reactions are usually self-limiting and do not require medication.

10. True/False: Urticaria is the formal term for excessive vomiting.

11. The leakage of contrast media from a vessel into the surrounding soft tissues is called _____

12. A reaction, based upon fear or anxiety, is called _____ .

13. An expected outcome to the introduction of contrast media is described as a _____ .

14. Indicate whether the following symptoms denote a side effect (SE), mild reaction (Mi R), moderate reaction (Mo R), or severe reaction (SR).

   _____ 1. Convulsions   _____ 10. Extravasation

   _____ 2. Metallic taste   _____ 11. Excessive urticaria

   _____ 3. Cyanosis

   _____ 4. Giant hives

   _____ 5. Itching

   _____ 6. Vasovagal response

   _____ 7. Temporary hot flash

   _____ 8. Difficulty in breathing

   _____ 9. Laryngeal spasm

15. What should the technologist do first when a patient is experiencing either a moderate or a severe contrast media reaction? _____

16. Intravenous contrast media may be administered by either:

   A. _____

   B. _____

17. True/False: The patient (or legal guardian) must sign an informed consent form before a venipuncture procedure.

18. For most IVUs, veins in the _____ are recommended for venipuncture.

A. Iliac fossa   C. Axillary fossa

B. Anterior, carpal region   D. Antecubital fossa

19. The most common size of needle used for bolus injections of contrast media is:

A. 23 to 25 gauge   C. 18 to 20 gauge

B. 14 to 16 gauge   D. 28 gauge

20. The two most common types of needles used for bolus injection of contrast media are

_____ and _____

21. In the correct order, list the four primary steps followed during a venipuncture procedure as listed and described in the textbook:

1. _____

2. _____

3. _____

4. _____

22. True/False: The bevel of the needle needs to be facing downward during the actual puncture into a vein.

23. True/False: If extravasation occurs during the puncture, the technologist should slightly retract the needle and then push it forward again.

24. True/False: If unsuccessful during the initial puncture, a new needle should be used during the second attempt.

25. True/False: The radiologist is responsible for documenting all aspects of the venipuncture procedure in the patient's chart.

REVIEW EXERCISE C: Radiographic Procedures, Contraindications, Pathologic Terminology, and Indications (see textbook pp. 555-565)

1. A. Why is the term *IVP* incorrect in describing a radiographic exam of the kidneys, ureters, and bladder following intravenous injection of contrast media?

_____

B. What is the correct term and correct initials for this exam? _____

2. Which specific aspect of the kidney is visualized during an IVU? _____

3. Which one of the following conditions is a common clinical indication for an IVU?

A. Sickle cell anemia   C. Hematuria

B. Multiple myeloma   D. Anuria

4. Which one of the following conditions is described as a rare tumor of the kidney?

A. Pheochromocytoma   C. Melanoma

B. Multiple myeloma   D. Renal cell carcinoma

5. Match the following urinary pathologic terms to the correct definition:

   _____ A. Pneumouria   1. Passage of large volume of urine

   _____ B. Urinary reflux   2. Presence of glucose in urine

   _____ C. Uremia   3. Excess in the blood of urea and creatinine

   _____ D. Anuria   4. Diminished amount of urine being excreted

   _____ E. Polyuria   5. Presence of gas in urine

   _____ F. Micturition   6. Indicated by presence of uremia, oliguria, or anuria

   _____ G. Retention   7. Constant or frequent involuntary passage of urine

   _____ H. Oliguria   8. Backward return flow of urine

   _____ I. Glucosuria   9. Absence of a functioning kidney

   _____ J. Urinary incontinence 10. Complete cessation of urinary secretion

   _____ K. Renal agenesis   11. Act of voiding

   _____ L. Acute renal failure   12. Inability to void

6. Match the correct pathologic indication to the following definitions:

   _____ A. Age-associated enlargement of the prostate gland   1. Vesicorectal fistula

   _____ B. Fusion of the kidney during the development of the fetus   2. Renal hypertension

   _____ C. Inflammation of the capillary loops of the glomeruli of the kidneys   3. Ectopic kidney

   _____ D. Artificial opening between the urinary bladder and aspects of the large intestine   4. Horseshoe kidney

   _____ E. A large stone that grows and completely fills the renal pelvis   5. Staghorn calculus

   _____ F. Increased blood pressure to the kidneys due to atherosclerosis   6. Polycystic kidney disease

   _____ G. Normal kidney that fails to ascend into the abdomen but remains in the pelvis   7. Benign Prostatic Hyperplasia

   _____ H. Multiple cysts in one or both kidneys   8. Glomerulonephritis

7. Match the following radiographic appearances to the correct pathologic indication:

    ____ A. Rapid excretion of contrast media   1. Malrotation

    ____ B. Mucosal changes within bladder   2. Vesicorectal fistula

    ____ C. Bilateral, small kidneys with blunted calyces   3. Renal cell carcinoma

    ____ D. Irregular appearance of renal parenchyma or collecting system   4. BPH

    ____ E. Signs of abnormal fluid collections   5. Renal hypertension

    ____ F. Abnormal rotation of the kidney   6. Renal calculi

    ____ G. Elevated or indented floor of bladder   7. Cystitis

    ____ H. Signs of obstruction of urinary system   8. Chronic Bright's disease

8. True/False: If an IVU and barium enema are both scheduled, the IVU should always be performed first.

9. True/False: The patient should void before an IVU to prevent possible rupture of the bladder if compression is applied.

10. What is the primary purpose of ureteric compression? _____

11. List the six conditions that could contraindicate the use of ureteric compression:

    A. _____   D. _____

    B. _____   E. _____

    C. _____   F. _____

12. When does the timing for and IVU exam start? _____

13. List the basic five-step timed imaging sequence for a routine IVU.

    A. _____   D. _____

    B. _____   E. _____

    C. _____

14. What is the primary difference between a standard and a hypertensive IVU?

_____

15. In what department are most retrograde urograms performed? _____

16. True/False: A retrograde urogram examines the anatomy and function of the pelvicalyceal system.

17. True/False: The Brodney clamp is used for male and female retrograde cystourethrograms.

18. Which of the following involves a direct introduction of the contrast media into the structure being studied?

    A. Retrograde urogram   C. Retrograde urethrogram

    B. Retrograde cystogram   D. All of the above

19. Which of the following alternative imaging modalities is NOT being utilized to diagnosed renal calculi?

    A. Nuclear medicine   C. Magnetic resonance imaging

    B. Sonography   D. Computed tomography

20. True/False: Urinary studies on pediatric patients should be scheduled early in the morning to minimize the risk of dehydration.

REVIEW EXERCISE D: Radiographic Positioning of the Urinary System (see textbook pp. 566-574)

1. What are the three reasons a scout projection is taken before an injection of contrast media for an IVU?

    A. _____   C. _____

    B. _____

2. What kVp range is recommended for an IVU? _____

3. Which ionization chambers should be activated for an AP scout projection? _____

4. True/False: Both the female midline dose and the female gonadal dose for an average unshielded AP projection for an IVU are in the 100 to 200 mrad range.

5. True/False: Male and female patients should have the gonads shielded for an AP scout projection.

6. True/False: Tomograms taken during an IVU with an exposure angle of 10° or less are called *zonography*.

7. How many tomograms (zonograms) are usually produced during an IVU? _____

8. At what stage of an IVU is the renal parenchyma best seen?

    A. 5 minutes following injection   C. During the post-void film

    B. 10 minutes following injection   D. Within 1 minute following injection

9. Where is the CR centered for a nephrotomogram?

    A. At xiphoid process   C. At iliac crest

    B. Midway between xiphoid process and iliac crest   D. At axillary costal margin

10. Which specific position, taken during an IVU, will place the left kidney parallel to the film?

    _____

11. How much obliquity is required for the LPO/RPO projections taken during an IVU? _____

12. Which position will best demonstrate possible nephroptosis? _____

13. How will an enlarged prostate gland appear on a post-void radiograph taken during an IVU?

    _____

14. Where should the pneumatic paddle be placed for the ureteric compression phase of an IVU?

    _____

15. What can be done to enhance filling of the calyces of the kidney if ureteric compression is contraindicated?

    _____

16. What specific anatomy is examined during a retrograde ureterogram?

    A. Primarily the ureters

    C. Entire urinary system

    B. Primarily the renal pelvis and calyces

    D. Urinary bladder

17. A retrograde pyelogram is primarily a nonfunctional study of the _____.

18. What CR angle is utilized for the AP projection taken during a cystogram?

    A. 20 to 25° caudad   C. 10 to 15° caudad

    B. 5 to 10° cephalad   D. 30 to 40° caudad

19 True/False: For a lateral cystogram, both the male and female dose are in the 100 (±50) mrad range.

20. Which specific position is recommended for a male patient during a voiding cystourethrogram?

_____

REVIEW EXERCISE E: Problem Solving for Technical and Positioning Errors (see textbook pp. 566-574)

1. **Situation:** A radiograph of an AP scout projection of the abdomen, taken during an IVU, reveals that the symphysis pubis is slightly cut off. The patient is too large to include the entire abdomen on a 35 x 43 cm (14 x 17 in.) IR. What should the technologist do in this situation?

_____

_____

2. **Situation:** A nephrogram is ordered as part of an IVU study. When the nephrogram image is processed, there is a minimal amount of contrast media within the renal parenchyma, and the calyces are beginning to fill with contrast media. What specific problem led to this radiographic outcome?

_____

_____

3. **Situation:** A 45° RPO radiograph taken during an IVU reveals that the left kidney is foreshortened. What modification is needed to improve this image during the repeat exposure?

_____

_____

4. **Situation:** An AP projection taken during the compression phase of an IVU reveals that the majority of the contrast media has left the collecting system. The technologist placed the pneumatic paddles near the umbilicus and ensured that they were inflated. What can the technologist do to ensure better retention of contrast media in the collecting system during the compression phase of future IVUs?

_____

_____

5. **Situation:** An AP projection radiograph taken during a cystogram reveals that the floor of the bladder is superimposed over the symphysis pubis. What can the technologist do to correct this problem during the repeat exposure?

_____

_____

6. **Situation:** A patient comes to the radiology department for an IVU. While taking the clinical history, the technologist learns the patient has renal hypertension. How must the technologist modify the IVU imaging sequence to accommodate this patient's condition?

_____

_____

7. **Situation:** A patient comes to the radiology department for an IVU. The AP scout reveals an abnormal density near the lumbar spine that the radiologist suspects is an abdominal, aortic aneurysm. What should the technologist do about the ureteric compression phase of the study that had been ordered?

_____

_____

8. **Situation:** A patient comes to the radiology department for an IVU. The patient history indicates that he may have an enlarged prostate gland. Which projection will best demonstrate this condition?

_____

9. **Situation:** A patient with a history of bladder calculi comes to the radiology department. A cystogram has been ordered. During the interview, the patient reports that he had a severe reaction to contrast media in the past. What other imaging modality (or modalities) can be performed to best diagnose this condition?

_____

10. **Situation:** The same patient described in question 9 may also have calculi in the kidney. What is the preferred imaging modality for this situation when iodinated contrast media cannot be used?

_____

PART III: Laboratory Exercises (see textbook pp. 555-574)

Although it is impossible to duplicate many aspects of urinary studies on a phantom in the lab, evaluation of actual radiographs and physical positioning is possible. You can get experience in positioning and radiographic evaluation of these projections by performing exercises using radiographic phantoms and practicing on other students (although you will not be taking actual exposures). Technologists must learn the positioning routine, room setup, and fluoroscopy procedure for their particular facility.

LABORATORY EXERCISE A: Radiographic Evaluation

1. Using actual radiographs of IVU, cystogram and retrograde urogram procedures provided by your instructor, evaluate each position for the following points (check off for each radiograph when completed):

_____   Evaluate the completeness of the study. (Are all pertinent anatomic structures included on the radiograph?)

_____   Evaluate for positioning or centering errors (e.g., rotation, off centering)

_____   Evaluate for correct exposure factors and possible motion. (Is the contrast media properly penetrated?)

_____   Determine whether patient obliquity is correct for specific positions.

_____   Determine whether markers and an acceptable degree of collimation and/or area shielding are visible on the images.

LABORATORY EXERCISE B: Physical Positioning

On another person, simulate performing all basic and special projections of the IVU as follows. (Check off each when completed satisfactorily.) Include the following six steps as described in the textbook.

Step 1.   Appropriate size and type of image receptor with correct markers
Step 2.   Correct CR placement and centering of part to CR and/or image receptor
Step 3.   Accurate collimation
Step 4.   Area shielding of patient where advisable
Step 5.   Use of proper immobilizing devices when needed
Step 6.   Approximate correct exposure factors, breathing instructions where applicable, and "making" exposure

Projections	Step 1	Step 2	Step 3	Step 4	Step 5	Step 6
• AP scout	____	____	____	____	____	____
• LPO and RPO	____	____	____	____	____	____
• AP cystogram	____	____	____	____	____	____
• Lateral cystogram	____	____	____	____	____	____

Answers to Review Exercises

Review Exercise A: Radiographic Anatomy of the Urinary System

1. D. Retroperitoneal
2. Suprarenal glands
3. Psoas muscles
4. Perirenal fat, or adipose capsule
5. 30°
6. Xiphoid process and iliac crest
7. Nephroptosis
8. A. Remove nitrogenous waste
   B. Regulate water levels
   C. Regulate acid-base balance
9. B. Uremia
10. Hilum
11. Cortex
12. Renal parenchyma
13. Nephron
14. Renal pyramids
15. Bowman's capsule
16. False (located in the cortex)
17. False (afferent)
18. A. Renal pelvis
    B. Major calyx
    C. Minor calyx
    D. Renal sinuses
    E. Cortex
    F. Medulla
    G. Ureter
19. A. Loop of Henle, medulla
    B. Distal convoluted tubule, cortex
    C. Afferent arteriole, cortex
    D. Efferent arteriole, cortex
    E. Glomerular capsule, cortex
    F. Proximal convoluted tubule, cortex
    G. Descending limb, medulla
    H. Ascending limb, medulla
    I. Collecting tubule, medulla
20. A. Peristalsis
    B. Gravity
21. C. Urinary bladder
22. Ureterovesical junction
23. Trigone
24. Prostate gland
25. C. 350 to 500 milliliters
26. D. Kidneys
27. A. Minor calyces
    B. Major calyces
    C. Renal pelvis
    D. Ureteropelvic junction (UPC)
    E. Proximal ureter
    F. Distal ureter
    G. Urinary bladder

Review Exercise B: Contrast Media, Contrast Media Reactions, and Venipuncture

1. A. Intravenous injection
   B. Catheterization

2. 1. I, 2. N, 3. I, 4. I, 5. N, 6. N, 7. N, 8. I, 9. N, 10. I
3. A. Diatrizoate or Iothalmate
4. A. Homeostasis
5. 0.6 to 1.5 mg/dl
6. 8 to 25 mg/100 ml
7. A. Diabetes mellitus
   B. 48 hours, 48 hours
8. A. Hypersensitivity toward iodinated contrast media
   B. Diabetes mellitus
   C. Asthma or other respiratory conditions
   D. Multiple myeloma
   E. Severe dehydration
   F. Chronic or acute renal failure or hepatic disease
9. True
10. False (it's the term for hives)
11. Extravasation
12. Vasovagal response
13. Side effect.
14. 1. SR, 2. SE, 3. SR, 4. Mo R, 5. Mi R, 6. Mi R, 7. SE, 8. SR, 9. SR, 10. Mi R, 11. Mo R
15. Call for medical assistance
16. A. Bolus injection
    B. Drip infusion
17. True
18. D. Antecubital fossa
19. C. 18 to 20 gauge
20. Butterfly and over-the-needle catheter
21. 1. Wash hands and put on gloves
    2. Select site and apply tourniquet
    3. Confirm puncture site and cleanse
    4. Initiate puncture
22. False (facing upward)
23. False (needle should be withdrawn and pressure applied)
24. True
25. False (technologist or the one doing the venipuncture is responsible)

Review Exercise C: Radiographic Procedures, Contraindications, Pathologic Terminology and Indications

1. A. An IVP implies a study of the renal pelvis (pyelo) (Intravenous Pyelogram)
   B. Intravenous urogram (IVU)
2. The collecting system of the kidney
3. C. Hematuria
4. A. Pheochromocytoma
5. A. 5
   B. 8
   C. 3
   D. 10

   E. 1
   F. 11
   G. 12
   H. 4
   I. 2
   J. 7
   K. 9
   L. 6
6. A. 7
   B. 4
   C. 8
   D. 1
   E. 5
   F. 2
   G. 3
   H. 6
7. A. 5
   B. 7
   C. 8
   D. 3
   E. 2
   F. 1
   G. 4
   H. 6
8. True
9. True
10. To enhance filling of the pelvicalyceal system with contrast media
11. A. Possible ureteric stones
    B. Abdominal mass
    C. Abdominal aortic aneurysm
    D. Recent abdominal surgery
    E. Severe abdominal pain
    F. Acute abdominal trauma
12. At start of injection of contrast media
13. A. 1-minute nephrogram or nephro-tomography
    B. 5-minute full KUB
    C. 15-minute full KUB
    D. 20-minute posterior R and L obliques
    E. Post-void (prone PA or erect AP)
14. A hypertensive IVU requires a shorter span of time between projections
15. In surgery
16. False (nonfunctional exam)
17. False (used for males only)
18. D. All of the above
19. C. Magnetic resonance imaging
20. True

Review Exercise D: Radiographic Positioning of the Urinary System

1. A. Verify patient preparation
   B. Determine if exposure factors are correct
   C. Detect any abnormal calcifications

2. 65 to 75 kVp
3. Upper right and left ionization chambers
4. False (in the 30 to 50 mrad range)
5. False (not female; would obscure essential anatomy)
6. True
7. Three
8. D. Within 1 minute following injection
9. B. Midway between xiphoid process and iliac crest
10. RPO
11. 30°
12. Erect position
13. The prostate gland will indent the floor of the bladder
14. Just medial to the ASIS
15. Place the patient in a 15° Trendelenburg position
16. A Primarily the ureters
17. Renal pelvis, major and minor calyces of the kidneys
18. C. 10 to 15° caudad
19. True
20. 30° RPO

Review Exercise E: Problem Solving for Technical and Positioning Errors

1. A second, smaller IR of the bladder should be taken placed crosswise to include this region. The larger IR should be centered 1 or 2 in. (2 to 5 cm) higher to include the upper abdomen.
2. Too long of a delay between the injection of contrast media and the filming of the nephrogram. The nephrogram needs to be taken close to 60 seconds following injection.
3. Decrease the obliquity of the RPO to no more than 30°.
4. Place the pneumatic paddles just medial to the ASIS to allow for compression of the distal ureters against the pelvic brim.
5. Increase caudad angulation of the central ray to project the symphysis pubis below the bladder.
6. Decrease the span of time between projections to capture all phases of the urinary system. (Take images at 1, 2, and 3 minutes rather than 1, 5, and 15 minutes.)
7. The technologist should not perform the compression phase of the study. Ureteric compression is contraindicated when an abdominal aortic aneurysm is suspected. (The technologist should consult with the radiologist or physician.)
8. The erect pre-void AP projection will best demonstrate an enlarged prostate gland.
9. Ultrasound or CT
10. CT is preferred but a nuclear medicine procedure could also be performed.

SELF-TEST

My Score = _____ %

Directions: This self-test should be taken only after completing **all** of the readings, review exercises, and laboratory activities for a particular section. The purpose of this test is not only to provide a good learning exercise but also to serve as a good indicator of what your final evaluation grade will be. It is strongly suggested that if you do not get at least a 90% to 95% grade on this self-test, you should review those areas in which you missed questions *before* going to your instructor for the final evaluation exam for this chapter. (There are 62 questions or blanks—each is worth 1.6 points.)

1. The kidneys are _____ structures.

    A. Retroperitoneal   B. Intraperitoneal   C. Infraperitoneal   D. Extraperitoneal

2. The ureters enter the _____ aspect of the bladder.

    A. Lateral   B. Anterolateral   C. Posterolateral   D. Superolateral

3. The kidneys lie on the _____ (anterior or posterior) surface of each psoas major muscle.

4. The kidneys lie at a _____ angle in relation to the coronal plane.

5. The three constricted points along the length of the ureters where a kidney stone is most likely to lodge are:

    A. _____   C. _____

    B. _____

6. An abnormal drop of more than _____ inches or _____ cm in the position of the kidneys when the patient is erect indicates a condition termed nephroptosis.

7. The buildup of nitrogenous waste in the blood creates a condition called _____ .

8. How much urine is normally produced by the kidneys in 24 hours?

    A. 2.5 liters   B. 180 liters   C. 0.5 liter   D. 1.5 liters

9. The renal veins connect directly to the:

    A. Abdominal aorta   C. Azygos vein

    B. Superior mesenteric vein   D. Inferior vena cava

10. The 8 to 18 conical masses found within the renal medulla are called the _____ .

11. The major calyces of the kidney unite to form the _____ .

12. The microscopic unit of the kidney (of which there are over a million in each kidney) is called the

    _____ .

13. True/False: The loop of Henle and collecting tubules are located primarily in the medulla of the kidney.

14. True/False: About 50% of the glomerular filtrate processed by the nephron is reabsorbed into the kidney's venous system.

15. The inner, posterior triangular aspect of the bladder that is attached to the floor of the pelvis is called the:

    _____ .

16. Identify the structures labeled on this radiograph (Fig. 17-4):

    A. _____

    B. _____

    C. _____

    D. _____

    E. _____

    F. _____

17. The term describing the radiographic procedure demonstrated on Fig. 17-4 radiograph is:

    _____

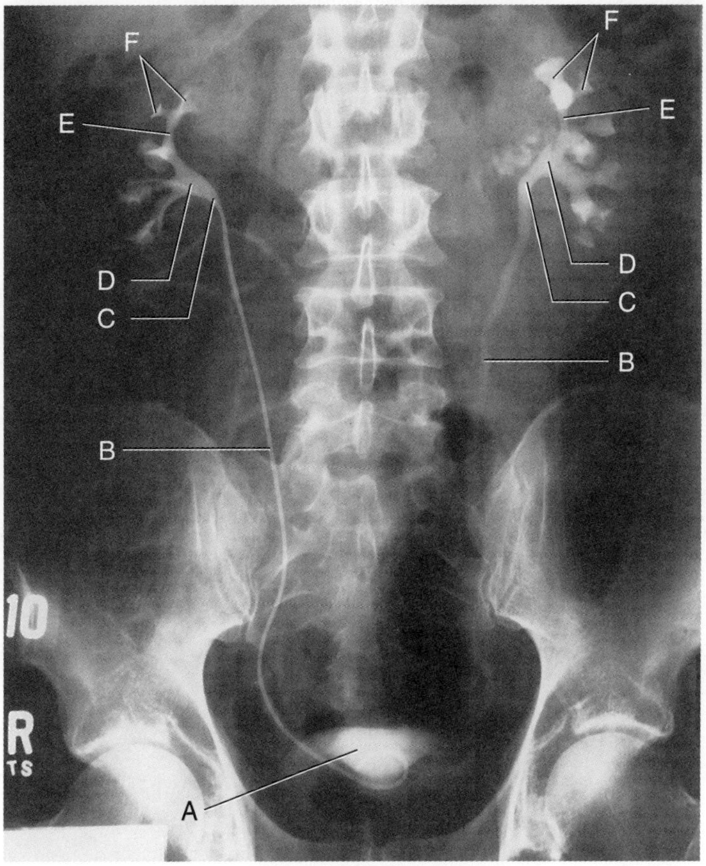

Fig. 17-4 Radiograph of the urinary system.

18. Under what circumstances should a pregnant patient have an IVU performed?

    _____

19. List the two types of iodinated contrast media used for urinary studies? _____

    _____

20. Match the following characteristics to the correct type of iodinated contrast media:

    _____   1.   Dissociates into two separate ions once injected   I.   Ionic

    _____   2.   Possesses low osmolality   N.   Nonionic

    _____   3.   Uses a salt as its cation

    _____   4.   Parent compound is a carboxyl group

    _____   5.   Less expensive as compared to the other type

    _____   6.   Produces a less severe contrast media reaction

    _____   7.   Diatrizoate is a common anion

    _____   8.   Does not contain a cation

    _____   9.   Creates a hypertonic condition in blood plasma

    _____   10. Creates a near isotonic solution

21.   The normal range of creatinine in an adult is:

   A.   2.0 to 3.4 mg/dl   C.   8 to 25 mg /100 ml

   B.   0.6 to 1.5 mg /dl   D.   0.1 to 1.25 mg /dl

22.   How long must a patient be withheld from Glucophage before having an iodinated contrast media procedure?

   A.   48 hours   C.   24 hours

   B.   2 hours   D.   72 hours

23.   Which one of the following conditions is considered high risk for an iodinated contrast media procedure?

   A.   Hematuria   C.   Diabetes mellitus

   B.   Renal failure   D.   Hypertension

24.   What is the best course of action for a patient experiencing a mild contrast media reaction?

   A.   Observe and reassure patient   C.   Inform your supervisor

   B.   Call for immediate medical attention   D.   Inform the referring physician

25.   A vasovagal reaction is classified as:

   A.   Side effect   C.   Moderate reaction

   B.   Mild reaction   D.   Severe reaction

26.   Extravasation is classified as a:

   A.   Side effect   C.   Moderate reaction

   B.   Mild reaction   D.   Severe reaction

27.   Profound shock is classified as a:

   A.   Side effect   C.   Moderate reaction

   B.   Mild reaction   D.   Severe reaction

28.   Tachycardia is classified as a:

   A.   Side effect   C.   Moderate reaction

   B.   Mild reaction   D.   Severe reaction

29.   Which one of the following veins is NOT normally selected for venipuncture during an IVU?

   A.   Basilic   C.   Axillary

   B.   Cephalic   D.   Radial

30.   At what angle is the needle advanced into the vein during venipuncture? _____

31.   The complete cessation of urinary secretion is called: _____

32.   A technique of using acoustic waves to shatter large kidney stones is called: _____

33.   The most common reason for urinary tract infection is:

   A.   Renal calculi   C.   Urinary incontinence

   B.   Uremia   D.   Vesicourethral reflux

34. Which one of the following conditions may produce hydronephrosis?

   A. Renal obstruction   C. Renal hypertension

   B. Glomerulonephritis   D. BPH

35. Which one of the following pathologic indications is an example of a congenital anomaly of the urinary system?

   A. Ectopic kidney   C. Polycystic kidney disease

   B. Pyelonephritis   D. BPH

36. True/False: The patient should void before the IVU to prevent dilution of the contrast media in the bladder.

37. True/False: The patient should complete a bowel cleansing procedure before the IVU.

38. Which one of the following conditions would contraindicate the use of ureteric compression?

   A. Hematuria   C. Hematuria

   B. Ureteric calculi   D. Multiple myeloma

39. Typically, at what timing sequence during an IVU are the oblique projections taken? _____

40. Which projection(s) best demonstrate the renal parenchyma, and when are they taken?

   _____

41. Which procedure may use a Brodney clamp? _____

42. Which specific body position will place the right kidney parallel to the film? _____

43. True/False: The gonadal dose for the AP post-void projection is higher for male patients than for female patients.

44. True/False: The retrograde ureterogram will demonstrate the ureters, renal pelvis, and major and minor calyces.

45. **Situation:** An AP projection taken during a retrograde cystogram reveals that the symphysis pubis is superimposed over the floor of the bladder. What can be done during the repeat exposure to correct this problem?

   _____

CHAPTER 18

Mammography

After you have completed **all** the activities of this chapter, you will be able to:

_____ 1. On drawings and radiographs, identify specific anatomy of the mammary glands.

_____ 2. Identify specific regions of the breast using the quadrant and the clock systems.

_____ 3. List the three general categories of breasts according to their tissue composition, age of the patient, and radiographic density.

_____ 4. List the technical considerations and equipment essential for quality images of the breast.

_____ 5. Identify the purpose of breast compression and the average pounds of force used when applying compression.

_____ 6. Identify alternative imaging modalities available to study the breast.   Include advantages and disadvantages of each system.

_____ 7. Define specific types of breast pathology.

_____ 8. List the American College of Radiology (ACR) nomenclature of terms and abbreviations for mammographic positioning.

_____ 9. Describe the basic and special projections most commonly performed in mammography; include patient positioning, CR placement, and structures best seen.

_____ 10. Describe the Eklund technique for imaging breasts with implants.

_____ 11. List the average skin dose and mean glandular dose (MGD) range for each projection of the breast as described in the textbook.

_____ 12. Given mammographic images, identify specific positioning and exposure factor errors.

POSITIONING AND FILM CRITIQUE

_____ 1. Using a peer in a simulated setting, position for basic and special mammographic projections.

_____ 2. Using appropriate radiographic phantoms, produce satisfactory radiographs of specific positions (if equipment is available).

_____ 3. Critique and evaluate mammographic images based on the four divisions of radiographic criteria: (1) structures shown, (2) position, (3) collimation and CR, and (4) exposure criteria.

_____ 4. Distinguish between acceptable and unacceptable mammographic images due to exposure factors, motion, collimation, positioning, or other errors.

Learning Exercises

Complete the following review exercises after reading the associated pages in the textbook as indicated by each exercise. Answers to each review exercise are given at the end of the review exercises.

PART I: Mammography Quality Standards, Anatomy, and Technical Considerations

REVIEW EXERCISE A: Mammography Quality Standards Act, Anatomy of the Breast, and Technical Considerations (see textbook pp. 576-584)

1. Radiographic examination of the mammary gland or breast is called _____.

2. In 1992 the American Cancer Society recommended that women over the age of _____ should have a screening mammogram performed.

    A. 35   C. 45

    B. 40   D. 50

3. The Mammographic Quality Standards Act (MQSA), which went into effect on October 1, _____, was passed to ensure high-quality mammography service requiring certification by the secretary of the Department of Health and Human Services (DHHS).

    A. 1992   C. 1994

    B. 1993   D. 1995

4. Women between the age of 40 and 49 years old should have a mammogram at least every:

    A. 1 year   C. 5 years

    B. 2 years   D. 6 months

5. As stated in the textbook, breast cancer accounts for _____ of all new cancers detected in women.

    A. 12%   C. 32%

    B. 15%   D. 50%

6. In Canada, mammography guidelines are set by the _____ .

7. The junction of the inferior part of the breast with the anterior chest wall is called the _____ .

8. The pigmented area surrounding the nipple is the _____ .

9. Breast tissue extending into the axilla is called the tail of the breast or the _____ .

10. In the average female breast, the _____ (craniocaudad or mediolateral) diameter is usually greater.

11. Five o'clock in the right breast would be in what quadrant? _____

12. Based on the clock system method, a suspicious mass at 2 o'clock on the right breast would be at _____ o'clock if it were in a similar position on the left breast.

13. What is the large muscle commonly seen on a mammogram that is located between the bony thorax and the mammary gland? _____

14. Two fibrous sheets of tissue join together just posterior to the breast to form the _____ space.

15. What is the function of the mammary gland?

_____

16. What are the three tissue types found in the mammary gland?

A. _____   B. _____   C. _____

17. Various small blood vessels, fibrous connective tissues, ducts, and other small structures seen on finished mammo-

grams are collectively called _____ .

18. Bands of connective tissue passing through the breast tissue are known as _____ .

19. Classify the following types of breasts into one of the three general categories: fibro-glandular (FG), fibro-fatty (FF),
or fatty (F).

_____ 1. 20 years, no children   _____ 5. 50 years, two children

_____ 2. 35 years, no children   _____ 6. Male

_____ 3. 35 years, three children   _____ 7. 35 years, lactating

_____ 4. 25 years, pregnant   _____ 8. 10 years

20. Which is the least dense of the following tissues: fibrous, glandular, or adipose? _____

21. Identify the labeled parts on this sagittal section drawing (Fig. 18-1):

A. _____

B. _____

C. _____

D. _____

E. _____

F. _____

G. _____

H. _____

I. _____

J. _____

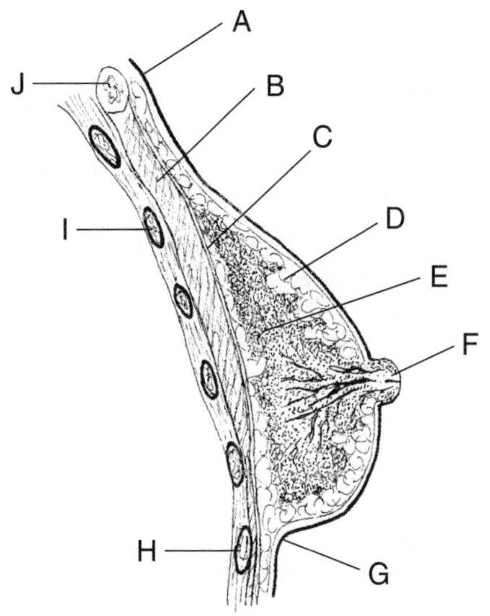

Fig. 18-1 Sagittal section of the breast.

22. Identify the labeled parts on Fig. 18-2:

    A. _____

    B. _____

    C. _____

    D. _____

    E. _____

    F. _____

    G. _____

    H. _____

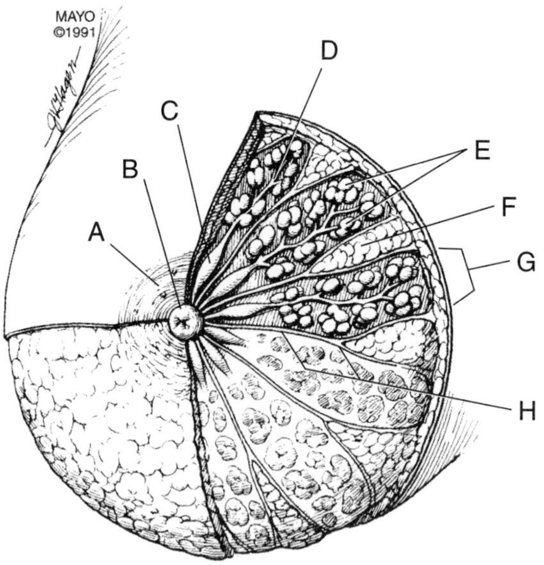

Fig. 18-2 Cutaway anterior view of the breast.

23. The glandular tissue of the breast is divided into _____ lobes.

24. Which portion of the breast is nearest to the chest wall (apex or base)? _____

25. Which portion of the breast is nearest to the nipple (apex or base)? _____

26. The central ray is usually directed through the _____ of the breast.

27. The ideal kilovoltage for mammography is between _____ and _____ kVp.

28. Name the target material used in mammography x-ray tubes. _____

29. The focal spot size on a dedicated mammography unit should be _____ mm or less.

30. Typically, compression applied to the breast is _____ to _____
    pounds of pressure.

31. List the two functions of compression during mammography:

    A. _____

    B. _____

32. What is the primary advantage of decreasing the thickness of the breast with compression?

    _____

33. The average required mAs range in mammography using 25 to 28 kVp is:

    A. 10 to 15   C. 40 to 60

    B. 20 to 30   D. 75 to 85

34. What is the typical skin dose for a mammographic projection?

    A. 100 to 200 mrad   C. 800 to 1000 mrad

    B. 400 to 600 mrad   D. 1200 to 1500 mrad

35. To minimize patient dose, the American College of Radiology (ACR) recommends a repeat rate of less than _____ .

    A. 2%   C. 10%

    B. 5%   D. 15%

36. True/False: MGD, as used in patient dose measurements in mammography, refers to mean gonadal dose.

37. True/False: Grids and AEC are used for most mammograms.

38. Which three image qualities need to be present in a good film mammogram?

    A. _____   B. _____   C. _____

39. What type of pathology is best diagnosed with ultrasound of the breast?

    _____

40. Which imaging modality is most effective in diagnosing problems related to breast implants?

    _____

41. True/False: Automatic exposure control cannot be used with breast implants.

42. List the two advantages of digital mammography over conventional film-screen systems:

    A. _____

    B. _____

43. Mammoscintigraphy utilizes the radionuclide called:

    A. Sulphur colloid   C. Technetium

    B. Iodine 131   D. Sestimibi

44. The most common form of benign tumor of the breast is:

    A. Fibroadenoma   C. Fibrocystic lesion

    B. Adenocarcinoma   D. Adenosarcoma

45. List the correct positioning term description for the following ACR abbreviations:

    A. MLO _____   F. LM   _____

    B. SIO _____   G. XCCL _____

    C. AT _____   H. LMO _____

    D. CC _____   I. ID   _____

    E. RL _____   J. CV   _____

PART II: Radiographic Positioning

REVIEW EXERCISE B: Positioning of the Breast (see textbook pp. 585-590)

1. What are the two basic projections performed for screening mammograms?

   A. _____   B. _____

2. What landmark determines the correct height for placement of the image receptor for the craniocaudad projection?

   _____

3. Anatomical markers and patient identification information need to be placed near the _____ side of the breast.

4. In the craniocaudad projection, what structure must be in profile? _____

5. In the craniocaudad projection, the head should be turned _____ (toward or away) from the side being radiographed.

6. Which basic projection will demonstrate more of the pectoral muscle? _____

7. How much CR/image receptor angulation is utilized for an average-size breast for the mediolateral oblique projection?

   _____

8. The patient with a small, thin breast would require _____ (more or less) CR angulation with the mediolateral oblique projection as compared with the average-size breast.

9. For the mediolateral oblique projection, the arm of the side being examined should be placed:

   A. On the hip   C. Resting on top of the head

   B. Forward, toward the front of the body   D. Behind the back, palm out

10. Which special projection is usually requested when a lesion is seen on the mediolateral oblique but not on the craniocaudad projection? _____

11. In both the craniocaudad and the mediolateral projections, the central ray is always directed to the

    _____ of the breast.

12. What is the most commonly requested special projection of the breast? _____

13. Which projection will most effectively show the axillary aspect of the breast? _____

14. How much is the CR/ image receptor angled from vertical for the mediolateral, true lateral projection?

    _____

15. Mark the following statements: **T** for True, **F** for False.

_____ 1. It is important for all skin folds to be smoothed out and all wrinkles and pockets of air removed on each projection for the breast.

_____ 2. Since the base of the breast is well-shown on the craniocaudad projection, this area does not need to be shown on the mediolateral oblique projection.

_____ 3. The axillary aspect of the breast is usually well-visualized on the craniocaudad projection.

_____ 4. Mammography is usually done in the standing position.

_____ 5. Because of a short exposure time, the patient does not need to be completely motionless during the exposure.

_____ 6. Use of AEC would result in underexposed films with breast implants.

_____ 7. In the craniocaudad projection, the chest wall must be pushed firmly against the image receptor.

_____ 8. Standard CC and MLO projections should be performed on patients who have implants.

_____ 9. Firm compression should not be used on patients with breast implants.

_____ 10. The patient skin dose for a true mediolateral projection is approximately 30% less than for the mediolateral oblique projection.

16. Which technique (method) is commonly used for the breast with an implant? _____

17. During the procedure mentioned in question 16, what must be done to allow the anterior aspect of the breast to be compressed and properly visualized? _____

18 If a lesion is too deep toward the chest wall and cannot be visualized with a laterally exaggerated craniocaudal projection, a _____ projection should be performed.
   A. Mediolateral oblique   C. Mediolateral
   B. Craniocaudal   D. Axillary tail

19. Telemammography is performed primarily to:
   A. Send digital images to remote locations   C. Reduce dose per projection
   B. Magnify specific regions of interest   D. Demonstrate the deep chest wall

20. What is the average mean glandular dose (MGD) dose for projections of the breast?
   A. 100 to 150 mrad   C. 500 to 700 mrad
   B. 200 to 400 mrad   D. 900 to 1000 mrad

REVIEW EXERCISE C: Critique Radiographs of the Breast (see textbook p. 591)

These questions relate to the radiographs found at the end of Chapter 18 of the textbook. Evaluate these radiographs for positioning accuracy as well as exposure factors, collimation, and correct use of anatomical markers. Describe the corrections needed to improve the overall image. The major, or "repeatable," errors imply that these specific errors require a repeat exposure regardless of the nature or degree of the other errors. Answers to each critique are given at the end of this chapter.

A.   CC Projection (Fig. C18-35)   *Description of possible error:*

   1.   Structures shown: _____

   2.   Part positioning: _____

   3.   Collimation and central ray: _____

   4.   Exposure criteria: _____

   5.   Markers: _____

   Repeatable error(s): _____

B .   MLO Projection (Fig. C18-36)   *Description of possible error:*

   1.   Structures shown: _____

   2.   Part positioning: _____

   3.   Collimation and central ray: _____

   4.   Exposure criteria: _____

   5.   Markers: _____

   Repeatable error(s): _____

C.   CC Projection (Fig. C18-37)   *Description of possible error:*

   1.   Structures shown: _____

   2.   Part positioning: _____

   3.   Collimation and central ray: _____

   4.   Exposure criteria: _____

   5.   Markers: _____

   Repeatable error(s): _____

D. MLO Projection (Fig. C18-38)   *Description of possible error:*

1. Structures shown: _____

2. Part positioning: _____

3. Collimation and central ray: _____

4. Exposure criteria: _____

5. Markers: _____

Repeatable error(s): _____

E. CC Projection (Fig. C18-39)   *Description of possible error:*

1. Structures shown: _____

2. Part positioning: _____

3. Collimation and central ray: _____

4. Exposure criteria: _____

5. Markers: _____

Repeatable error(s): _____

F. CC Projection (Fig. C18-40)   *Description of possible error:*

1. Structures shown: _____

2. Part positioning: _____

3. Collimation and central ray: _____

4. Exposure criteria: _____

5. Markers: _____

Repeatable error(s): _____

PART III: Laboratory Exercises

This part of the learning activity exercise needs to be carried out in the radiology department where the mammography machine is located. Part B can be carried out in a classroom or any room where illuminators are available.

LABORATORY EXERCISE A: Positioning

For this section you need another person to act as your "patient." Male and female students should be separated for this exercise, and students can be fully clothed for the simulated positioning. A clinical instructor must be present.
Include each of the following during this exercise. (Check off when completed.)

_____   Manipulate the x-ray machine into all the positions and become familiar with the locks and devices.

_____   Place or exchange the cone on the machine.

_____   Place a cassette into the cassette holder.

_____   Place a fist on the image receptor tray and compress it by using the compression device.
(This should be performed so the student can sense the pressure of the device.)

_____   Place another student in position and *simulate* the CC, MLO, XCCL, and ML positions.

_____   **Optional:** If the department or school possesses a breast phantom, perform the basic and special mammogram positions.

LABORATORY EXERCISE B: Film Critique and Evaluation

Your instructor will provide various breast radiographs for these exercises.   Some will be optimal quality radiographs that meet all or most of the evaluation criteria described for each projection in the textbook. Others will be less than optimal quality, and others will be unacceptable, requiring a repeat exam. You should evaluate each radiograph as specified below.

Radiographs

1	2	3	4	5	6	
____	____	____	____	____	____	a. Correct alignment and centering of part
____	____	____	____	____	____	b. Pectoral muscle is included
____	____	____	____	____	____	c. Tissue thickness is distributed evenly
____	____	____	____	____	____	d. Optimal compression is noted
____	____	____	____	____	____	e. Dense areas are adequately penetrated
____	____	____	____	____	____	f. High tissue contrast and optimal resolution noted
____	____	____	____	____	____	g. Absence of artifacts
____	____	____	____	____	____	h. Marker is in proper position; patient identification, including date, is accurate
____	____	____	____	____	____	i. Based on acceptable variances to criteria factors, determine which of these radiographs are acceptable and which are unacceptable and should have been repeated. (Place a check if the radiograph needs to be repeated.)

Answers to Review Exercises

Review Exercise A: Mammography Quality Standards Act, Anatomy of the Breast, and Technical Considerations

1. Mammography
2. B. 40
3. C. 1994
4. B. 2 years
5. C. 32%
6. Canadian Association of Radiologists
7. Inframammary crease
8. Areola
9. Axillary prolongation
10. Mediolateral
11. Lower inner quadrant (LIQ)
12. 10 o'clock
13. Pectoralis major muscle
14. Retromammary
15. Lactation or secretion of milk
16. A. Glandular
    B. Fibrous or connective
    C. Adipose (fatty)
17. Trabeculae
18. Cooper's ligaments
19. 1. FG, 2. FG, 3. FF, 4. FG, 5. F,
    6. F, 7. FG, 8. F
20. Adipose
21. A. Skin
    B. Pectoralis major muscle
    C. Retromammary space
    D. Adipose (fatty) tissue
    E. Glandular tissue
    F. Nipple
    G. Inframammary crease
    H. 6th rib (lower breast margin - varies among individuals)
    I. 2nd rib (upper breast margin)
    J. Clavicle
22. A. Areola
    B. Nipple
    C. Ampulla
    D. Ducts
    E. Alveoli
    F. Mammary fat
    G. Lobe
    H. Cooper's ligament
23. 15 to 20
24. Base
25. Apex
26. Base
27. 25 and 28 kVp
28. Molybdenum
29. 0.3 mm
30. 25 to 40
31. A. Decrease thickness of breast
    B. Bring breast structures closer to IR
32. Reducing the amount of scatter radiation produced from the breast
33. D. 75 to 85
34. C. 800 to 1000 mrad
35. B. 5%
36. False (mean glandular dose)
37. True
38. A. Fine detail
    B. Edge sharpness
    C. Soft tissue visibility
39. Distinguishing a cyst from a solid mass
40. Magnetic resonance imaging (MRI)
41. True
42. A. Mammographic images can be digitally enhanced, modified, or enlarged without additional exposure
    B. Digital mammographic images can be sent to remote locations by telephone or satellite
43. D. Sestimibi
44. A. Fibroadenoma
45. A. Mediolateral oblique
    B. Superolateral-inferomedial oblique
    C. Axillary tail view
    D. Craniocaudal
    E. Rolled lateral
    F. Lateromedial
    G. Laterally exaggerated craniocaudal
    H. Inferolateral-superomedial
    I. Implant displaced
    J. Cleavage view

Review Exercise B: Positioning of the Breast

1. A. Craniocaudal (CC)
   B. Mediolateral oblique (MLO)
2. Inframammary crease
3. Axillary
4. Nipple
5. Away
6. Mediolateral oblique (MLO) projection
7. 45 degrees from vertical
8. More
9. B. Forward, toward front of body
10. Laterally exaggerated craniocaudal (XCCL) projection
11. Base
12. Laterally exaggerated craniocaudal (XCCL) projection
13. Laterally exaggerated craniocaudal (XCCL) projection
14. 90°
15. 1. T, 2. F, 3. F, 4. T, 5. F,
    6. F, (overexposed) 7. T, 8. T,
    9. T, 10. F (is the same)
16. Ecklund technique
17. The breast implant needs to be "pinched" or pushed posterior toward the chest wall out of the exposure field

18. D. Axillary tail
19. B. Magnify specific regions of interest
20. A. 100 to 150 mrad

Review Exercise C: Critique Radiographs of the Breast

A. CC projection (Fig. C18-36)
1. *Folds of fatty tissue superimpose breast tissue
2. Breast not pulled away from chest wall and folds of tissue not pulled back
3. Collimation not applicable for mammography. CR centering is acceptable
4. Exposure factors are acceptable
5. Anatomical side marker visible
   Repeatable error(s): Criteria #1

B. MLO projection (Fig. C18-37)
1. *Pertinent muscle not seen to nipple level, and outer tissue is not compressed
2. Lower part of breast not pulled away from chest wall onto film sufficiently
3. Collimation not applicable for mammography. CR centering is acceptable
4. Exposure factors are acceptable
5. Anatomical side marker visible
   Repeatable error(s): Criteria #1

C. CC projection (Fig. C18-37)
1. *Part of lateral posterior breast is cut off
2. *Medial posterior breast not included, and shoulder is superimposed over the lateral posterior tissue
3. Collimation not applicable for mammography. CR centering is acceptable
4. Exposure factors are acceptable
5. Anatomical side marker visible
   Repeatable error(s): Criteria #1 and #2

D. MLO projection (Fig. C18-38)
1. *Posterior medial breast cut off, no pectoral muscle visible. (White specks are calcium; they are not dust artifacts.)
2. *Breast not pulled out away from chest wall
3. Collimation not applicable for mammography. CR centering is acceptable
4. Exposure factors are acceptable
5. Anatomical side marker visible
   Repeatable error(s): Criteria #1 and #2

E. CC projection (Fig. C18-39)
1. *Motion is present, which obliterates all detail
2. Acceptable (dark half circle indicates posterior breast is included)
3. Collimation not applicable for mammography. CR centering is acceptable
4. Exposure factors are acceptable
5. Anatomical side marker visible
   Repeatable error(s): Criteria #1

F. CC projection (Fig. C18-40)
1. *Hair artifacts evident on posterior breast tissue, obscures breast tissue detail
2. Acceptable
3. Collimation not applicable for mammography. CR slightly off-centered toward medial side
4. Exposure factors are acceptable
5. Anatomical side marker visible
   Repeatable error(s): Criteria #1

SELF-TEST

Directions: This self-test should be taken only after completing **all** of the readings, review exercises, and laboratory activities for a particular section.   The purpose of this test is not only to provide a good learning exercise but also to serve as a good indicator of what your final evaluation grade will be. It is strongly suggested that if you do not get at least a 90% to 95% grade on this self-test, you should review those areas in which you missed questions *before* going to your instructor for the final evaluation exam for this chapter. (There are 58 questions or blanks—each is worth 1.7 points.)

1. What does the acronym *MQSA* represent, and what year did it go into effect? _____

2. Which health facilities (if any) are exempt from the MQSA requirements? _____

3. In 1992, the American Cancer Society recommended that all women over age _____ undergo screening mammography.

4. Currently, 1 in _____ American women develops breast cancer sometime in her life.

5. The junction between the inferior aspect of the breast and chest wall is called the _____ .

6. In which quadrant of the breast would the tail or axillary prolongation be found? _____

7. One o'clock in the left breast would relate to _____ in the right breast using the clock system.

8. Which large muscle is directly located posterior to the mammary gland? _____

9. What is the function of the mammary gland? _____

10. Name the bands of connective tissue passing through the breast tissue to provide support.

    _____

11. Which of the three breast tissues is radiographically the least dense? _____

12. What is the term used by radiologists for various small structures seen on the mammogram?

    _____

13. Which term describes the thickest portion of the breast near the chest wall? _____

14. Which one of the following tissue types would be found in the breasts of a 25-year-old pregnant female?

    A. Fibro-glandular   C. Fatty

    B. Fibro-fatty   D. Cystic

15. Which one of the following tissue types would be found in the breasts of a 35-year-old female who has borne two children?

    A. Fibro-glandular   C. Fatty

    B. Fibro-fatty   D. Cystic

16. The male breast would be classified as:

    A. Fibro-glandular   C. Fatty

    B. Fibro-fatty   D. Cystic

17. Which one of the following tissue types requires more compression during mammography as compared with the others?

    A. Fibro-glandular   C. Fatty

    B. Fibro-fatty   D. Cystic

18. Identify the anatomy on Fig. 18-3:

    A. _____

    B. _____

    C. _____

    D. _____

    E. Which basic mammogram projection is demonstrated

    in Fig. 18-3? _____

    F. The right marker on this mammogram is correctly placed on

    the _____ side of the breast.

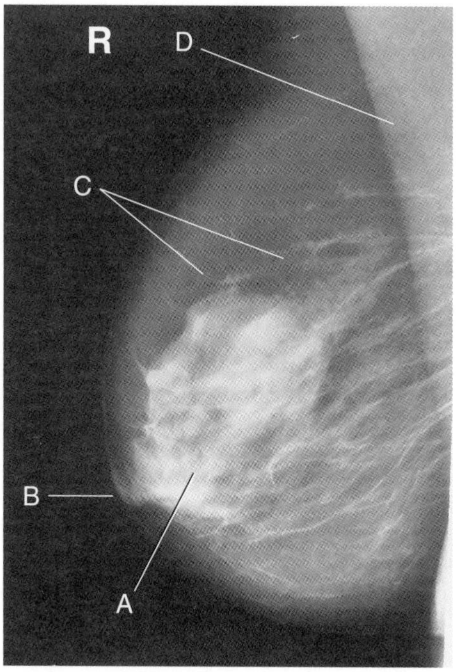

Fig. 18-3 Breast anatomy on a mammogram.

19. The target material used in mammography x-ray tubes is _____ .

20. To utilize the maximum advantage of the anode-heel effect, the anode side of the x-tube should be over the

    _____ (base or apex) of the breast.

21. True/False: Automatic exposure control (AEC) can be used for most mammographic projections.

22. True/False: Compression of the breast will improve image quality by reducing scatter radiation.

23. True/False: A grid is generally not used for mammography.

24. What size focal spot should be used for telemammography of small breast nodules or tissue samples?

    _____

25. What is the magnification factor for an exposure with a source-object distance (SOD) of 20 inches and source

    image-receptor distance (SID) of 40 inches? _____

26. The average MGD (mean glandular dose) received by the patient during a basic two-projection mammogram exami-

    nation is in the _____ range.

    A. 50 to 150 mrad   C. 400 to 600 mrad

    B. 200 to 300 mrad   D. 800 to 1100 mrad

27. Which imaging modality is best suited to distinguish a cyst from a solid mass within the breast?

_____

28. Which imaging modality is best suited to diagnose an extracapsular rupture of a breast implant?

_____

29. True/False: A radiolucent breast implant is being designed that will permit AEC to be used with these devices.

30. True/False: The principal way to reduce patient dose during mammography is to use higher kVp techniques.

31. True/False: One reason that mammoscintigraphy is not ordered more frequently is the high number of false positives reported with this procedure.

32. Which one of the following radionuclides is used for sentinal node studies?

    A. Sulphur colloid   C. Technetium

    B. Sestimibi   D. Iodine 131

33. Carcinoma of the breast is divided into two categories: _____ and _____ .

34. Which one of the following ACR abbreviations refers to the _laterally exaggerated craniocaudal_ projection?

    A. LECC   C. LCC

    B. LXCC   D. XCCL

35. What is the ACR abbreviation for a _mediolateral oblique_ projection? _____

36. List the two basic projections taken during a screening mammogram:

    A. _____   B. _____

37. Which of the basic projections taken during a mammogram will best demonstrate the pectoral muscle?

_____

38. The typical kVp range for mammography is _____ .

39. Which projection best demonstrates the axillary aspect of the breast? _____

40. What are the ACR abbreviations for the special projection, inferolateral-superomedial, used with a pacemaker?

_____

41. The use of automatic exposure control (AEC) when performing a projection with a breast implant in place can lead

    to _____ (over or under) exposure of the breast.

42. A. The technique of "pinching" the breast to push an implant posteriorly to the chest wall is known as the

        _____ technique.

    B. What is the correct ACR term and abbreviation for this technique? _____

43. What other special projection can be taken if a lesion is too deep into the axillary tail aspect of the chest wall to be seen with an XCCL, laterally exaggerated craniocaudal projection? (Include the correct ACR term and abbreviation.)

_____

44. Identification markers should always be placed near the _____ .

45. How is the opposite breast prevented from superimposing the breast being examined on the MLO projection?

_____

46. With a large breast, which of the two basic projections is most likely to require two images to include all the breast tissue?

_____

47. Which projection is usually requested when a lesion is seen on the MLO (mediolateral oblique) but not on the CC (craniocaudad) projection?

_____

48. What landmark determines the correct height for placement of the image receptor for the CC (craniocaudad) projection?

_____

49. Which one of the following projections is recommended for demonstrating inflammation of the breast?

   A. Craniocaudal

   B. Mediolateral oblique

   C. Mediolateral (true lateral)

   D. Laterally exaggerated craniocaudal

50. **Situation:** A mammogram is performed for a patient with breast implants. The resultant images are overexposed. The following factors were used: 28 kVp, AEC, grid, and gentle compression. Which one of the following modifications would produce more diagnostic images during the repeat study?

   A. Lower kVp

   B. Do not use a grid

   C. Use manual exposure factors

   D. Do not use breast compression

CHAPTER 19

Trauma and Mobile Radiography

This chapter has been divided into the following four main sections:

1. **Trauma and Fracture Terminology.** Radiographers should know the more common fracture terms included in this chapter to better understand patient histories and to ensure that the most appropriate projections are taken to demonstrate these fracture sites.
2. **Positioning Principles and Grid Use.** Understanding certain positioning principles, including correct use of portable grids, is essential in trauma and mobile radiography as it is described in this section.
3. **Mobile X-ray Equipment and Radiation Protection.** Understanding the various types of mobile x-ray and fluoroscopy equipment used in trauma radiography (including use in surgery) is essential for radiographers. Knowing and following safe radiation protection practices for workers around mobile equipment is especially important due to the unshielded environments where mobile equipment is generally used (such as in the emergency room, surgery, or in patients' rooms.
4. **Trauma and Mobile Positioning and Procedures.** This section describes specific positioning for each body part in which the patient cannot be moved from the supine position. Adaptation of CR angles and film placement as required is demonstrated and described for each body part.

CHAPTER OBJECTIVES

After you have completed **all** the activities of this chapter, you will be able to:

_____ 1. Define and apply terms for specific types of fractures and soft-tissue injuries.

_____ 2. List the projections taken for a post-reduction study of the limbs, including open and closed reductions.

_____ 3. Explain the two positioning principles that must be observed during trauma radiography.

_____ 4. List the three grid use rules to prevent grid cutoff.

_____ 5. Describe the two primary types of mobile radiographic units and their operating principles.

_____ 6. Explain the features, operating principles, and uses of mobile fluoroscopy units.

_____ 7. List the three methods for maintaining a sterile field with C-arm type equipment.

_____ 8. List the three cardinal rules of radiation protection as they apply to trauma and mobile radiography.

_____ 9. Describe the difference in exposure field levels with different orientations of the x-ray tube and intensifiers with the C-arm.

_____ 10. Explain why the AP projection orientation of the C-arm is not recommended.

_____ 11. List projections for trauma and mobile procedures of the chest, bony thorax, and abdomen.

_____ 12. List projections for trauma and mobile procedures for various parts of the upper and lower limbs.

_____ 13. List projections for trauma and mobile procedures of the cervical, thoracic, and lumbar spine.

_____ 14. List trauma and mobile procedures for the skull and facial bones.

Learning Exercises

The following review exercises should be completed only after careful study of the associated pages in the textbook as indicated by each exercise.

   After completing each of these individual exercises, check your answers with the answer sheets that follow before continuing to the next exercise.

REVIEW EXERCISE A: Radiographic Trauma and Fracture Terminology (see textbook pp. 595-600)

1. True/False: Mobile CT units are available for use in emergency and surgical situations.

2. True/False: Nuclear medicine is effective in diagnosing certain emergency conditions such as pulmonary emboli.

3. True/False: For trauma patients who cannot be moved for conventional diagnostic imaging, other modalities, such as ultrasound or nuclear medicine, may be used rather than trying to move the patient into specific positions.

4. List the two terms for describing displacement of a bone from a joint:

   A. _____   B. _____

5. List the four regions of the body most commonly dislocated during trauma:

   A. _____   C. _____

   B. _____   D. _____

6. What is the correct term for a partial dislocation? _____

7. A forced wrenching or twisting of a joint that results in a tearing of supporting ligaments is a

   _____ .

8. An injury in which there is no fracture or breaking of the skin would describe a _____ .

9. What is the correct term that describes the relationship of the long axes of fracture fragments?

   _____

10. Which term describes a type of fracture in which the fracture fragment ends are overlapped and not in contact?

    _____

11. A. Which term describes the angulation of a distal fracture fragment toward the midline? _____

    B. Would this fracture angulation be described as a medial or lateral apex? _____

12. What is the primary difference between a simple and compound fracture?

    _____

13. List two types of incomplete fractures:

    A. _____   B. _____

14. Which type of comminuted fracture produces several wedge-shaped separate fragments? _____

15. What is the name of the fracture in which one fragment is driven into the other? _____

16. List the secondary name for the following fractures:

  A.   Hutchinson's fracture: _____

  B.   Baseball fracture: _____

  C.   Compound fracture: _____

  D.   Depressed fracture: _____

  E.   Simple fracture: _____

17. True/False: An avulsion fracture is the same as a chip fracture.

18. What type of reduction fracture does *not* require surgery? _____

19. Match the following types of fractures to the correct definition (use each choice only once):

  _____ 1.   Greenstick   A.   Fracture of proximal half of ulna with dislocation of radial head

  _____ 2.   Comminuted   B.   Fracture of the base of the 1st metacarpal

  _____ 3.   Monteggia's   C.   Fracture of the pedicles of C2

  _____ 4.   Boxer's   D.   Fracture of distal radius with anterior displacement

  _____ 5.   Smith's   E.   Complete fracture of distal fibula, frequently with fracture of medial malleolus

  _____ 6.   Hutchinson's   F.   Fracture of lateral malleolus, medial malleolus, and distal posterior tip of tibia

  _____ 7.   Bennett's   G.   Incomplete fracture with broken cortex on one side of bone only

  _____ 8.   Avulsion   H.   Fracture resulting in multiple (two or more) fragments

  _____ 9.   Depressed   I.   Fracture of distal 5th metacarpal

  _____ 10.   Stellate   J.   Intra-articular fracture of radial styloid process

  _____ 11.   Trimalleolar   K.   Fracture of distal radius with posterior displacement

  _____ 12.   Compression   L.   Indented fracture of the skull

  _____ 13.   Pott's   M.   Fracture due to a severe stress to a tendon

  _____ 14.   Colles'   N.   Fracture with fracture lines radiating from center point

  _____ 15.   Hangman's   O.   Fracture producing a reduced height of the anterior vertebral body

20. A. Fig. 19-1 illustrates which specific "named fracture?"

_____

  B. Which bone is most commonly fractured, and which displacement commonly occurs with this fracture?

_____

  C. Describe the type of injury or fall that commonly results

  in this type of fracture? _____

_____

21. A. Fig. 19-2 illustrates which specific "named" fracture?

_____

  B. Which bone(s) is(are) commonly fractured with this

  type of fracture? _____

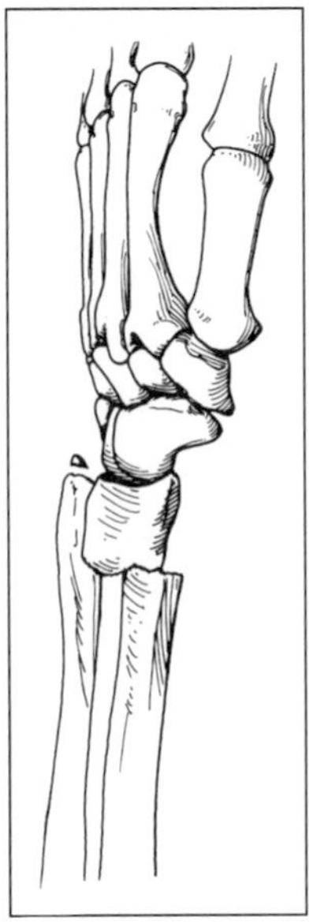

Fig. 19-1 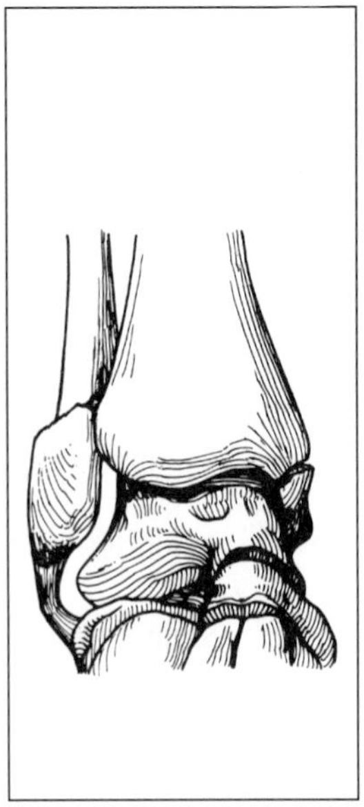   **Fig. 19-2**

REVIEW EXERCISE B: Positioning Principles and Grids (see textbook pp. 600-602)

1. Which single term best describes the primary difference between trauma positions and standard positioning?

_____

2. What should be done to achieve specific projections if the patient cannot move due to trauma?

_____

3. What is the minimum number of projections generally required for any trauma study? _____

4. How many joints must be included for an initial study of a long bone? _____

5. True/False: A follow-up post reduction radiograph of the middle portion of long bones should be collimated closely to the fracture region.

6. Grids are required for any body part measuring greater than _____ cm.

7. List the three factors that must be met to avoid grid cutoff (three limitations or rules to prevent grid cutoff):

  A. _____   B. _____   C. _____

8. True/False: Lead grid lines usually run parallel to the centerline of the long axis of the grid.

9. True/False: To avoid grid cutoff, the angulation of the CR must be perpendicular to the length of the grid.

10. What does "grid focal range" mean? _____

11. What is the preferred grid ratio for a grid used for portable procedures? _____

12. What is considered to be a medium grid focal range? _____

13. A typical long focal range portable grid has a focal range of _____ .

14. What happens to the radiographic image if the SID exceeds a grid's focal range? _____

15. True/False: One particular surface of a focused grid must always be facing the x-ray tube to prevent grid cutoff.

16. A common grid ratio used for mobile work is:

    A.   4:1   B.   6:1 or 8:1   C.   10:1 or 12:1   D.   16:1

REVIEW EXERCISE C: Mobile X-ray Equipment and Radiation Protection (see textbook pp. 603-606)

1. List the two primary types of mobile x-ray units:

    A. _____   B. _____

2. Which type of mobile unit is lighter in weight? _____

3. With battery-powered types, how long does recharging take if the batteries are fully discharged?

    _____

4. True/False: A fully charged battery-powered mobile unit has a driving range of up to 10 miles on level ground.

5. What is the common term for a mobile fluoroscopy unit? _____

6. What are the two primary components of a mobile fluoroscopy unit (located on each end of the structure from which it gets its name)?

    A. _____   B. _____

7. Why shouldn't the mobile fluoroscopy unit be placed in the AP projection ("tube on top" position)?

    _____

8. With the tube and intensifier in a horizontal position, at which side of the patient should the surgeon stand if he or

    she must remain near the patient—the x-ray tube side or the intensifier side? _____ .

    Why? _____

9. Of the two monitors found on most mobile fluoroscopy units, which one is generally considered the "active"

    monitor—the right or the left? _____

10. True/False: Image orientation on the mobile fluoroscopy monitors must be determined by the operator *before* the patient is brought into the room.

11. True/False: All mobile digital type fluoroscopy units have the ability to magnify the image on the monitor during fluoroscopy.

12. True/False: The pulse mode with mobile fluoroscopy units is helpful during procedures to produce brighter images, but it results in significantly increased patient exposure.

13. True/False: Standard cassettes with conventional single-exposure radiographs can be used with most mobile fluoroscopy units.

14. True/False: AEC exposure systems are not feasible with mobile fluoroscopy.

15. Name the feature that allows an image to be held on the monitor while also providing continuous fluoroscopy imaging?

    _____

16. List the three methods for maintaining a sterile field with the mobile fluoroscopy unit.

    A. _____   C. _____

    B. _____

17. List the three terms describing the cardinal rules of radiation protection:

    A. _____   B. _____   C. _____

18. Which cardinal rule is *most* effective in reducing occupational exposure? _____

19. Which one of the following measures is most effective (and practical) in limiting exposure with mobile fluoroscopy?

    A. Limit C-arm procedures to surgery cases only

    B. Prevent non-radiologists from using the C-arm

    C. Use intermittent or "foot-tapping" fluoroscopy

    D. Limit all fluoroscopy procedures to no more than 10 minutes

   For Questions 20 to 24, review exposure field information on Figs. 19-3 and 19-4. Also see the textbook, p. 606.

20. **Situation:** The C-arm is in position for a PA projection. What exposure field range would the operator receive at waist level standing 3 feet from the patient?

    A. 20 to 25 mR/hr   C. 50 to 100 mR/hr

    B. 25 to 50 mR/hr   D. 100 to 300 mR/hr

21. Approximately how much exposure at waist level would the operator receive with 5 minutes of fluoroscopy exposure standing 3 feet from the patient? (Hint: first convert mR/hr to mR/min by dividing by 60, then multiply by minutes of fluoroscopy time.)

    A. 5 mR   C. 25 mR

    B. 60 mR   D. 2 mR

22. If a radiographer receives 50 mR/ hr standing 3 feet from the mobile fluoroscopy unit, what would be the exposure rate if he or she moved back to a distance of 4 feet?

    A. 10 mR/hr

    B. 25 mR/hr

    C. 100 mR/hr

    D. No significant difference

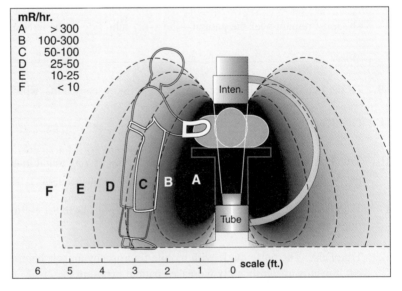

Fig. 19-3 Occupational exposure during mobile fluoroscopy, PA projection.

23. A radiographer standing 1 foot from a mobile fluoroscopy unit is receiving approximately 400 mR/hr. What is the *total* exposure to the radiographer if the procedure takes 10 minutes of fluoroscopy time to complete?

_____

24. **Situation:** An operator receives 25 mR/hr to the facial and neck region with the C-arm in position for a PA projection (intensifier on top). Approximately how much would the operator receive at the same distance if the C-arm were reversed to an AP projection position (tube on top)?

    A. 25 to 50 mR/hr

    B. 50 to 100 mR/hr

    C. 100 to 300 mR/hr

    D. 300 to 500 mR/hr

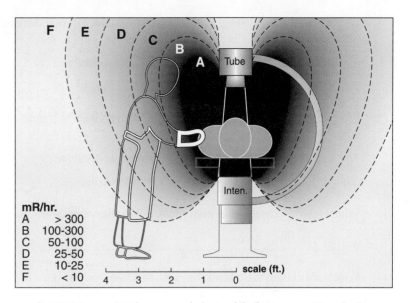

mR/hr.
A   > 300
B   100-300
C   50-100
D   25-50
E   10-25
F   < 10

scale (ft.)
4   3   2   1   0

Fig. 19-4 Occupational exposure during mobile fluoroscopy, AP projection.

25. A 30° C-arm tilt from the vertical perspective will increase exposure to the head and neck regions of the operator by

    a factor of _____.

REVIEW EXERCISE D: Trauma and Mobile Positioning and Procedures (see textbook pp. 607-628)

1. How is the CR centered and aligned in relationship to the sternum for an AP portable projection of the chest?

   _____

2. True/False: Focused grids are recommended for mobile chest projections.

3. Which way (crosswise or lengthwise) should a 35 x 43 cm (14 x 17 in.) IR be placed for an AP portable chest on an

   average or large patient? _____ Why? _____

   _____

4. What specific position should be performed to demonstrate a possible pneumothorax in the left lung for a patient

   who cannot stand or sit erect? _____

5. Which position can be used to replace the RAO of the sternum for the patient who cannot lie prone on the table but

   can be rotated into a semi-supine position? _____

6. How must the grid be aligned to prevent grid cutoff when angling the CR mediolaterally for an oblique projection

   of the sternum when the patient cannot be rotated or moved at all from the supine position?

   _____

7. Other than the straight AP, what other projection of the ribs can be taken for the supine immobile patient who can-

   not be rotated into an oblique position?_____

8. Which one of the following positions or projections will best demonstrate free intra-abdominal air on the patient who cannot stand or sit erect?

   A. Left lateral decubitus   C. Right lateral decubitus

   B. AP KUB   D. Dorsal decubitus

9. Which one of the following projections of the abdomen will most effectively demonstrate a possible abdominal aortic aneurysm?

   A. Left lateral decubitus   C. Right lateral decubitus

   B. AP KUB   D. Dorsal decubitus

10. What is the disadvantage of performing a PA rather than an AP projection of the thumb?

   _____

11. Which projections are taken for a post-reduction study of the wrist?

   _____

12. **Situation:** A study of a fractured wrist was taken with the following exposure factors: 60 kVp, 10 mAs, detail screens. A fiberglass cast is placed on the wrist and a post-reduction study is ordered. Which one of the following techniques would be ideal for the post-reduction study?

   A. 70 kVp and 10 mAs   C. 65 kVp and 10 mAs

   B. 80 kVp and 10 mAs   D. 55 kVp and 15 mAs

13. True/False: A PA horizontal beam projection of the elbow can be taken for a patient with multiple injuries.

14. True/False: For a trauma lateral projection of the elbow, the CR must be kept parallel to the interepicondylar plane.

15. **Situation:** A patient with a possible fracture of the proximal humerus enters the emergency room. Because of multiple injuries, the patient is unable to stand or sit erect. What positioning routine should be performed to diagnose the extent of the injury?

   _____

16. **Situation:** A patient with a possible dislocation of the proximal humerus enters the emergency room. Because of multiple injuries, the patient is unable to stand or sit erect. In addition to a basic AP projection, what second projection will demonstrate whether it is an anterior or posterior dislocation?

   _____

17. How much CR angulation should be used for an AP axial projection of the clavicle on a hypersthenic patient?

   A. 10°   B. 15°   C. 20°   D. 25°

18. A lateral "Y" projection taken AP for a trauma patient usually requires a _____ degree rotation of the body away from the image receptor.

   A. 20 to 30   B. 45   C. 50 to 60   D. 70

19. To ensure that the joints are opened up for an AP projection of the foot, how is the CR aligned?

   A. Perpendicular to the long axis of the tibia

   B. Perpendicular to the plantar surface

   C. 10° posteriorly from perpendicular to plantar surface

   D. 10° posteriorly from perpendicular to dorsal surface

20. **Situation:** An orthopedic surgeon orders a mortise projection of the ankle, but the patient has a severely fractured ankle and cannot rotate the ankle medially for the mortise projection. What can the radiographer do to provide this projection without rotating the ankle?

_____

21. **Situation:** A patient with a possible dislocation of the patella enters the emergency room. What type of positioning routine should be performed on this patient that would safely demonstrate the patella?

_____

22. **Situation:** A patient with a possible fracture of the proximal tibia and fibula enters the emergency room. The basic AP and lateral projections are inconclusive. Because of severe pain, the patient is unable to rotate the leg from the AP position. What position or projection could be performed that would provide an unobstructed view of the fibular head and neck?

_____

23. Which one of the following positions would be performed on a trauma patient to provide a lateral view of the proximal femur?

    A. Danelius-Miller method   C. Waters method

    B. Fuchs method   D. Ottonello method

24. Which lateral projection can be taken of the proximal femur without having to abduct or flex the unaffected limb?

_____

25. How is the CR aligned for the method identified in question 24?

_____

26. **Situation:** A patient with injuries suffered in a motor vehicle accident enters the emergency room.   The ER physician orders a lateral C-spine projection to rule out a fracture or dislocation. Because of the thickness of the shoulders, C6-7 is not visualized. What additional projection can be taken safely to demonstrate this region of the spine?

_____

27. **Situation:** A patient with a possible C2 fracture enters the emergency room on a backboard. The AP projection does not demonstrate C2. In addition, the patient cannot open his mouth because of a mandible fracture. Which projection can be performed safely to demonstrate this region of the spine?

    A. Fuchs   C. Vertebral arch projection

    B. Judd   D. 35 to 40° cephalad axial projection

28. Which projection will best demonstrate (with only minimal distortion) the pedicles of the cervical spine on a severely injured patient?

_____

29. Identify the two CR angles for the double angle Method Two for the oblique cervical spine.

    A. _____° medial   B. _____° cephalad

30. When using the Method Two, double angle technique, how is the cassette positioned for an oblique cervical spine to minimize distortion?

_____

31. **Situation:** A patient with a possible basilar skull fracture enters the emergency room. The ER physician wants a projection that best demonstrates a sphenoid effusion. The patient cannot stand or sit erect. Which one of the following projections would achieve this goal?

    A. AP skull   C. Horizontal beam lateral skull

    B. Lateral recumbent skull   D. Modified Waters projection

32. Which one of the following projections of the skull would project the petrous ridges in the lower one third of the orbits on a supine trauma patient?

    A. AP skull, CR 0° to OML   C. AP skull, CR 15° cephalad to OML

    B. AP skull, CR 15° caudad to OML   D. AP skull, CR 30° caudad to OML

33. True/False: AP projections of the skull and facial bones will increase exposure to the thyroid gland as compared to PA projections.

34. True/False: The CR should not exceed a 30° caudad angle for the AP axial projection of the cranium to avoid excessive distortion of the cranial bones.

35. How is the CR angled and where is it centered for the AP acanthioparietal (reverse Waters) projection of the facial bones?

_____

36. What type of CR angulation is required for the trauma version of an axiolateral projection of the mandible?

_____

37. **Situation:** A patient with a Monteggia's fracture enters the emergency room. Which one of the following positioning routines should be performed on this patient?

    A. AP and lateral thumb   C. AP and horizontal beam lateral lower leg

    B. PA and horizontal beam lateral wrist   D. PA or HP and horizontal beam lateral forearm

38. **Situation:** A patient with a possible Greenstick fracture enters the emergency room. What age group does this type of fracture usually affect?

    A. Pediatric   C. Middle age

    B. Young adult   D. Elderly

39. **Situation:** A patient with a possible Pott's fracture enters the emergency room. Which one of the following positioning routines should be performed on this patient?

    A. AP and horizontal beam lateral lower leg   C. AP and lateral thumb

    B. PA and horizontal beam lateral wrist   D. Three projections of the hand

40. **Situation:** A patient is struck directly on the patella with a heavy object, shattering it. The resultant fracture most likely would be described as a:

    A. Burst fracture   C. Stellate fracture

    B. Compression fracture   D. Smith's fracture

Answers to Review Exercises

Review Exercise A: Radiographic Trauma and Fracture

1. True
2. True
3. False. It is important to rotate the x-ray tube and image receptor around patients if they are unable to move.
4. A. Dislocation
   B. Luxation
5. A. Shoulder
   B. Fingers or thumb
   C. Patella
   D. Hip
6. Subluxation
7. Sprain
8. Contusion
9. Apposition
10. Bayonet apposition
11. A. Varus (deformity) angulation
    B. Lateral apex
12. A simple fracture does not break through the skin, but a compound fracture protrudes through the skin.
13. A. Torus fracture
    B. Greenstick fracture
14. Butterfly fracture
15. Impacted fracture
16. A. Chauffeur's
    B. Mallet
    C. Open
    D. Ping-pong
    E. Closed
17. False. (A chip fracture involves an isolated fracture not associated with a tendon or ligament.)
18. Closed reduction
19. 1. G, 2. H, 3. A, 4. I, 5. D, 6. J, 7. B, 8. M, 9. L, 10. N, 11. F, 12. O, 13. E, 14. K, 15. C
20. A. Colles' fracture
    B. Distal radius, posterior displacement of distal fragment
    C. Fall on outstretched arm
21. A. Pott's fracture
    B. Distal fibula and occasionally the distal tibia or medial malleolus

Review Exercise B: Positioning Principles and Grids

1. Adaptation
2. Move the CR and IR around the patient to produce similar projections rather than moving the patient
3. Two. Two projections should be taken 90° to each other
4. Two. Both joints must be included on the initial study
5. False (must include at least one joint nearest injury)
6. 10
7. A. Correct CR centering
   B. Correct CR angling
   C. Correct grid focal range
8. True
9. False (parallel to)
10. The SID range in which the x-ray beam can pass through the grid without excessive absorption
11. 6:1 or 8:1 grid ratio
12. 34 to 46 in. (86 to 117 cm)
13. 48 to 72 in. (122 to 183 cm)
14. It will create "off-distance" grid cut-off
15. True
16. B. 6:1 or 8:1

Review Exercise C: Mobile X-ray Equipment and Radiation Protection

1. A. Battery powered, battery driven type
   B. Standard AC power source, non-motor drive
2. Standard power source, non-motor drive
3. 8 hours
4. True
5. C-arm
6. A. X-ray tube
   B. Image intensifier
7. Because it results in a significant increase in exposure to the head and neck region of the operator
8. Intensifier side; the radiation field pattern extends out farther on the x-ray tube side
9. Left monitor
10. True
11. True
12. False (reduces exposure to patient)
13. True
14. False (can be used)
15. Roadmapping
16. A. Draping the total C-arm, tube, and intensifier
    B. Draping the patient
    C. Using a "shower curtain" type arrangement to maintain a sterile field
17. A. Time
    B. Distance
    C. Shielding
18. Distance
19. C. use intermittent or "foot-tapping" fluoroscopy
20. C. 50 to 100 mR/hr
21. A. 5 mR (60 mR ÷ 60 min = 1 mR × 5 min = 5)
22. B. 25 mR/hr
23. 67 mR (400 ÷ 60 x 10 = 67)
24. C 100 to 300 mR/hr
25. Four

Review Exercise D: Trauma and Mobile Positioning and Procedures

1. Centered 3 to 4 in. (7 to 10 cm) below jugular notch, angled caudad so as to be perpendicular to sternum
2. False (not recommended due to probable grid cutoff)
3. Crosswise, to prevent side cutoff of the right or left lateral margins of the chest. More important with portable chests due to increased divergence of x-ray beam at the shorter SID.
4. Right lateral decubitus
5. 15 to 20° LPO
6. Crosswise
7. 30 to 40° cross-angled mediolateral projection (Note: This results in image distortion and should be done as a last resort)
8. A. left lateral decubitus
9. D. dorsal decubitus
10. Increase OID of the thumb (increases distortion)
11. PA and lateral projections
12. C. 65 kVp and 10 mAs
13. True
14. True
15. AP and horizontal beam, transthoracic lateral
16. A horizontal beam transthoracic lateral
17. B. 15°
18. A. 20 to 30
19. C. 10° posteriorly from perpendicular to plantar surface (Note: This would also be 10° posteriorly from plane of IR)
20. Angle the CR 15 to 20° lateromedially to the long axis of the foot
21. AP and horizontal beam lateral with no flexion of knee
22. 45° lateromedial cross-angle AP projection of the knee and proximal tibia/fibula
23. A. Danelius-Miller method
24. Mediolateral (Sanderson) projection
25. Cross-angled mediolaterally to be near perpendicular to the long axis of the foot
26. Swimmer's lateral using a horizontal beam CR

27. D. 35 to 40° cephalad axial projection
28. 45° oblique using the double-angle method with IR perpendicular to CR
29. A. 45° medial
    B. 15° cephalad
30. Cassette placed on a stool under the table and patient, set at a 45° angle, perpendicular to CR
31. C. horizontal beam lateral skull
32. C. AP skull, CR 15° cephalad to OML
33. True
34. False (should not exceed 45°)
35. Parallel to the mentomeatal line, centered to acanthion
36. 25 to 30° cephalad and possibly 5 to 10° posterior to clear the shoulder
37. D. PA or AP and horizontal beam lateral forearm
38. A. Pediatric
39. A. AP and horizontal beam lateral lower leg
40. C. Stellate fracture

SELF-TEST

My Score = _____%

Directions: This self-test should be taken only after completing **all** of the readings, review exercises, and laboratory activities for a particular section.   The purpose of this test is not only to provide a good learning exercise but also to serve as a strong indicator of what your final evaluation grade will be. It is strongly suggested that if you do not get at least a 90% to 95% grade on this self-test, you should review those areas in which you missed questions before going to your instructor for the final evaluation exam for this chapter. (There are 68 questions or blanks—each is worth 1.5 points.)

1. From the list of possible fracture types on the left, indicate which fracture is represented on each drawing or radiograph by writing in the correct term where indicated (A through I):

   • Single (closed) fracture

   • Compound (open) fracture

   • Torus fracture

   • Greenstick fracture

   • Plastic fracture

   • Transverse fracture

   • Oblique fracture

   • Spiral fracture

   • Comminuted fracture

   • Impacted fracture

   • Baseball (mallet) fracture

   • Barton's fracture

   • Bennett fracture

   • Colles' fracture

   • Monteggia's fracture

   • Nursemaid's elbow fracture

   • Pott's fracture

   • Avulsion fracture

   • Chip fracture

   • Compression fracture

   • Stellate fracture

   • Tuft fracture

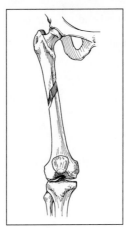

A. _____

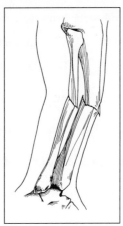

B. _____

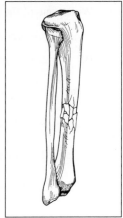

C. _____

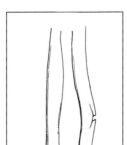

D. _____

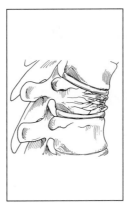

E. _____

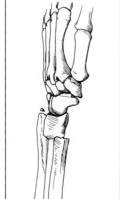

F. _____

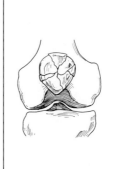

G. _____

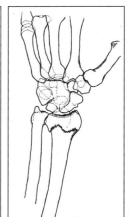

H. _____

I. _____

2. A.   What is the correct term for the displacement of a bone from a joint? _____

    B.   What is the correct term for a partial displacement? _____

3. What region of the body encounters partial dislocations most frequently? _____

4. Which one of the following terms describes a poor alignment between the ends of a fractured bone?
    A. Dislocation   C. Apex angulation
    B. Lack of apposition   D. Anatomical apposition

5. Which one of the following terms describes a bending of a distal fracture away from the midline?
    A. Valgus angulation   C. Apex angulation
    B. Varus angulation   D. Bayonet apposition

6. Match the following definitions to the correct type of fracture (use each answer only once):

    _____   1. Fracture through the pedicles of C2   A. Nursemaid's elbow

    _____   2. Fracture of proximal half of ulna with dislocation of radial head   B. Bennett's

    _____   3. Fracture due to a disease process   C. Baseball

    _____   4. Fracture resulting in an isolated bone fragment   D. Pathological

    _____   5. Subluxation of the radial head of a child   E. Hangman's

    _____   6. Fracture along base of 1st metacarpal   F. Hutchinson's

    _____   7. Fracture of distal phalanx with finger extended   G. Stress or fatigue

    _____   8. Also called a *March fracture*   H. Chip

    _____   9. Also called a *Chauffeur's fracture*   I. Monteggia's

7. True/False: Any trauma study requires at least two projections as close to 90° opposite from each other as possible.

8. True/False: On an initial study of a long bone, both joints should be included for each projection.

9. Which one of the following projections (on a sthenic adult) would require the use of a grid?
    A. AP leg (tibia-fibula)   C. Lateral elbow
    B. Lateral ankle   D. AP shoulder

10. What is the preferred grid ratio for trauma radiography?
    A. 5:1   C. 10:1 to 12:1
    B. 6:1 to 8:1   D. 16:1

11. List the two factors that determine a grid's focal range:

    A. _____   B. _____

12. True/False: Using an SID greater than the established focal range will produce grid cutoff.

13. Which type of mobile radiography x-ray unit is self-propelled? _____

14. Which type of mobile x-ray unit is lighter weight? _____

15. True/False: C-arms are most generally stationary fluoroscopy units used in surgery.

16. True/False: The C-arm fluoroscopy unit can be rotated 180°.

17. True/False: The AP projection during a C-arm procedure is recommended to minimize OID.

18. True/False: Digital C-arm units can store images on video tape or computer hard disk memory.

19. What is the term for the process of holding one image on the C-arm monitor while also providing continuous fluo-

    roscopy? _____

20. What is the primary benefit of the "pulse mode" on a digital C-arm unit? _____

21. List the three cardinal rules of radiation protection:

    A. _____   B. _____   C. _____

22. Which one of the cardinal rules is most effective in reducing occupational exposure?

    _____

23. **Situation:** A radiographer using a C-arm fluoroscope receives 125 mR/hr standing 2 feet from the patient. What is
    the exposure rate if the radiographer moves to a distance of 6 feet?

    A. Less than 10 mR/hr   C. 30 to 50 mR/hr

    B. 15 to 30 mR/hr   D. 50 to 75 mR/hr

24. **Situation:** A radiographer receives 30 mR/hr during a C-arm fluoroscopic procedure. What is the *total* exposure

    dose if the procedure takes 8 minutes of fluoroscopy time? _____

25. True/False: The exposure dose is greater on the image intensifier side as compared with the x-ray tube side with the
    C-arm in the horizontal configuration.

26. True/False: A 30° tilt of C-arm from the vertical perspective will increase the dose by a factor of three to the head
    and neck region.

27. **Situation:** A patient with a possible pleural effusion in the right lung enters the emergency room. The patient is un-
    able to stand or sit erect. What position would best demonstrate this condition?

    A. Right lateral decubitus   C. Dorsal decubitus

    B. AP supine   D. Semi-erect AP

28. Where is the CR centered for an AP semi-erect projection of the chest? _____

29. **Situation:** A patient with a crushing injury to the thorax enters the emergency room. The patient is on a backboard
    and cannot be moved. Which projections can be performed to determine if the sternum is fractured?

    _____

30. **Situation:** A patient with possible ascites (fluid accumulation in peritoneal cavity of the abdomen) enters the emergency room. The patient is unable to stand or sit erect. Which one of the following positions would best demonstrate this condition?

    A. AP supine KUB

    B. Dorsal decubitus

    C. Left lateral decubitus

    D. Prone KUB

31. How many projections are required for a post-reduction study of the wrist? _____

32. How is the CR aligned for a trauma lateral projection of the elbow? _____

33. Which lateral projection would best demonstrate the mid-to-distal humerus without rotating the limb?

    _____

34. How much obliquity of the body is generally required for a lateromedial scapula projection with a trauma patient

    who can be turned up partially on her side? _____

35. To ensure that the CR is aligned properly for an AP trauma projection of the foot, the CR is angled:

    _____ .

36. **Situation:** A patient with a possible fracture of the ankle enters the emergency room. The patient cannot rotate the lower limb. What can be done to provide the orthopedic surgeon with a mortise projection of the ankle?

    _____

37. Which one of the following statements is *not* true about the Sanderson method?

    A. The unaffected leg does not need to be moved at all.

    B. The patient is obliqued into a 15 to 20° posterior oblique position.

    C. The affected leg is rotated 10 to 15° internally if possible.

    D. The CR is angled to be perpendicular to the long axis of the foot of the affected limb.

38. Which one of the following projections will demonstrate the C1-2 vertebra if the patient cannot open his mouth?

    A. 35 to 40° cephalad, AP axial projection

    B. Swimmer's lateral

    C. 15 to 20° cephalad, AP axial projection

    D. Articular pillar projection

39. **Situation:** A patient with a possible fracture of the cervical spine pedicles enters the emergency room. Which one of the following projections will best demonstrate this region of the spine with the least distortion without moving the patient?

    A. Perform a Swimmer's lateral

    B. Perform an articular pillar projection

    C. Perform a double angle oblique projection with IR perpendicular to CR

    D. Perform a 45° CR oblique projection with IR flat on table-top

40. What are the two advantages of angling the cassette 45° for the trauma oblique cervical, which also results in a long OID for the Method Two double angle projection?

    A. _____

    B. _____

41. Which one of the following facial bone projections will best demonstrate air-fluid levels in the maxillary sinuses for a patient unable to stand or sit erect?

    A. AP acanthioparietal   C. AP modified acanthioparietal

    B. Trauma, horizontal beam lateral   D. AP axial

42. A. On a horizontal beam lateral trauma skull projection, should the cassette be placed lengthwise or crosswise to

        the patient? _____

    B. Where should the CR be centered for this lateral skull projection? _____

43. **Situation:** A patient with a possible compression fracture of the lumbar spine enters the emergency room. Which specific position of the lumbar spine series would best demonstrate this?

    A. AP   C. Lateral

    B. LPO and RPO   D. AP L5-S1 projection

44. **Situation:** A patient with a possible Barton's fracture comes to the radiology department. Which one of the following positioning routines would best demonstrate this?

    A. AP or PA and lateral wrist   C. AP and lateral foot

    B. AP, mortise, and lateral ankle   D. AP and lateral lower leg

45. Radiologists often use the Salter-Harris system to classify _____ fractures.

    A. Pathologic   C. Stellate

    B. Trimalleolar   D. Epiphyseal

CHAPTER 20

Pediatric Radiography

Positioning considerations are unique to pediatric radiography and present a definite challenge for all radiographers. Children cannot be handled and positioned like miniature adults. They have special needs and require patience and understanding. Their anatomical makeup is vastly different from that of adults, especially the skeletal system. The bony development (ossification) of children goes through specific growth stages from infancy to adolescence. These need to be understood by radiographers so that the appearance of the normal growth stages can be recognized. Examples of normal bone development patterns at various ages are included in this chapter and in the textbook.

The basic and optional projections and positions are much different for children than for adults. You need to know and understand these differences to be able to visualize the essential anatomy on children of various ages.

The most obvious differences for children when compared with adults are the methods of positioning and immobility. Small children cannot just be instructed to hold still in certain positions or to hold their breath during the exposure. You will need to learn how to relate to children and communicate with them to get their cooperation without forceful immobilization.

Special immobilization techniques need to be learned along with the use of various types of commonly available immobilization paraphernalia. Specialized restraining devices available in many departments will be explained and demonstrated in this chapter.

Radiation protection for these small patients must also be a major concern, because the younger the child, the more sensitive that child's tissues are to radiation. Thus **accurate collimation and gonadal shielding** are absolutely essential. High-speed screens and films should also be used, and **repeats must be minimized.** Specific patient doses in icon boxes for each projection are not provided in this chapter because of the many variables involved. However, **keeping all child doses as low as possible** is even more important than in adult radiography. Therefore, careful study of this chapter and related clinical experience are essential **before** you attempt a radiographic examination on a small child or infant. As a student, you may have limited opportunity to observe and assist with pediatric patients during your training. This makes learning and mastering the information provided in this chapter of the textbook and this workbook-laboratory manual even more important.

CHAPTER OBJECTIVES

After you have completed **all** the activities of this chapter, you will be able to:

_____ 1. List the steps and process of the technologist's introduction to the child and parent and the potential role of the parent during the child's examination.

_____ 2. Define the term *nonaccidental trauma (NAT)* and describe the role of technologists if they suspect child abuse based on individual state guidelines.

_____ 3. Identify the more common commercial immobilization devices and explain their function.

_____ 4. List the most common types of paraphernalia used for immobilization.

_____ 5. List the six steps of "mummifying" an infant. Perform this procedure on a simulated patient.

_____ 6. Define terms relating to bone development or ossification and identify the radiographic appearance and the normal stages of development of secondary growth centers.

_____ 7. Identify methods of reducing patient and parent doses and repeat exposures during pediatric procedures.

_____ 8. Identify alternative imaging modalities and procedures performed on pediatric patients.

_____ 9. List the common pathologic indications for radiographic examinations of the chest, upper and lower limbs, pelvis and hips, skull, and pediatric abdomen procedures.

_____ 10. For select forms of pathology of the pediatric skeletal system, determine whether manual exposure factors would increase, decrease, or remain the same.

_____ 11. Describe positioning, technical factors, shielding requirements, and immobilization techniques for procedures of the chest, skeletal system, and abdomen.

———— 12. List general patient preparation requirements for procedures of the pediatric abdomen, including specific minimum patient preparation requirements for the upper GI, lower GI, and IVU procedures.

———— 13. List the types and quantities of contrast media based on age as recommended for upper GI, lower GI, and IVU procedures.

———— 14. Using an articulated pediatric mannequin, correctly immobilize and position a patient. Using gonadal shielding, perform examinations of the chest, abdomen, upper limb, lower limb, pelvis and hips, and skull.

———— 15. According to established evaluation criteria, critique and evaluate radiographs provided by your instructor for each of the previously mentioned examinations.

———— 16. Discriminate between acceptable and unacceptable radiographs and describe how positioning or technical errors can be corrected.

Learning Exercises

Complete the following review exercises after reading the associated pages in the textbook as indicated by each exercise. Answers to each review exercise are given at the end of the review exercises.

PART I: Introduction to Pediatric Radiography

REVIEW EXERCISE A: Immobilization, Ossification, Radiation Protection, Pre-examination Preparation, and Pathologic Indications (see textbook pp. 630-639)

1. List the two important general factors that produce a successful pediatric radiographic procedure:

   A. _____

   B. _____

2. List the three possible roles for the parent during a pediatric procedure.

   A. _____

   B. _____

   C. _____

3. True/False: Parents should never be in the radiographic room with their child.

4. True/False: Battered child syndrome (BCS) is the acceptable term for child abuse.

5. True/False: The technologist is responsible for reporting potential signs of child abuse to the police.

6. True/False: The technologist should always use as short an exposure time as possible during pediatric procedures.

7. List the correct term for the following pediatric immobilization devices:

   A. A piece of Plexiglas with short Velcro straps for immobilization of upper and lower limbs: _____

   B. A device used to hold down upper or lower limbs without obscuring essential anatomy: _____

   C. A device with an adjustable-type bicycle seat and two clear plastic body clamps: _____

8. Which of the immobilization devices just mentioned is most commonly used for erect chests and abdomens?

    _____

9. True/False: Sandbags completely filled with fine sand should be used to immobilize pediatric patients.

10. If stockinettes are used for immobilization, what size should be used for a larger pediatric patient?

    A. 1 inch   C. 3 inch

    B. 2 inch   D. 4 inch

11. Which type of tape is *not* recommended for immobilization purposes on children (because it may create an artifact
    on the radiograph when placed over the region being radiographed)?

    _____

12. When adhesive tape is used to immobilize (if not placed directly over parts to be radiographed), what two methods
    are used to prevent the adhesive tape from injuring the fragile skin of infants?

    A. _____

    B. _____

13. A. If Ace bandages are used for immobilization of the legs, which size should be used on infants and smaller chil-

        dren: 3 inch, 4 inch, or 6 inch? _____

    B. What size should be used on older children? _____

14. Briefly describe the six steps for "mummifying" a child.

    1. _____

        _____

    2. _____

        _____

    3. _____

        _____

    4. _____

        _____

    5. _____

        _____

    6. _____

        _____

15. Primary centers of bone formation (ossification) involving the midshafts of long bones are called

    _____ .

16. Secondary centers of ossification of the long bones are called _____.

17. The spaces between the primary and secondary areas of ossification are called _____.

18. At approximately what age does the epiphysis of the fibular apex first become clearly visible (see textbook, p. 634)?

   A. 1 or 2 years old   C. 5 or 6 years old

   B. 3 or 4 years old   D. Teens

19. At approximately what age does the skeleton reach full ossification?

   A. 12 years old   C. 25 years old

   B. 18 years old   D. 40 years old

20. List three safeguards to help reduce repeat exposures during pediatric procedures:

   A. _____   C. _____

   B. _____

21. List three safeguards to reduce the patient dose during pediatric procedures (in addition to gonadal shielding):

   A. _____   C. _____

   B. _____

22. When two technologists are working together, match the following duties with the primary or assisting technologist:

   ____ 1. Makes exposures   A. Primary technologist

   ____ 2. Positions the patient   B. Assisting technologist

   ____ 3. Processes the images

   ____ 4. Positions the tube and collimates

   ____ 5. Sets exposure factors

   ____ 6. Instructs the parents

23. True/False: Clothing, bandages, and diapers generally do not need to be removed from the regions being radiographed on pediatric patients since they do not cause artifacts on the radiographs (if metallic fasteners are not present).

24. Which one of the following imaging modalities is most effective in diagnosing pyloric stenosis in children?

   A. Sonography   C. Functional MRI

   B. Spiral/helical CT   D. Nuclear medicine

25. Functional MRI may be used to detect disorders in all the following conditions *except:*

   A. Autism   C. Hydrocephalus

   B. Tourette's syndrome   D. Attention deficient hyperactivity disorder

26. Match the following pathologic indications of the pediatric chest with the best definition and/or statement (use each choice only once):

_____ A. Meconium aspiration

_____ B. Hyaline membrane disease

_____ C. Neonate Graves' disease

_____ D. Epiglottitis

_____ E. Cystic fibrosis

_____ F. Croup

_____ G. Hemoptysis

1. Bacterial infection can lead to closure of the upper airway

2. Also known as *respiratory distress syndrome*

3. Inherited disease leading to clogging of bronchi

4. Condition may develop during stressful births

5. Viral infection leading to labored breathing and dry cough

6. Coughing up blood

7. A form of hyperthyroidism

27. Match the following pathologic indications of the pediatric skeletal system to the best definition and/or statement:

_____ A. Meningocele

_____ B. Kohler's bone disease

_____ C. Legg-Calve-Perthes disease

_____ D. Talipes equinus

_____ E. Osteogenesis imperfecta

_____ F. Achondroplasia

_____ G. Myelocele

_____ H. Osteochondroses

1. Most common form of short-limbed dwarfism

2. Hereditary disorder characterized by soft and fragile bones

3. Congenital defect where the spinal cord protrudes through an opening in the vertebral column

4. A common lesion at the hip

5. Group of diseases affecting the epiphyseal plates of long bones

6. Congenital defect in which the meninges of the spinal cord protrude through an opening in the vertebral column

7. Inflammation of the navicular bone in the foot

8. Congenital deformity of the foot involving plantar flexion

28. Match the following pathologic indications of the pediatric abdomen to the best definition and/or statement:

_____ A. Hydronephrosis

_____ B. Pyloric stenosis

_____ C. NEC

_____ D. Atresias

_____ E. Hypospadias

_____ F. Hirshsprung's disease

_____ G. Celiac disease

1. May result in repeated, forceful vomiting

2. Rhythmic contractions of large intestine are absent

3. Condition characterized by absence of on opening in an organ

4. Condition resulting from an allergic reaction to gluten

5. Enlarged renal collection system due to obstruction

6. Inflammation of the inner lining of the intestine

7. Congenital defect in male urethra

29. Indicate whether the following pathologic conditions require that manual exposure factors be increased (+), decreased (−), or remain the same (0):

    A.   Pneumonia   _____

    B.   Pneumothorax   _____

    C.   Osteogenesis imperfecta   _____

    D.   Legg-Calve- Perthes disease   _____

    E.   Osteomalacia   _____

    F.   Osteopetrosis   _____

    G.   Volvulus   _____

30. True/False: Malignant bone tumors are rare in young children.

PART II: Radiographic Positioning

REVIEW EXERCISE B: Pediatric Positioning of the Chest, Skeletal System, and Skull (see textbook pp. 641-652)

1. Complete the following technical factors for an AP or PA pediatric chest:

    A.   Grid or non-grid: _____   D.   SID, AP supine chest: _____

    B.   kVp range: _____   E.   SID, PA erect chest: _____

    C.   Image receptor lengthwise or crosswise: _____

2. What kVp range is generally used for a lateral chest? _____

3. Should a grid be used for a lateral chest (yes or no)? _____

4. The Pigg-O-Stat can be used effectively for an erect PA and lateral chest from infancy to approximately age

    _____.

5. When should a chest exposure be made for a crying child?

    _____

6. Which radiographic structures are evaluated to determine rotation on a PA projection of the chest?

    _____

7. How is the x-ray tube aligned for a lateral projection of the chest if the patient is on a Tam-em board?

    _____

8. True/False: If available, the Pigg-O-Stat should be used rather than relying on parental assistance during a pediatric chest examination.

9. True/False: A well-inspired, erect chest radiograph taken on a young pediatric patient will visualize only six to seven ribs above the diaphragm.

10. True/False: The entire upper limb is commonly included on an infant rather than individual exposures of specific parts of the upper limb.

11. True/False: Except for survey exams, individual projections of the elbow, wrist, and shoulder should generally be taken on older children rather than including these regions on a single projection.

12. Match the following pathologic indicators with the correct radiographic procedure:

    _____ 1. Atelectasis   A. Chest

    _____ 2. Kohler's disease   B. Upper or lower limb

    _____ 3. Cystic fibrosis

    _____ 4. Talipes

    _____ 5. RDS

13. Which single radiographic position will provide a lateral projection of bilateral lower limbs for the nontraumatic pediatric patient?

    _____

14. Which radiographic projections (and method) are performed for the infant with congenital club feet?

    _____

15. True/False: It is important to place the foot into true AP and lateral positions when performing a clubfoot study.

16. True/False: It is possible to provide gonadal shielding for both male and female pediatric patients for AP and lateral projections of hips.

17. What size image receptor should be used for a skull routine on a 6-year-old patient? _____

18. Which one of the following CR angulations will place the petrous ridges in the lower one third of the orbits with an AP reverse Caldwell projection of the skull?

    A. 15° cephalad to OML   C. CR perpendicular to OML

    B. 15° caudad to OML   D. 30° cephalad to OML

19. Which one of the following pathologic indicators would apply to a pediatric skull series?

    A. Osteomyelitis   B. CHD   C. Mastoiditis   D. Hyaline membrane disease

20. Which skull positioning line is placed perpendicular to the film for an AP Towne 30° caudal projection of the skull?

    A. IOML   B. OML   C. MML   D. AML

21. True/False: Parental assistance for skull radiography is preferred rather than using head clamps and a mummy wrap on a pediatric patient.

22. True/False: Children more than 5 years old can usually hold their breath after a practice session.

23. Correct centering for the following can be achieved by placing the central ray at the level of which structure or landmark?

    A. AP, PA, or lateral chest _____

    B. AP abdomen (infants and small children) _____

    C. AP supine abdomen (older children) _____

    D. AP skull _____

REVIEW EXERCISE C: Positioning of the Pediatric Abdomen and Contrast Media Procedures (see textbook pp. 653-662)

1. True/False: The chest and abdomen are generally almost equal in circumference in the newborn.

2. True/False: Bony landmarks in infants are easy to palpate and locate.

3. True/False: It is difficult to distinguish the small bowel from the large bowel on a plain abdomen on an infant.

4. True/False: The radiographic contrast on a pediatric abdominal radiograph is high compared with that of an adult abdominal radiograph.

5. Complete the recommended NPO fasting before the following pediatric contrast media procedures:

    A. Infant to 1-year-old upper GI: _____   C. Infant lower GI _____

    B. 1 year and older upper GI: _____   D. Pediatric IVU _____

6. List five conditions that contraindicate the use of laxatives or enemas in preparation for a lower GI study:

    A. _____

    B. _____

    C. _____

    D. _____

    E. _____

7. Indicate which of the following pathologic indicators apply for an AP abdomen (KUB) by placing an X in the corresponding column. Place an X by only those indicators that apply to the abdomen.

    _____   A. Croup   _____   E. Mastoiditis

    _____   B. NEC   _____   F. Hepatomegaly

    _____   C. Intussusception   _____   G. Appendicitis

    _____   D. Foreign body localization   _____   H. Hydrocephalus

8. Where is the CR centered for a small child erect abdomen? _____

9. A. What is the minimum kVp for an AP abdomen projection of a newborn without a grid? _____

    B. A grid is recommended for a pediatric AP abdomen if the abdomen measures more than _____ cm.

10. Which one of the following projections of the abdomen will best demonstrate the prevertebral region?

    A. AP supine KUB   B. PA prone KUB   C. Dorsal decubitus abdomen   D. AP erect abdomen

11. Which one of the following conditions is caused by inflammation of the inner lining of the large or small bowel, resulting in tissue death?

    A. NEC   B. CHD   C. Intussusception   D. Meconium ileus

12. Which of the following procedures or projections should be performed for a possible meconium ileus?

    A. IVU procedure   B. Barium enema   C. AP supine abdomen   D. AP erect abdomen

13. List the amount of barium that should be given to the following patients for an upper GI series:

   A. Newborn to 1 year old: _____   C. 3 to 10 years old: _____

   B. 1 to 3 years old: _____   D. Over 10 years old: _____

14. What is the only recourse if a pediatric patient refuses to drink barium for an upper GI series?

   _____

15. True/False: A piece of lead vinyl should be placed beneath the child's lower pelvis during conventional fluoroscopy to reduce the gonadal/mean bone marrow dose.

16. True/False: The transit time of the contrast media for reaching the cecum during a pediatric small bowel series is approximately 2 hours.

17. True/False: Latex enema tips should be used for barium enemas for children under the age of 1 year.

18. True/False: Small retention enema tips can be used on infants during a barium enema to help barium retention.

19. What type of contrast media is recommended for reducing an intussusception? _____

20. What is the maximum height of the barium enema bag before the beginning of the procedure? _____

21. A backward flow of urine from the bladder into the ureters and kidneys is called _____ .

22. A malignant tumor of the kidney common in children under the age of 5 years is:

   A. Wilms' tumor   B. Adenocarcinoma   C. Ewing's sarcoma   D. Teratoma

23. What is the most common pathologic indication for a voiding cystourethrogram? _____

24. True/False: A radionuclide study for vesicourethral reflux provides a smaller patient dose compared to a fluoroscopic voiding cystourethrogram.

25. Indicate the suggested contrast media dosages for IVU procedures for the following weight categories of pediatric patients:

   A. 0 to 12 lb   _____

   B. 13 to 25 lb   _____

   C. 26 to 50 lb   _____

   D. 51 to 100 lb   _____

   E. >100 lb   _____

26. What are the suggested contrast media dosages for the following metric weight measurements?

   A. 0 to 11 kg   _____

   B. 12 to 23 kg   _____

   C. 24 to 45 kg   _____

   D. >45 kg   _____

27. True/False: The lower abdomen can be shielded for the 3-minute film taken during an IVU for both males and females.

28. True/False: To help depress the large bowel and create a radiolucent window to better visualize the kidneys, a carbonated drink should be given to pediatric patients before an IVU.

29. True/False: Most radiologists prefer their pediatric patients to be dehydrated before an IVU.

30. True/False: Since allergic reactions to iodinated contrast agents are rare in pediatric patients, the use of ionic contrast media is recommended for IVUs.

PART III: Laboratory Exercises (see textbook pp. 630-662)

Exercises A and B need to be carried out in a radiographic laboratory or a general diagnostic room in the radiology department. General immobilization paraphernalia need to be available (i.e., tape, sheets or large towels, sandbags, various sizes and shapes of positioning sponge blocks, retention bands, head clamps, stockinettes, and Ace bandages). More common commercial immobilization devices such as the Tam-em Board or the Pigg-O-Stat (or similar devices) are optional if such are available. However, at least one of these devices should be made available for student use.

Exercise C can be carried out in a classroom or any room where illuminators (view boxes) are available.

LABORATORY EXERCISE A: Immobilization

For this section you will need some type of large articulate doll mannequin to use as your patient. The doll should have arms and legs that are flexible (similar to that of a child). This does not need to be a phantom-like doll since radiographs will not be taken, but it will be used to simulate immobilization techniques and positioning for various body parts.

Check each of the following as you complete that activity.

_____ 1. Complete the six steps of "mummifying."

_____ 2. Use a tubular-type stockinette of appropriate size to immobilize the "patient's" arms and hands placed above and behind the head.

_____ 3. Use the appropriate size Ace bandage to immobilize the lower limbs by wrapping with appropriate tension from the hips to the ankles.

_____ 4. Apply a retention band correctly across the abdomen and upper and lower limbs to completely immobilize these parts of the "patient."

_____ 5. Use sandbags under and over the legs and over each arm to immobilize for an AP abdomen.

_____ 6. Apply tape correctly in combination with sandbags to immobilize the head and the upper and lower limbs.

_____ 7. Apply head clamps to immobilize the head in combination with mummification of the patient and the use of sandbags or a retention band to prevent limb or body movement.

Tam-em Board if available:

_____ 8. Immobilize your patient correctly with the Velcro straps to restrain the upper and lower limbs and across the pelvic region.

Pigg-O-Stat if available:

_____ 9. Immobilize your "patient" correctly with the arms above the head using the plastic side body clamps to restrain the arms and head.

LABORATORY EXERCISE B: Physical Positioning

This section again requires the use of a large articulated doll mannequin. Practice the following projections or positions until you can perform them accurately and without hesitation. Place a check by each when you have achieved this.

Include the following details as you simulate the basic projections for each exam as follows. Assume the patient will not cooperate and that forceful immobilization is required. Use suggested immobilization techniques.

_____ Correct size and type of image receptor (appropriate for size of "patient")

_____ Correct centering of part to image receptor

_____ Correct SID, and location and angle of central ray

_____ Selection of appropriate restraining devices and application of the same

_____ Correct placement of markers

_____ Correct use of contact gonadal shield

_____ Accurate collimation to body part of interest

_____ Approximate correct exposure factors

EXAMINATION	IMMOBILIZATION
_____ 1. AP chest, supine	Tam-em-Board or sand bags and/or stockinette and "Ace" bandages
_____ 2. Lateral chest, patient recumbent in lateral position	Sandbags and tape, or retention band

If Tam-em Board is available:

_____ 3. Lateral chest, patient supine, horizontal beam CR	Tam-em Board (see textbook, p. 631)

If Pigg-O-Stat is available:

_____ 4. PA chest erect, 72 in. (180 cm) SID	Pigg-O-Stat (see textbook, p. 642)
_____ 5. Lateral chest erect, 72 in. (180 cm) SID	Pigg-O-Stat (see textbook, p. 644)
_____ 6. AP abdomen, erect	Pigg-O-Stat (see textbook, p. 655)
_____ 7. AP abdomen, supine	Tam-em Board, or tape, sandbags and retention band (see textbook, p. 654)
_____ 8. AP and lateral upper limb (from shoulder to hand)	Tape, sandbags and/or retention band (see textbook, p. 645)
_____ 9. AP and lateral lower limb (from hips to feet)	Tape, sandbags and/or retention band (see textbook, p. 647)
_____ 10. AP and lateral feet (such as follow-up exams for clubfeet)	Sitting on pad using tape (see textbook, p. 648)
_____ 11. AP pelvis and hips	Tape and sandbags and/or retention band (see textbook, p. 649)
_____ 12. Lateral hips	Tape and sandbags and/or retention band (see textbook, p. 652)
_____ 13. AP skull, 15° AP and 30° Towne	Head clamps or tape for head. Mummification and sandbags or retention band for limbs and body (see textbook, p. 651)
_____ 14. Lateral skull, turned into lateral position	Head clamps or tape for head. Mummification and sandbags or retention band for limbs and body (see textbook, p. 652)
_____ 15. Lateral skull, horizontal beam in supine position	Tam-em Board and tape for head (see textbook, p. 652)

LABORATORY EXERCISE C: Anatomy Review and Critique Radiographs of the Abdomen

Use those radiographs provided by your instructor. These should include optimal-quality and less-than-optimal quality radiographs of each of the following: chest, supine and erect abdomen, AP and lateral upper limb, AP and lateral pelvis and hips, AP and lateral lower limb, and AP and lateral skull radiographs.

Radiographs of the pelvis and upper and lower limbs of patients of various ages should be included to demonstrate the normal ossification or growth stages from infancy to adolescence.

Place a check by each of the following when completed.

_____ 1. Examine normal stages of growth by the appearance of the epiphyses in the pelvis and the long bones of the upper and lower limbs. Estimate the approximate age of the patient by the appearance of such epiphyses.

_____ 2. Critique each radiograph based on evaluation criteria provided for each projection in the textbook. Pediatric radiographs require a wider range of acceptable positioning criteria than for adults. Part centering and specific central ray locations are not as critical for pediatric radiographs because multiple anatomical parts or bones are included on one film. This is possible because detailed views of joint areas are not as important since these secondary growth areas are not yet fully developed. Thus complete limbs can be included on one film.

The following criteria guidelines can be used and checked as each radiograph is evaluated. Determine the corrections or adjustments in positioning or exposure factors necessary to bring those less-than-optimal radiographs up to a more desirable standard.

	Radiographs		*Criteria Guidelines*			
1	*2*	*3*	*4*	*5*	*6*	
____	____	____	____	____	____	a. Correct image receptor size as appropriate for age and size of patient?
____	____	____	____	____	____	b. Correct orientation of part to image receptor?
____	____	____	____	____	____	c. Acceptable alignment and/or centering of part to image receptor?
____	____	____	____	____	____	d. Correct collimation and correct CR angle where appropriate (such as for an AP skull)?
____	____	____	____	____	____	e. Evidence of gonadal shield correctly placed (if this should be visible)?
____	____	____	____	____	____	f. Pertinent anatomy well visualized?
____	____	____	____	____	____	g. Evidence of motion?
____	____	____	____	____	____	h. Optimal exposure (density and/or contrast)?
____	____	____	____	____	____	i. Patient ID with date and side markers visible without superimposing essential anatomy?

Answers to Review Exercises

Review Exercise A: Introduction, Immobilization, Ossification, Radiation Protection, Pre-exam Preparation, and Pathologic Indications

1. A. Technologist's attitude and approach to a child
   B. Technical preparation of the room
2. A. Serve as an observer in the room to lend support and comfort to their child
   B. Serve as a participator to assist with immobilization
   C. Remain in the waiting room, and do not accompany the child into the room
3. False (may be permissible with proper lead shielding if not pregnant)
4. False (correct term is *nonaccidental trauma, NAT*)
5. False (should report to radiologist or superior)
6. True
7. A. Tam-em board
   B. Plexiglass hold-down paddle
   C. Pigg-o-stat
8. Pigg-o-stat
9. False (should not be overfilled so as to be soft and pliable)
10. D. 4 inch
11. Adhesive
12. A. Twisting the tape so the adhesive surface is not against the skin
    B. Placing a gauze pad between the tape and the skin
13. A. 4 in.
    B. 6 in.
14. 1. Place the sheet on the table folded in half or thirds lengthwise
    2. Place patient in middle of sheet with the right arm down to the side. Fold sheet across the patient's body and pull sheet across the body keeping the arm against the body.
    3. Place the patient's left arm along the side of the body and on top of the sheet. Bring the free sheet over the left arm to the right side of the body. Wrap the sheet around the body as needed.
    4. Pull the sheet tightly so the patient cannot free arms.
    5. Place a long piece of tape from the right to the left wrapped arm to prevent the patient from breaking out of the sheet.
    6. Place a piece of tape around the patient's knees.
15. Diaphysis
16. Epiphyses
17. Epiphyseal plates
18. C. 5- or 6-year-old
19. C. 25 years old
20. A. Proper immobilization
    B. Short exposure times
    C. Accurate technique charts
21. A. Close collimation
    B. Low-dosage techniques
    C. Minimum number of images
22. 1. B, 2. A, 3. B, 4. A, 5. B, 6. A
23. False (Should be removed, may cause artifacts)
24. A. Sonography
25. C. Hydrocephalus
26. A. 4, B. 2, C. 7, D. 1, E. 3, F. 5, G. 6
27. A. 6, B. 7, C. 4, D. 8, E. 2, F. 1, G. 3, H. 5
28. A. 5, B. 1, C. 6, D. 3, E. 7, F. 2, G. 4
29. A. (+), B. (-), C. (-), D. (0), E. (-), F. (+), G. (-)
30. True

Review Exercise B: Pediatric Positioning of the Chest, Skeletal System, and Skull

1. A. Non-grid
   B. 70 to 80 kVp
   C. Crosswise
   D. 50 to 60 in. (127 to 212 cm)
   E. 72 in. (180 cm)
2. 75 to 80 kVp
3. No
4. Two
5. As the child fully inhales and holds his or her breath
6. The sternoclavicular joints and lateral rib margins should be equidistant from the vertebral column
7. Horizontally
8. True
9. False (9 or 10)
10. True
11. True
12. 1. A, 2. B, 3. A, 4. B, 5. A
13. Bilateral frogleg
14. AP and lateral feet, Kite method
15. False (Take two projections 90° from each other)
16. True (if correctly placed)
17. 10 x 12 in. (24 x 30 cm) (a child's skull is near adult size)
18. A. 15° cephalad to OML
19. C. Mastoiditis
20. B. OML
21. False
22. True
23. A. Mammillary (nipple) line
    B. 1 in. (2.5 cm) above umbilicus
    C. At level of iliac crest
    D. Glabella

Review Exercise C: Positioning of the Pediatric Abdomen and Contrast Media Procedures

1. True
2. False (most bony landmarks are nonexistent in infants)
3. True
4. False (contrast is low)
5. A. 4 hours
   B. 6 hours
   C. No prep required
   D. 4 hours
6. A. Hirschsprung's disease
   B. Extensive diarrhea
   C. Appendicitis
   D. Obstruction
   E. Dehydration (patients who cannot withstand fluid loss)
7. B, C, D, F, G
8. One inch (2.5 cm) above the umbilicus
9. A. 65
   B. 9 cm
10. C. dorsal decubitus abdomen
11. A. NEC
12. D. AP erect abdomen
13. A. 2 to 4 ounces
    B. 4 to 6 ounces
    C. 6 to 12 ounces
    D. 12 to 16 ounces
14. Insert a nasogastric tube into the stomach
15. True
16. False (usually 1 hour)
17. False (latex tips should not be used because of possible allergic response to latex)
18. False (retention tips should not be used on small children)
19. Air for the pneumatic reduction of intussusception
20. 3 feet
21. Vesicoureteral reflux
22. A. Wilms' tumor
23. Urinary tract infection (UTI)
24. True
25. A. 2 cc/lb
    B. 25 cc
    C. 1 cc/lb
    D. 50 cc
    E. 1/2 cc/lb
26. A. 3 ml/kg
    B. 2 ml/kg
    C. 50 ml
    D. 1 ml/kg
27. True
28. False (not recommended by pediatric radiologists)
29. False (should *not* be dehydrated)
30. False (not recommended)

SELF-TEST

Directions: This self-test should be taken only after completing all of the readings, review exercises, and laboratory activities for a particular section. The purpose of this test is not only to provide a good learning exercise but also to serve as a good indicator of what your final evaluation grade will be. It is strongly suggested that if you do not get at least a 90% to 95% grade on this self-test, you should review those areas where you missed questions before going to your instructor for the final evaluation exam for this chapter. (There are 73 questions or blanks—each is worth 1.4 points.)

1. At what age can most children be talked through a radiographic examination without forceful immobilization?

   A. 1 year　　C. 3 years

   B. 2 years　　D. 5 years

2. At the first meeting between the technologist and the patient (accompanied by an adult), which of the following generally should *not* be done?

   A. Introduce yourself

   B. Take the necessary time to explain what you will be doing

   C. Discuss the possible forceful immobilization that will be needed if the child will not cooperate

   D. Describe the total amount of radiation the patient will receive with that specific exam if it has to be repeated because of a lack of cooperation

   E. All of the above should be done

3. If child abuse is suspected by the technologist, he or she should:

   A. Ask the parent when the abuse occurred

   B. Report the abuse immediately to the necessary state officials as required by the state

   C. Refuse to do the examination or to touch the child until a physician has examined the patient

   D. Do none of the above

4. The following is *not* the name of a known commercially available immobilization device

   A. Posi-Tot　　　C. Pigg-O-Stat

   B. Tam-em Board　　D. Hold-em Tiger

5. The most suitable immobilization device for erect chests and/or the abdomen is:

   A. Posi-Tot　　　C. Pigg-O-Stat

   B. Tam-em Board　　D. Hold-em Tiger

6. List the three factors that will reduce the number of repeat exposures with pediatric patients.

   A. _____　　C. _____

   B. _____

7. What important question should a female parent be asked before allowing her to assist with holding her child during an exposure? _____

8. Which immobilization device or method should be used for an erect 1-year-old chest procedure? Assume these devices are available.

    A. Tam-em board   C. Pigg-O-Stat

    B. Hold- down paddle   D. Parent holding child

9. Which one of the following procedures can be performed to diagnose possible genetic fetal abnormalities?

    A. Nuclear medicine fetal scan   C. Functional MRI

    B. Spiral/helical CT   D. 3-D ultrasound

10. Which of the procedures can be performed to evaluate children for attention deficient hyperactivity disorder?

    A. Spiral/helical CT   C. 3-D ultrasound

    B. Functional MRI   D. Nuclear medicine

11. Match the following conditions to the correct definition or statement (use each choice only once):

    _____ A. Croup   1. Due to an allergic reaction to gluten

    _____ B. Respiratory distress syndrome   2. Group of diseases affecting the epiphyseal growth plates

    _____ C. Epiglottitis   3. Abnormally enlarged ventricles in brain

    _____ D. Osteochondroses   4. A common condition in children between the ages of 1 to 3 due to a viral infection

    _____ E. Osteogenesis imperfecta   5. Enlargement of the liver

    _____ F. Hydrocephalus   6. Second most common form of cancer in children under 5 years of age

    _____ G. Osteomalacia   7. Bacterial infection of the upper airway that may be fatal if untreated

    _____ H. Hirschsprung's disease   8. Congenital defect in which an opening into an organ is missing

    _____ I. Celiac disease   9. Condition where the alveoli and capillaries of the lungs are injured or infected

    _____ J. Neuroblastoma   10. Bacterial infection of the kidney

    _____ K. Pyelonephritis   11. Also known as *congenital megacolon*

    _____ L. Atresia   12. Also known as *rickets*

    _____ M. Hepatomegaly   13. Inherited condition that produces very fragile bones

12. Indicate whether the following pathologic conditions require that manual exposure factors be increased (+), decreased (-), or remain the same (0):

    A. Cystic fibrosis _____

    B. Hyaline membrane disease _____

    C. Osteogenesis imperfecta _____

    D. Hydrocephalus _____

    E. Idiopathic juvenile osteoporosis _____

    F. Osteopetrosis _____

    G. Volvulus _____

13. Which one of the following techniques will help remove the scapulae from the lung fields during chest radiography?

    A. Make exposure upon the second inspiration   C. Extend arms upward

    B. Extend the chin   D. Place arms behind the patient's back

14. What is the typical kVp range for a pediatric study of the upper limb? _____

15. True/False: A hand routine for a 7-year-old would be the same as for an adult patient.

16. True/False: For a bone survey of a young child, both limbs are commonly radiographed for comparison.

17. Which technique or method is performed to radiographically study congenital clubfoot?

    _____

18. Where is gonadal shielding placed for a bilateral hip study on a female pediatric patient?

    _____

19. Complete the following related to ossification by matching the correct term with the description. More than one choice per blank is possible.

    E = Epiphysis, **D** = Diaphysis, **EP** = Epiphyseal plate.

    _____ 1. Primary centers

    _____ 2. Secondary centers

    _____ 3. Space between primary and secondary centers

    _____ 4. Occurs before birth

    _____ 5. Continues to change from birth to maturity

20. Match the examination in the right column most likely associated with the pathologic indicators in the left column. Answers may be used more than once.

    _____ 1. Intussusception   A. Chest

    _____ 2. NEC   B. Abdomen

    _____ 3. Hydrocephalus   C. Upper and lower limbs

    _____ 4. Atelectasis   D. Pelvis and hips

    _____ 5. Premature closure of fontanelles   E. Skull

    _____ 6. CHD

    _____ 7. Cystic fibrosis

    _____ 8. Meconium ileus

    _____ 9. Legg-Calve-Perthes disease

    _____ 10. Hemoptysis

    _____ 11. Shunt check

    _____ 12. Bronchiectasis

    _____ 13. Hyaline membrane disease

21. How much is the CR angled from the OML for an AP Towne projection of the skull?

A. 15°   C. 25°

B. None   D. 30°

22. Where is the CR centered for a lateral projection of the skull?

A. At the EAM   C. 1 in.   (2.5 cm) above the EAM

B. Midway between the glabella and inion   D. 3/4 in.   (2 cm) anterior and superior to EAM

23. The NPO fasting period for a 6-month-old before an upper GI is:

A. 4 hours   C. 1 hour

B. 6 hours   D. 8 hours

24. Other than preventing artifacts in the bowel, what is the other reason that solid food is withheld for 4 hours before a pediatric IVU?

    _____

25. Which one of the following conditions would contraindicate the use of laxatives before a contrast media procedure?

A. Gastritis   C. Appendicitis

B. Blood in stool   D. Diverticulosis

26. Where is the CR centered for a KUB on:

A. An 8-year-old child? _____

B. A 1-year-old child? _____

27.   At what level is the CR centered for a PA and lateral pediatric chest? _____

28.   What is the recommended amount of barium for an 8-year-old child having an upper GI?

_____

29.   How is barium instilled into the large bowel for a barium enema study on an infant?

_____

30.   What is the bowel prep for a pediatric voiding cystourethrogram (VCUG)? _____

31.   When is urinary reflux most likely to occur during a VCUG? _____

32.   For a pediatric small bowel study, the barium normally reaches the ileocecal region in_____
      hour(s).

33.   A VCUG on a child is most commonly performed to evaluate for (A) _____ and is gener-

      ally scheduled to be completed (B) _____ (before or after) an IVU or ultrasound study of

      the kidneys.

34.   True/False: Gonadal shielding should only be used in supine positions due to the difficulty in keeping the shield in
      place.

35.   True/False: There should be no attempt to straighten out the abnormal alignment of the foot during a clubfoot study.

Angiography and Interventional Procedures

This chapter, which includes extensive detailed and somewhat complex anatomy and procedural information, is an excellent introduction to angiography. It provides effective preparation for the additional clinical training and experience that a special procedures technologist will need.

CHAPTER OBJECTIVES

After you have completed **all** the activities of this chapter, you will be able to:

_____ 1. List the divisions and components of the circulatory system.

_____ 2. List the three functions of the cardiovascular system.

_____ 3. On drawings, identify the components of the pulmonary and general systemic circulation.

_____ 4. Identify the four chambers of the heart, associated valves, and coronary circulation.

_____ 5. List and identify the four arteries supplying blood to the brain and the three branches arising from the aortic arch.

_____ 6. List the major branches of the external and internal carotid arteries and the primary divisions of the brain supplied by each.

_____ 7. On drawings, identify the major veins of the neck draining blood from the head and neck region.

_____ 8. List the major venous sinuses found in the cranium.

_____ 9. List the four segments of the thoracic aorta and describe the three common variations of the aortic arch.

_____ 10. List and identify the five major branches of the abdominal aorta.

_____ 11. List and identify the major abdominal veins.

_____ 12. List and identify the major arteries and veins of the upper and lower limbs.

_____ 13. List four functions of the lymphatic portion of the circulatory system.

_____ 14. Identify the six steps related to the Seldinger technique

_____ 15. Identify the equipment generally found in a neuroangiographic room.

_____ 16. Identify the pathologic indications, contraindications, and general procedure for cerebral angiography.

_____ 17. Identify the indications, catheterization technique, and general procedure for thoracic and abdominal aortography.

_____ 18. Identify the pathologic indications, contraindications, and general procedure for peripheral angiography.

_____ 19. Identify specific examples of vascular and nonvascular interventional procedures.

132   REVIEW EXERCISE A: Radiographic Anatomy of Cardiovascular System, Pulmonary and Systemic Circulation, and Cerebral Arteries and Veins

CHAPTER 21

Learning Exercises

Complete the following review exercises after reading the associated pages in the textbook as indicated by each exercise. Answers to each review exercise are given at the end of the review exercises.

REVIEW EXERCISE A: Radiographic Anatomy of Cardiovascular System, Pulmonary and Systemic Circulation, and Cerebral Arteries and Veins (see textbook pp. 666-672)

1. List the two major divisions or components of the circulatory system:

    A. _____   B. _____

2. List the body system or part supplied by the following four divisions of the circulatory system:

    A. Cardio _____   C. Pulmonary _____

    B. Vascular _____   D. Systemic _____

3. List the three functions of the cardiovascular system:

    A. _____

    B. _____

    C. _____

4. Identify the major components of the general cardiovascular circulation as labeled on this drawing (Fig. 21-1):

    A. _____

    B. _____

    C. _____

    D. _____

    E. _____

    F. _____

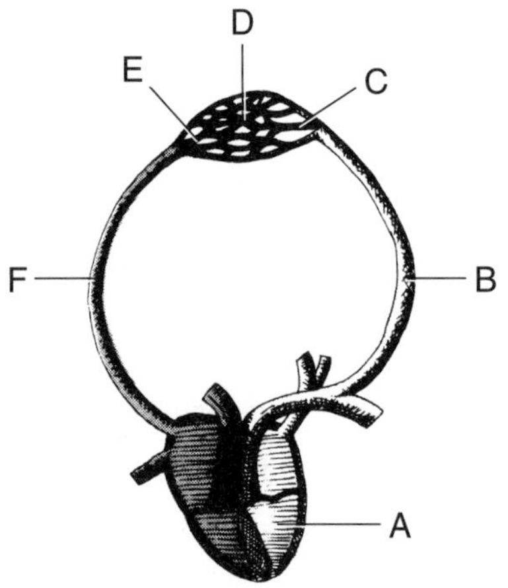

Fig. 21-1 Components of cardiovascular circulation.

5. Which of the six general components of the circulatory system, identified in question 4 above, carry oxygenated blood to body tissue?

    _____

6. Which of the six general components of the circulatory system carry deoxygenated blood?

    _____

7. List the common term (where indicated) and the function for the following three blood components:

COMMON TERM   *FUNCTION*

1. Erythrocytes   A. _____   B. _____

2. Leukocytes   A. _____   B. _____

3. Platelets   A. (No other term given)   B. _____

8. Plasma, the liquid portion of blood, consists of (A) ____% water and (B) ____% plasma protein and salts, nutri-ents, and oxygen.

9. Identify the chambers of the heart and the associated blood vessels (arteries and veins) as labeled on Fig. 21-2.

A. _____ (chamber)

B. _____ (chamber)

C. _____ (chamber)

D. _____

E. _____

F. _____

G. _____

H. _____

I. _____

J. _____ (chamber)

K. _____

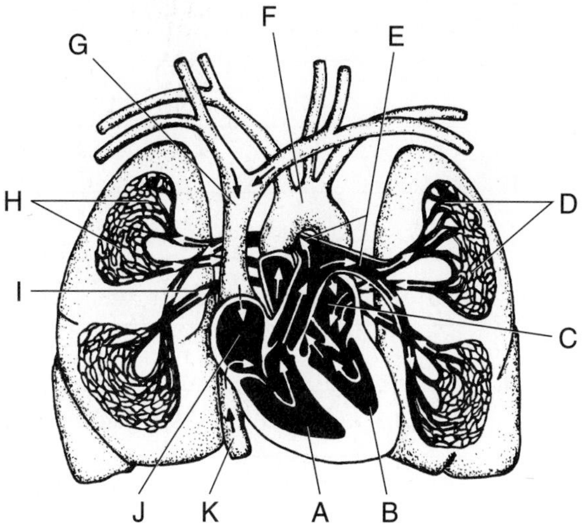

Fig. 21-2 Heart and pulmonary circulation (frontal view).

Questions 10 and 11 relate to Fig. 21-2

10. In general, arteries carry oxygenated blood, and veins carry deoxygenated blood. The exceptions to these are:

A. The _____ , which carry deoxygenated blood to the lungs.

B. The _____ , which carry oxygenated blood back to the atrium of the heart.

11. A. Blood from the upper body returns to the heart through the _____ .

B. Blood from the abdomen and the lower limbs returns through the _____ .

C. Both of these major veins enter the _____ of the heart.

12. Identify the four major valves between the following heart chambers and associated vessels.

A. Between right atrium and right ventricle: _____

B. Between right ventricle and pulmonary arteries: _____

C. Between left atrium and left ventricle: _____

D. Between left ventricle and aorta: _____

13.   A. The arteries that deliver blood to the heart muscle are the _____ .

B.   These arteries originate at the _____ .

14.   List the three major branches of the coronary sinus:

A.   _____   C.   _____

B.   _____

15.   Identify the labeled arteries on this drawing (Fig. 21-3):

A.   _____

B.   _____

C.   _____

D.   _____

E.   _____

F.   _____

G.   _____

H.   _____

I.   _____

J.   _____

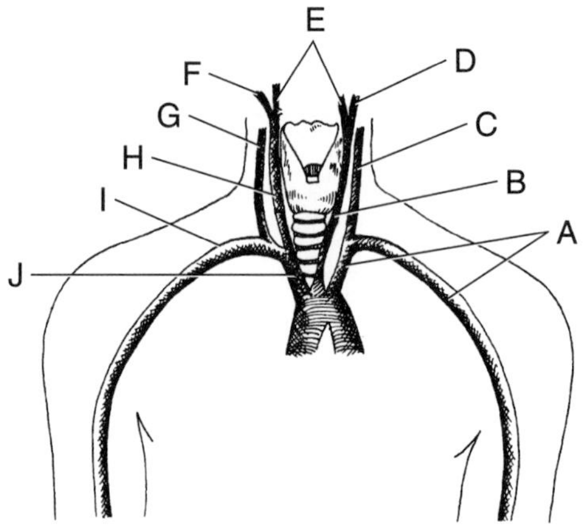

Fig. 21-3 Arterial branches of the aortic arch.

16.   List the three major branches of arteries arising from the arch of the aorta that supply the brain with blood:

A.   _____   C.   _____

B.   _____

17.   List the four major arteries supplying blood to the brain (important radiographically on a four-vessel angiogram):

A.   _____   C.   _____

B.   _____   D.   _____

18.   True/False: The brachiocephalic artery bifurcates to form the right common and right vertebral arteries.

19.   True/False: The level for bifurcation of the common carotid artery into the internal and external carotid arteries is at
the level of C3-4.

20.   Any injection of the common carotid inferior to the bifurcation would result in filling both the

_____ and _____ arteries.

21.   What is the name of the "S-shaped" portion of the internal carotid artery near the petrous portion of the temporal
bone?

A.   Carotid sinus   C.   Carotid body

B.   Carotid canal   D.   Carotid siphon

CHAPTER 21   REVIEW EXERCISE A: Radiographic Anatomy of Cardiovascular System, Pulmonary and Systemic Circulation, and Cerebral Arteries and Veins

135

22. List the two end branches of the internal carotid artery:

    A. _____   B. _____

23. The _____ artery supplies much of the forebrain with blood.

24. The _____ supply the posterior circulation of the brain.

25. The two vertebral arteries unite to form the single _____ artery.

26. Which of the two major branches of each internal carotid artery (anterior cerebral or middle cerebral) supply the lateral aspects of the cerebral hemispheres? _____

27. The anterior and middle cerebral arteries superimpose one another to a greater extent on the

    _____ (lateral or frontal) view.

28. Identify which one of the following four drawings (Fig. 21-4) demonstrate the following:

    1. Middle cerebral artery and branches of the internal carotid artery   _____

    2. Anterior cerebral artery and branches of the internal carotid artery   _____

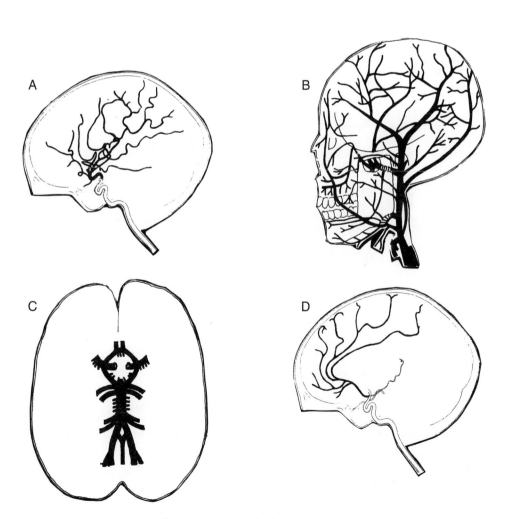

Fig. 21-4 Major cerebral arterial systems.

136 REVIEW EXERCISE A: Radiographic Anatomy of Cardiovascular System, Pulmonary and Systemic Circulation, and Cerebral Arteries and Veins

CHAPTER 21

29. The posterior brain circulation communicates with the anterior circulation at the base of the brain in an arterial circle configuration called the circle of Willis (Fig. 21-5). Identify the five arteries or branches that make up the circle of Willis, the left half of which are labeled on this drawing.

    1. _____

    2. _____

    3. _____

    4. _____

    5. _____

    6. A. Identify the major structure (labeled A) that would be located in the center of the circle of Willis.

       _____

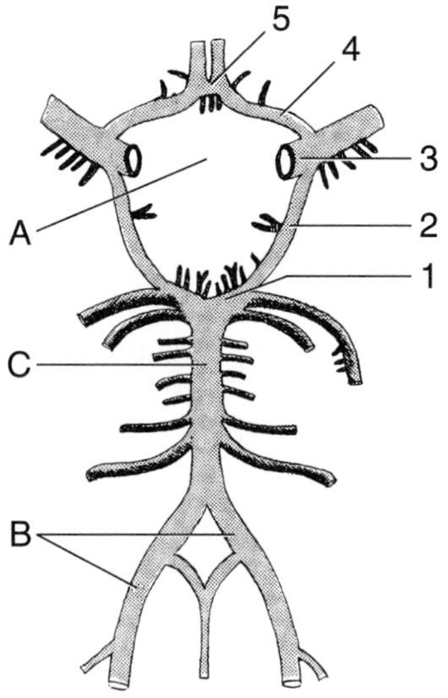

Fig. 21-5 Structure identification of the Circle of Willis.

    B. The right and left _____ enter the cranium through the foramen magnum.

    C. They then unite to form this single _____ artery.

30. List the three pairs of major veins draining the head, face, and neck region:

    A. _____

    B. _____

    C. _____

31. A. The three pairs of major veins, described in question 30, join the subclavian vein to form the

       _____ vein.

    B. This vein joins the equivalent vein on the other side to form the _____, which returns

       blood to the _____ of the heart.

32. True/False: The sinuses found in the brain are situated between layers of the dura mater.

33. True/False: All veins found in the brain possess no valves and are extremely thin.

34. Which one of the following dura mater sinuses is located in the superior portion of the falx cerebri?

    A. Superior sagittal sinus   C. Straight sinus

    B. Inferior sagittal sinus   D. Sigmoid sinus

35. Which bony landmark signifies the location of the confluence of venous sinuses?

    A. Foramen magnum   C. Internal occipital protuberance

    B. Petrous portion of temporal bone   D. Sella turcica

REVIEW EXERCISE B: Radiographic Anatomy of Thoracic and Abdominal Arteries and Veins, Portal System,
Upper and Lower Arteries and Veins, and Lymphatic System (see textbook pp. 673-677)

1. List the four segments of the aorta as labeled on Fig. 21-6.

    A. _____

    B. _____

    C. _____

    D. _____

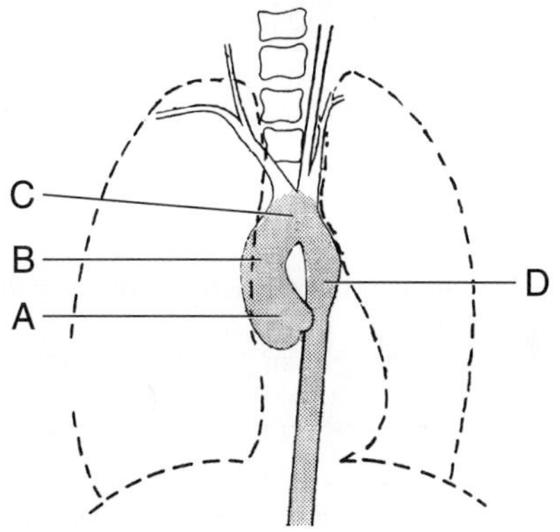

Fig. 21-6 Four segments of the aorta.

2. List the three common variations of the aortic arch that may
    be visualized on aortograms and are demonstrated in Fig. 21-7.

    A. _____

    B. _____

    C. _____

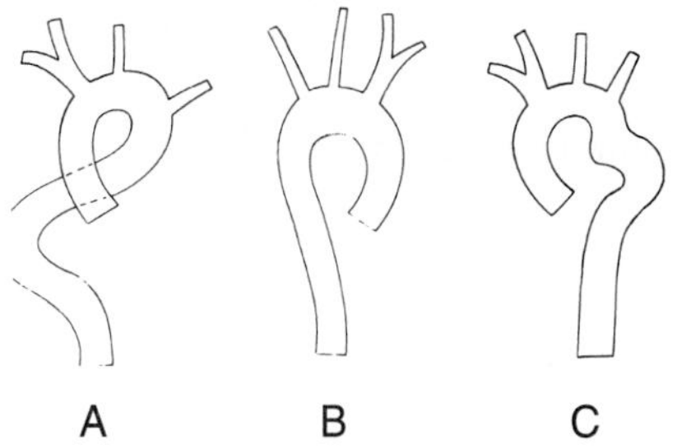

Fig. 21-7 Variations of the aortic arch.

3. Which one of the following veins receives blood from the intercostal, bronchial, esophageal, and phrenic veins?

    A. Pulmonary veins   B. Azygos vein   C. Inferior vena cava   D. Superior vena cava

4. List the five major branches of the abdominal aorta as labeled 1 through 5 on this drawing (Fig. 21-8):

    They are listed in order from the top down.

    1. _____

    2. _____

    3. _____

    4. _____

    5. _____

5. List the three branches of the celiac artery labeled A-C.

    A. _____

    B. _____

    C. _____

    List the divisions of the abdominal aorta as it enters the
    pelvic region labeled D-F.

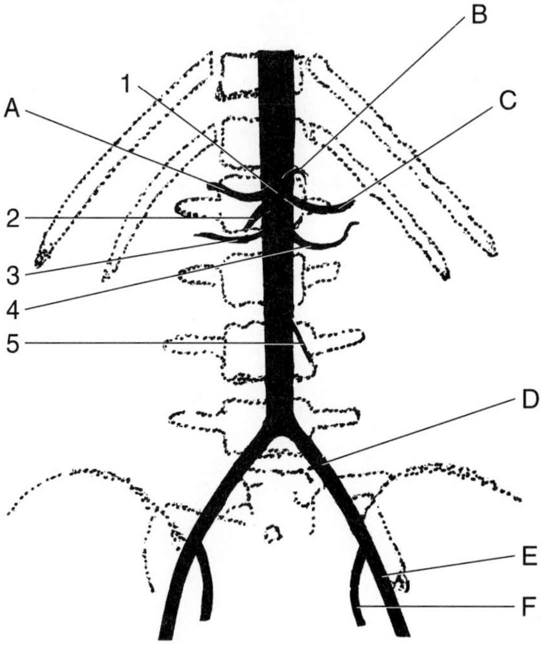

Fig. 21-8 Branches and divisions of the abdominal aorta.

    D. _____

    E. _____   F. _____

6. At what level does the descending aorta pass through the diaphragm to become the abdominal aorta?

    A. T10   C. L1

    B. T12   D. L2

7. The distal abdominal aorta bifurcates at the level of _____ vertebra.

8. Venous blood is returned to the heart from structures below the diaphragm through the inferior vena cava. Identify the major venous tributaries to the inferior vena cava as labeled on Fig. 21-9:

    A. _____

    B. _____

    C. _____

    D. _____

    E. Inferior vena cava

    F. _____

    G. _____

    H. _____

    I. _____

    J. _____

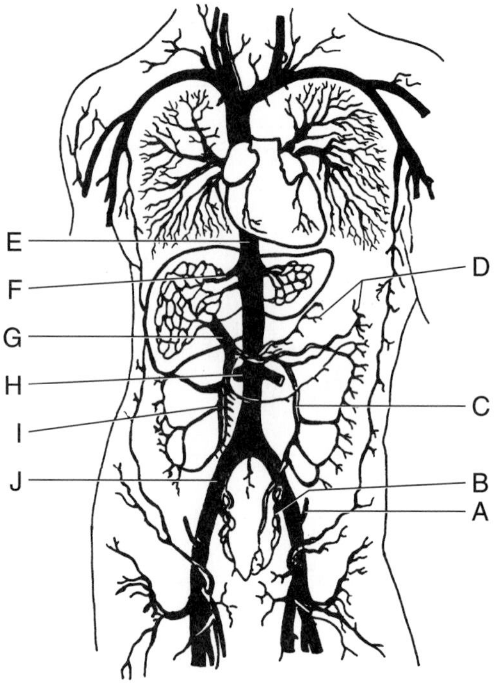

Fig. 21-9 Tributaries to the inferior vena cava.

9. Identify the following veins (*A, B, D,* and *E*) that make up the portal system as labeled on Fig. 21-10:
    Hint: *A* and *B* are the two major veins that unite to form the hepatic portal vein (*C*).

    A. _____

    B. _____

    C. Hepatic portal vein

    D. _____ drain "filtered" blood from the liver and return it to the

    E. _____

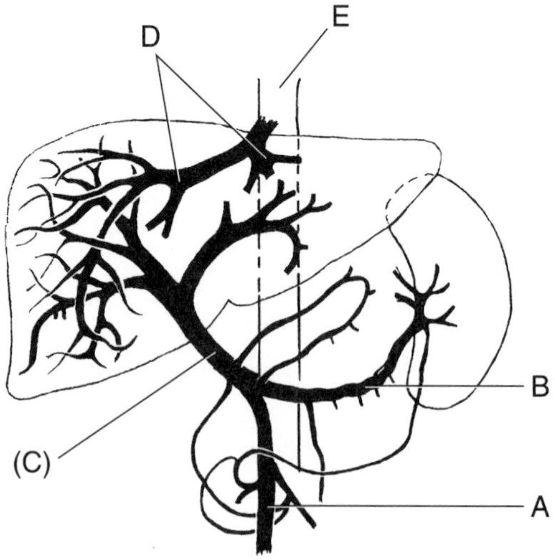

Fig. 21-10 Portal system.

10. Identify the following upper limb arteries (Fig. 21-11):

On the right side of the body, the *"A"* _____

artery gives rise to the *"B"* _____ artery.

Identify the following primary arteries of the upper limb labeled *C-F*.

C. _____

D. _____

E. _____

F. _____

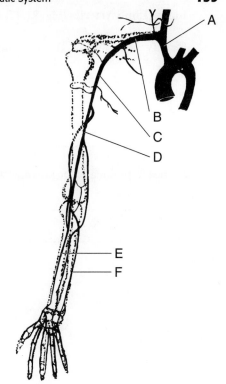

Fig. 21-11 Upper limb arteries.

11. Identify the following upper limb veins (Fig. 21-12):

The venous system of the upper and lower limbs may be divided into two sets. For the upper limb these begin with:

A. _____ and

B. _____ , which

form two parallel drainage channels.

Label the veins *C-G* returning blood to the heart:

C. _____

D. _____

E. _____

F. _____

G. _____

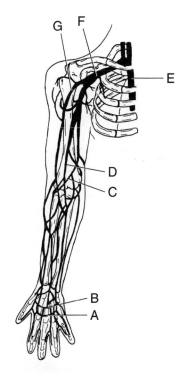

Fig. 21-12 Upper limb veins.

12. The vein most commonly used to draw blood at the elbow is

the _____ .

(Hint: This is one of the veins [*A-G*] as identified in Fig. 21-12.)

140   REVIEW EXERCISE B: Radiographic Anatomy of Thoracic and Abdominal Arteries and Veins, Portal System, Upper and Lower
Arteries and Veins, and Lymphatic System
CHAPTER 21

Lower Limb Arteries (Fig. 21-13)

13. Identify the following: The lower limb arterial system begins at the

   "A" _____ artery and continues as the

   "B" _____ artery until it divides into the

   "C" _____ and "D" _____

   arteries in the area of the proximal and mid femur. At the knee this becomes the

   "E" _____ artery, which continues into the foot as the

   "F" _____ artery.

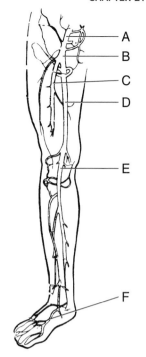

Fig. 21-13 Lower limb arteries.

Lower Limb Veins (Fig.   21-14)

14. Identify the following labeled veins of the lower limb:

   A. _____

   B. _____

   C. _____

   D. _____

   E. _____

   F. _____

   G. _____

   H. _____

   I. _____

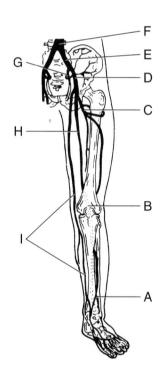

Fig. 21-14 Lower limb veins.

15. The longest vein in the body is the _____ of the lower limb. (Hint: This is one of the labeled veins in Fig. 21-14.)

16. Which duct in the lymphatic system receives interstitial fluid from the left side of the body, lower limbs, pelvis and abdomen and drains this fluid into the left subclavian vein?

   _____

17. List the four functions of the lymphatic system:

A. _____

B. _____

C. _____

D. _____

18. The general term describing radiographic examination of the lymphatic **vessels and nodes** following injection of

contrast media is _____ .

19. The term frequently used to study the lymph **vessels** specifically following injection of contrast media is

_____ .

20. True/False: It may take up to 24 hours following injection of the contrast medium to visualize the lymph nodes during a lymphogram.

21. True/False: Oil-based contrast media should never be used during a lymphogram.

REVIEW EXERCISE C: Cerebral Angiographic Procedures and Equipment and Supplies (see textbook pp. 678-685)

1. True/False: Computed tomography angiography (CTA) does not require the use of iodinated contrast media to demonstrate vascular structures.

2. True/False: Magnetic resonance angiography (MRA) does not require the use of any type of contrast media or vessel puncture.

3. True/False: Rotational angiography units move around the anatomy up to 360° during the procedure.

4. True/False: Nuclear medicine complements other angiographic modalities even though it provides little anatomical detail.

5. True/False: Most pediatric angiographic procedures require patient sedation.

6. Which of the following individuals is (are) not part of the angiographic team?

A. Scrub nurse   C. Technologist

B. Respiratory therapist   D. Radiologist

7. A common method or technique of introducing a needle and/or catheter into the blood vessel for angiographic pro-

cedures is called the _____ .

8. List the six steps to the previously mentioned technique (in the correct order).

A. _____   D. _____

B. _____   E. _____

C. _____   F. _____

9. Other than the method listed above, what are two other techniques for accessing a vessel during angiography?

   A. _____

   B. _____

10. Which one of the following is not a common risk or complication of angiography?

    A. Embolus formation   C. Hypertension

    B. Dissection of a vessel   D. Contrast media reaction

11. Which one of the following vessels is preferred for arterial vessel access during angiography?

    A. Femoral artery   C. Axillary artery

    B. Brachial artery   D. Common carotid artery

12. True/False: Angiographic rooms need to be considerably larger than conventional radiographic rooms.

13. The purpose of the heating device on an electromechanical injector is _____.

14. Outlets for _____ and _____ should be located on the room walls near the work area.

15. True/False: The use of digital and/or digital subtraction angiography (DSA), as part of a PAC system, can eliminate the need for hard-copy images.

16. True/False: The older photographic image subtraction method resulted in superior quality images compared to the newer digital subtraction system but was too time consuming to be used for most procedures.

17. List three post processing options with digital imaging to improve or modify the image:

    A. _____

    B. _____

    C. _____

18. True/False: Magnetic resonance angiography requires the use of special contrast media to demonstrate vasculature.

19. True/False: Carbon dioxide can be used instead of iodinated contrast media during angiography when iodinated agents are contraindicated.

20. List the five common pathologic indicators for cerebral angiography.

    A. _____

    B. _____

    C. _____

    D. _____

    E. _____

21. The point of bifurcation is of special interest to the radiologist and at this point, the internal carotid artery is more

    _____ (medial or lateral) when compared with the external carotid on an AP projection.

22. List those vessels commonly demonstrated during cerebral angiography:

    A. _____

    B. _____

    C. _____

    D. _____

REVIEW EXERCISE D: Radiographic Procedures and Positioning for Thoracic, Angiocardiography, Abdominal, Peripheral, and Interventional Angiography (see textbook pp. 685-697)

1. List specific pathologies that are common indications for thoracic and pulmonary angiography.

    A. _____

    B. _____

    C. _____

    D. _____

    E. _____

2. The most common pathologic indicator for **pulmonary** arteriography is _____.

3. The preferred puncture site for a thoracic aortogram is the:

    A. Femoral vein   C. Pulmonary artery

    B. Pulmonary vein   D. Femoral artery

4. The preferred puncture site for a pulmonary arteriogram is:

    A. Femoral vein   C. Pulmonary artery

    B. Pulmonary vein   D. Femoral artery

5. What is the average amount of contrast media injected during a thoracic angiogram?

    A. 5 to 8 ml   C. 20 to 25 ml

    B. 10 to 15 ml   D. 30 to 50 ml

6. To prevent superimposition of the aortic arch with surrounding structures during a thoracic aortogram, a _____ degree RPO is often performed.

    A. 5 to 10   C. 45

    B. 15 to 20   D. 60

7. Coronary angiography is typically a study of the:

    A. Coronary arteries   C. Coronary veins

    B. Aortic arch   D. Chambers of the heart

8. What type of catheter is typically used for a left ventriculogram? _____

144   REVIEW EXERCISE D: Radiographic Procedures and Positioning for Thoracic, Angiocardiography, Abdominal, Peripheral, and Interventional Angiography

CHAPTER 21

9. The average imaging rate during angiocardiography is:

   A. 2 to 3 frames per second   C. 15 to 30 frames per second

   B. 8 to 10 frames per second   D. 45 to 60 frames per second

10. Which one of the following terms describes the pumping efficiency of the left ventricle?

    A. Ejection fraction   C. Ejection coefficient

    B. Systolic contraction ratio   D. Myocardial perfusion ratio

11. List five common pathologic indicators for abdominal angiography.

    A. _____

    B. _____

    C. _____

    D. _____

    E. _____

12. The common puncture site for selective abdominal angiography is the _____ artery using the Seldinger technique.

13. Selective abdominal angiography can be performed to visualize specific branches (and associated organs) of the abdominal aorta.   Which three branches are most commonly catheterized for this purpose?

    A. _____   C. _____

    B. _____

14. List the term for an angiographic study of the superior and inferior vena cava. _____

15. True/False: Venograms are rarely performed today due to increased use of color duplex ultrasound.

16. To study the left upper limb arteries, the catheter is passed from the aortic arch into the:

    A. Left common carotid   C. Left vertebral artery

    B. Left brachiocephalic vein   D. Left subclavian artery

17. True/False: Lymphography can be performed to diagnose Hodgkin's lymphoma.

18. Which one of the following conditions may contraindicate a lymphogram?

    A. Advanced pulmonary disease   C. Cervical cancer

    B. Prostate cancer   D. Peripheral swelling

19. What type of contrast agent is most often used for a lymphogram?

    A. Water-soluble iodinated-nonionic   C. Oil-based

    B. Water-soluble iodinated-ionic   D. Negative-CO_2

20. Why is a blue dye injected subcutaneously at the beginning of a lower limb lymphogram?

    A. Helps to identify lymph vessels   C. Anesthetizes lymph vessels

    B. Increases transit time of contrast media   D. Reduces risk of contrast media reaction

21. Indicate whether the following interventional procedures are vascular or nonvascular procedures.

_____ 1. Percutaneous transluminal angioplasty (PTA)   A. Vascular procedure

_____ 2. Infusion therapy   B. Nonvascular procedure

_____ 3. Percutaneous biliary drainage (PBD)

_____ 4. Percutaneous gastrostomy

_____ 5. Stent placement

_____ 6. Embolization

_____ 7. Percutaneous abdominal drainage

_____ 8. Nephrostomy

_____ 9. Thrombolysis

_____ 10. Percutaneous needle biopsy

_____ 11. Percutaneous vertebroplasty

_____ 12. Transjugular intrahepatic portosystemic shunt (TIPS)

22. What vasoconstrictor is commonly given during infusion therapy to control bleeding?

_____

23. What type of catheter is often used to retrieve urethral stones? _____

24. What type of catheter is used for transluminal angioplasty? _____

25. What is the correct term describing the interventional procedure for dissolving a blood clot?

_____

26. Which one of the following pathologic indications is most common for performing a percutaneous biliary drainage (PBD)?

   A. Biliary obstruction   C. Posttraumatic biliary leakage

   B. Suppurative cholangitis   D. Unresectable malignant disease

27. True/False: Percutaneous abdominal drainage procedures have a success rate of only 50%.

28. True/False: Percutaneous gastrostomy is performed primarily for patients who are unable to eat orally.

29. True/False: Interventional angiographic procedures are used primarily for providing diagnostic information and secondarily for treatment of disease.

30. True/False: Interventional imaging procedures are most commonly performed by technologists in surgery with the assistance of a radiologist.

Answers to Review Exercises

Review Exercise A: Radiographic Anatomy of Cardiovascular System, Pulmonary and Systemic Circulation, and Cerebral Arteries and Veins

1. A. Cardiovascular
   B. Lymphatic
2. A. Heart
   B. Blood vessels
   C. Heart to lungs
   D. Throughout the body
3. A. Transportation of oxygen, nutrients, hormones, and chemicals
   B. Removal of waste products
   C. Maintenance of body temperature, water, and electrolyte balance
4. A. Heart
   B. Artery
   C. Arteriole
   D. Capillary
   E. Venule
   F. Vein
5. B (artery) and C (arteriole)
6. E (venule) and F (vein)
7. 1. A. Red blood cells
      B. Transports oxygen
   2. A. White blood cells
      B. Defends against infection and disease
   3. A. (No other term given)
      B. Repairs tears in blood vessels and promotes blood clotting
8. (A) 92, (B) 7
9. A. Right ventricle
   B. Left ventricle
   C. Left atrium
   D. Capillaries of left lung
   E. Pulmonary arteries
   F. Aorta (arch)
   G. Superior vena cava
   H. Capillaries of right lung
   I. Pulmonary veins
   J. Right atrium
   K. Inferior vena cava
10. A. Pulmonary arteries
    B. Pulmonary veins
11. A. Superior vena cava
    B. Inferior vena cava
    C. Right atrium
12. A. Tricuspid valve
    B. Pulmonary (pulmonary semilunar) valve
    C. Mitral (bicuspid) valve
    D. Aortic (aortic semilunar) valve
13. A. Right and left coronary arteries
    B. Aortic bulb
14. A. Great cardiac vein
    B. Middle cardiac vein
    C. Small cardiac vein

15. A. Left subclavian
    B. Left common carotid
    C. Left vertebral
    D. Left internal carotid
    E. Right and left external carotids
    F. Right internal carotid
    G. Right vertebral
    H. Right common carotid
    I. Right subclavian
    J. Brachiocephalic
16. A. Brachiocephalic artery
    B. Left common carotid artery
    C. Left subclavian artery
17. A. Right common carotid artery
    B. Left common carotid artery
    C. Right vertebral artery
    D. Left vertebral artery
18. False (right common carotid and right subclavian)
19. True
20. Internal and external carotid
21. D carotid siphon
22. A. Anterior cerebral artery
    B. Middle cerebral artery
23. Anterior cerebral
24. Vertebrobasilar arteries
25. Basilar
26. Middle cerebral arteries
27. Lateral
28. 1. A
    2. D
29. 1. Posterior cerebral arteries
    2. Posterior communicating arteries
    3. Internal cerebral arteries
    4. Anterior cerebral arteries
    5. Anterior communicating artery
    6. A. Hypophysis (pituitary) gland
       B. Vertebral arteries
       C. Basilar
30. A. Right and left internal jugular veins
    B. Right and left external jugular veins
    C. Right and left vertebral veins
31. A. Brachiocephalic
    B. Superior vena cava, right atrium
32. True
33. True
34. A superior sagittal sinus
35. C internal occipital protuberance

Review Exercise B: Radiographic Anatomy of Thoracic and Abdominal Arteries and Veins, Portal System, Upper and Lower Arteries and Veins, and Lymphatic System

1. A. Aortic bulb
   B. Ascending aorta
   C. Aortic arch
   D. Descending aorta

2. A. Left circumflex
   B. Inverse aorta
   C. Pseudocoarctation
3. B (azygos vein)
4. 1. Celiac axis
   2. Superior mesenteric artery
   3. Right renal artery
   4. Left renal artery
   5. Inferior mesenteric artery
5. A. Common hepatic artery
   B. Splenic artery
   C. Left gastric artery
   D. Left common iliac artery
   E. Left external iliac artery
   F. Left internal iliac artery
6. B (T12)
7. L4
8. A. Left external iliac vein
   B. Left internal iliac vein
   C. Inferior mesenteric vein
   D. Splenic vein
   E. (Inferior vena cava)
   F. Hepatic vein
   G. Portal vein
   H. Right renal vein
   I. Superior mesenteric vein
   J. Right common iliac vein
9. A. Superior mesenteric vein
   B. Splenic vein
   C. (Hepatic portal vein)
   D. Hepatic veins
   E. Inferior vena cava
10. A. Brachiocephalic
    B. Subclavian
    C. Axillary
    D. Brachial
    E. Radial
    F. Ulnar
11. A. Superficial palmar arch vein
    B. Deep palmar arch vein
    C. Median cubital
    D. Brachial
    E. Superior vena cava
    F. Subclavian
    G. Cephalic
12. Median cubital
13. A. External iliac artery
    B. Common femoral
    C. Deep femoral
    D. Femoral
    E. Popliteal
    F. Dorsalis pedis
14. A. Anterior tibial
    B. Popliteal
    C. Deep femoral
    D. External iliac
    E. Left common iliac
    F. Inferior vena cava
    G. Internal iliac
    H. Femoral
    I. Great saphenous

15. Great saphenous vein
16. Thoracic duct
17. A. Fight diseases by producing lymphocytes and microphages
    B. Return proteins and other substances to the blood
    C. Filter lymph in the lymph nodes
    D. Transfer fats from the intestine to the blood
18. Lymphography
19. Lymphangiography
20. True
21. False (are commonly used)

Review Exercise C: Equipment and Supplies and Cerebral Angiographic Procedures

1. False (does require)
2. True
3. False (only 180°)
4. True
5. True
6. B. Respiratory therapist
7. Seldinger technique
8. A. Insertion of needle
   B. Placement of needle in lumen of vessel
   C. Insertion of guide wire
   D. Removal of needle
   E. Threading of catheter to area of interest
   F. Removal of guide wire
9. A. Cutdown
   B. Translumbar approach
10. C. Hypertension
11. A. Femoral artery
12. True

13. To maintain temperature of contrast media at body temperature
14. Oxygen and suction
15. True
16. False. (older film method resulted was not superior and was more time consuming)
17. A. Pixel-shifting or remasking
    B. Magnified or zooming
    C. Quantitative analysis of image to measure size or distances
18. False (does not require contrast media)
19. True
20. A. Vascular stenosis including arterial occlusions
    B. Aneurysms
    C. Arteriovenous malformations
    D. Trauma
    E. Neoplastic disease
21. Lateral
22. A. Internal carotid arteries
    B. Common carotid arteries
    C. External carotid arteries
    D. Vertebral arteries

Review Exercise D: Radiographic Procedures and Positioning for Thoracic, Angiocardiography, Abdominal, Peripheral, and Interventional Angiography

1. A. (Aneurysm)
   B. Congenital abnormalities
   C. Vessel stenosis
   D. Embolus
   E. Trauma
2. Pulmonary embolus

3. D. Femoral artery
4. A. Femoral vein
5. D. 30 to 50 ml
6. C. 45
7. A. Coronary arteries
8. Pigtail catheter
9. C. 15 to 30 frames per second
10. A. Ejection fraction
11. A. Aneurysm
    B. Congenital abnormality
    C. GI bleed
    D. Stenosis/occlusion
    E. Trauma
12. Femoral
13. A. Renal arteries
    B. Celiac artery
    C. Superior and inferior mesenteric arteries
14. Venacavagraphy
15. True
16. D. Left subclavian artery
17. True
18. A. Advanced pulmonary disease
19. C. Oil-based
20. A. Helps to identify lymph vessels
21. 1. A, 2. A, 3. B, 4. B, 5. A, 6. A, 7. B, 8. B, 9. A, 10. B, 11. B, 12. A
22. Vasopressin (Pitressin)
23. Basket catheter or loop snare
24. Balloon catheter
25. Thrombolysis
26. D (unresectable malignant disease)
27. False (70% to 80%)
28. True
29. False (primarily for treatment of disease)
30. False (performed primarily in angiographic suite)

SELF-TEST

Directions: This self-test should be taken only after completing all of the readings, review exercises, and laboratory activities for a particular section.   The purpose of this test is not only to provide a good learning exercise but also to serve as a good indicator of what your final evaluation grade will be. It is strongly suggested that if you do not get at least a 90% to 95% grade on this self-test, you should review those areas in which you missed questions before going to your instructor for the final evaluation exam for this chapter. (There are 73 questions or blanks—each is worth 1.4 points.)

1. The two arteries that deliver blood to the heart muscle are:

   A. Right and left pulmonary veins   C. Right and left pulmonary arteries

   B. Right and left brachiocephalic arteries   D. Right and left coronary arteries

2. Which of the following arteries does not originate from the arch of the aorta?

   A. Brachiocephalic   C. Left common carotid

   B. Left subclavian   D. Right common carotid

3. Each common carotid artery bifurcates into the internal and external arteries at the level of:

   A. Lower margin of thyroid cartilage   C. Upper margin of thyroid cartilage

   B. C6 vertebra   D. C2 vertebra

4. Which vessels carry oxygenated blood from the lungs back to the heart?

   A. Pulmonary veins   C. Coronary arteries

   B. Pulmonary arteries   D. Aorta

5. The _____ artery arises from the brachiocephalic artery rather than the aortic arch.

   A. Right vertebral   C. Right common carotid

   B. Left vertebral   D. Left common carotid

6. The external carotid does not supply blood to the:

   A. Anterior portion of brain   C. Anterior neck

   B. Facial area   D. Greater part of the scalp and meninges

7. Two branches of each internal carotid artery, which are well visualized with an internal carotid arteriogram, are the:

   A. Posterior and middle cerebral arteries   C. Right and left vertebral arteries

   B. Anterior and middle cerebral arteries   D. Facial and maxillary arteries

8. The two vertebral arteries enter the cranium through the foramen magnum and unite to form the:

   A. Brachiocephalic artery   C. Circle of Willis

   B. Vertebrobasilar artery   D. Basilar artery

9. The basilar artery rests upon the clivus of the _____ bone.

   A. Ethmoid   B. Parietal   C. Temporal   D. Sphenoid

10. Which of the following veins does not drain blood from the head, face, and neck regions?

    A. Right and left internal jugular veins   C. Internal and external cerebral veins

    B. Right and left vertebral veins   D. Right and left external jugular veins

11. The superior and inferior sagittal sinuses join certain other sinuses such as the transverse sinus at the base of the

    brain to become the _____ .

    A. External jugular vein   C. Subclavian vein

    B. Internal jugular vein   D. Vertebral vein

12. Which vein receives blood from the intercostal, esophageal, and phrenic veins?

    A. Superior vena cava   C. Azygos vein

    B. Inferior vena cava   D. Brachiocephalic veins

13. Match the following abdominal arteries with the labeled parts on Fig. 21-15.

    _____ 1. Inferior mesenteric

    _____ 2. Superior mesenteric

    _____ 3. Left renal

    _____ 4. Right renal

    _____ 5. Common hepatic

    _____ 6. Celiac (trunk) axis

    _____ 7. Left common iliac

    _____ 8. Left internal iliac

    _____ 9. Left external iliac

    _____ 10. Left gastric

    _____ 11. Abdominal aorta

    _____ 12. Splenic

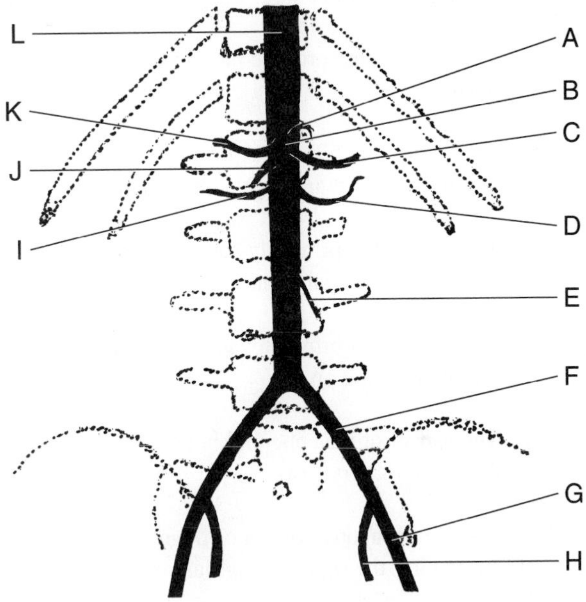

Fig. 21-15 Abdominal arteries.

14. True/False: The right subclavian artery arises directly from the aortic arch.

15. True/False: The cephalic vein is most commonly used for venipuncture.

16. True/False: The great saphenous vein is the longest vein in the body.

17. True/False: The thoracic duct is the largest lymph vessel in the body.

18. Which one of the following functions is *not* performed by the lymphatic system?

    A. Produce lymphocytes and microphages   C. Filter the lymph

    B. Synthesize simple carbohydrates   D. Return proteins and other substances to the blood

19. Solid food should be withheld for approximately _____ hours before an angiographic procedure.

    A. 1   C. 8

    B. 4   D. 24

20. Match the correct term best describing each of the following definitions:

    _____ 1. Also known as *red blood cells*

    _____ 2. Component of blood that helps repair tears in blood vessel walls and promotes blood clotting

    _____ 3. Carries deoxygenated blood from the right ventricle of the heart to the lungs

    _____ 4. Heart valve found between the left atrium and left ventricle

    _____ 5. Heart valve found between the right atrium and right ventricle

    _____ 6. The vessels that provide blood to the heart muscle

    _____ 7. The artery that bifurcates to form the right common carotid and right subclavian artery

    _____ 8. The artery that primarily supplies blood to the anterior neck, scalp, and meninges

    _____ 9. The artery that bifurcates into the anterior and middle cerebral artery

    _____ 10. The aspect of the sphenoid bone upon which the basilar artery rests

    _____ 11. The membranous portion of the dura mater containing the superior sagittal sinus

    _____ 12. The artery that forms the left gastric, hepatic, and splenic arteries

    _____ 13. The vein created by the splenic and superior mesenteric veins

    _____ 14. The vessel that carries oxygenated blood from the lungs to the left atrium of the heart

    _____ 15. A radiographic study of the lymph vessels

    A. Brachiocephlaic artery

    B. Pulmonary veins

    C. Celiac artery

    D. Coronary arteries

    E. Superior vena cava

    F. Portal vein

    G. Falx cerebri

    H. Lymphangiogram

    I. Inferior mesenteric artery

    J. Coronary sinus

    K. External carotid artery

    L. Tricuspid valve

    M. Clivus

    N. Mitral (bicuspid) valve

    O. Erythrocytes

    P. Pulmonary artery

    Q. Platelets

    R. Internal carotid artery

21. Injection flow rate in angiography is not affected by:

    A. Viscosity of contrast media   C. Body temperature

    B. Length and diameter of catheter   D. Injection pressure

22. Which one of the following imaging modalities will best demonstrate absence or presence of blood flow within a vessel?

    A. Computed tomography angiography   C. Magnetic resonance imaging

    B. Color duplex ultrasound   D. CO_2 angiography

23. True/False: Contrast media must be used during magnetic resonance angiography.

24. True/False: CO_2 angiography requires the use of a special injector.

25. Which of the following is not a pathologic indicator for cerebral angiography?

    A. Vascular lesions   C. Coarctation

    B. Aneurysm   D. Arteriovenous malformation

26. The imaging sequence during cerebral angiography, to include all phases of circulation, will typically require:

    A. 1 to 3 seconds   C. 8 to 10 seconds

    B. 4 to 6 seconds   D. 12 to 15 seconds

27. Pulmonary arteriography is usually performed to diagnose:

    A. Heart valve disease   C. Arteriovenous malformation

    B. Pulmonary emboli   D. Coarctation of the aorta

28. The most common vascular approach during pulmonary arteriography is the:

    A. Femoral vein   C. Superior vena cava

    B. Femoral artery   D. Axillary artery

29. Which one of the following positions will prevent superimposition of the proximal aorta during a thoracic aortogram?

    A. 45° RPO   C. AP

    B. 45° LPO   D. Lateral

30. During angiocardiography, the catheter is advanced from the aorta into the:

    A. Superior vena cava   C. Left ventricle

    B. Right ventricle   D. Brachiocephalic artery

31. The imaging rate during angiocardiography is between:

    A. 1 to 3 frames per second   C. 10 to 12 frames per second

    B. 4 to 8 frames per second   D. 15 to 30 frames per second

32. Which of the following would not be a common pathologic indicator for abdominal angiography?

    A. Aneurysm   C. Trauma

    B. Stenosis or occlusions of aorta   D. Malabsorption syndrome

33. The average amount of contrast media injected during a venacavagram is:

    A. 6 to 8 ml   C. 30 to 40 ml

    B. 10 to 15 ml   D. 50 to 70 ml

34. True/False: For peripheral angiography, imaging is commonly unilateral for both upper and lower limb exams.

35. True/False: Venograms of the extremity are rarely performed today because of the increased sensitivity of ultrasound.

36. Why is a blue dye injected during a lymphogram?

    A. Helps to visualize the lymph vessels   C. Helps to identify the veins of the limb

    B. Anesthetizes the vessels   D. Reduces spasm of the lymph vessels

37. True/False: Images are often taken 24 hours following injection during a lymphogram.

38. True/False: The most common contrast agent used during lymphography is water-soluble, non-ionic.

39. The most common pathologic indication for chemo-embolization is to treat:

    A. Brain aneurysm   C. AV malformation

    B. Stenosed vessels   D. Hepatic malignancies

40. Match the following descriptions to the correct term or interventional procedure.

    _____ 1. Infusion of therapeutic drugs   A. Embolization

    _____ 2. Device to extract urethral stones   B. Nephrostomy

    _____ 3. Procedure to dissolve blood clots   C. Infusion therapy

    _____ 4. Technique to restrict uncontrolled hemorrhage   D. Basket or loop snare catheter

    _____ 5. Technique to decompress obstructed bile duct   E. Percutaneous gastrostomy

    _____ 6. Direct puncture and catheterization of the renal pelvis   F. Thrombolysis

    _____ 7. Placement of an extended feeding tube into the stomach   G. Percutaneous biliary drainage

41. True/False: A vena cava filter is placed superior to the renal veins to prevent renal vein thrombosis.

42. True/False: The TIPS procedure involves placement of an intrahepatic stent.

CHAPTER 22

Computed Tomography

This chapter presents the general principles of computed tomography (CT) and the various equipment systems in use today. A study of soft tissue anatomy of the central nervous system (CNS) as viewed in axial sections is included. An introduction into the purpose, pathologic indications, and procedure of cranial, thoracic, abdominal, and pelvic computed tomography is also covered in this chapter. Selected sectional images of these three regions are presented.

CHAPTER OBJECTIVES

After you have completed **all** the activities of this chapter, you will be able to:

_____ 1. List three advantages of computed tomography over conventional radiography.

_____ 2. Identify the generational changes and advances in computed tomography systems.

_____ 3. List the major components of a computed tomographic system.

_____ 4. Explain the basic operating principles of computed tomography imaging to include x-ray transmission, data acquisition, image reconstruction, window width, window level, and slice thickness.

_____ 5. Identify the variables or image parameters controlled by the computed tomography technologist.

_____ 6. Calculate the pitch ratio for a helical CT scan using different variables.

_____ 7. List the two general divisions of the central nervous system (CNS).

_____ 8. Identify the specialized cells (neurons) of the nervous system and describe their specific parts and functions.

_____ 9. List the specific membranes or coverings of the CNS and identify the meningeal spaces or potential spaces associated with them.

_____ 10. List the three primary divisions of the brain.

_____ 11. List the four major cavities of the ventricular system and identify specific structures and passageways of the ventricular system.

_____ 12. Identify select gray and white matter structures in the brain.

_____ 13. Describe the concept of the "blood-brain barrier."

_____ 14. List the twelve cranial nerves.

_____ 15. List the common pathologic indicators for cranial, thoracic, abdominal, and pelvic computed tomography studies.

_____ 16. Identify specific structures of the brain, thorax, abdomen, and pelvis on axial drawings and CT images.

_____ 17. Identify the imaging parameters for cranial, thoracic, abdominal, and pelvic computed tomography studies.

Learning Exercises

Complete the following review exercises after reading the associated pages in the textbook as indicated by each exercise. Answers to each review exercise are given at the end of the review exercises.

REVIEW EXERCISE A: Basic Principles of Computed Tomography (see textbook pp. 700-704)

1. List the three advantages of CT over conventional radiography:

    A. _____

    B. _____

    C. _____

2. Match the following characteristics with the correct generation of CT scanner:

    _____ 1. Fan-shaped beam with 30 or more detectors   A. First-generation

    _____ 2. 1 to 2 detector system   B. Second-generation

    _____ 3. 8 times faster than a 1 second, single-slice scanner   C. Third-generation

    _____ 4. First scanner to rotate a full 360° around patient   D. Fourth-generation

    _____ 5. Capable of helical-type volume scanning (multiple answers)   E. Multi-slice CT

    _____ 6. Capable of 1-second or less scan times (multiple answers)

    _____ 7. Contains a bank of up to 960 detectors

    _____ 8. Scan times of 4 1/2 minutes per slice

    _____ 9. Up to 4800 detectors on a fixed ring

    _____ 10. Helical or continuous volume scanning (CVS) (multiple answers)

    _____ 11. The first type with fixed detectors rather than detectors rotating with x-ray tube

    _____ 12. Capable of acquiring 4 slices simultaneously

    _____ 13. First scanner with larger aperture, which permitted full body scanning

3. True/False: Noninvasive studies of the cardiovascular system are possible with multi-slice CT.

4. True/False: Helical CT scanners are limited to one 360° rotation per slice in the same direction.

5. Which of the following is *not* an advantage of multi-slice CT scanners?

    A. Fast imaging speed   C. Minimizes patient motion

    B. Acquires large number of slices rapidly   D. Low-cost system to maintain

6. The actual thickness of tomographic slices with CT systems is:

   A.　1 to 3 or 4 centimeters　　　　C.　1/4 to 1 or more centimeters

   B.　0.5 or more millimeters　　　　D.　10 to 40 or more millimeters

7. The actual thickness of a tomographic slice is controlled by:

   A.　Detectors　　　　　　　　　　C.　Effective focal spot

   B.　Filament of x-ray tube　　　　　D.　Source collimator

8. Define the term *voxel.* _____

9. What do the detectors measure in a CT system? _____

10. A voxel is a _____ dimensional image of the tissue while a pixel represents only _____ dimensions.

11. The depth of the voxels is determined by:

    A.　Slice thickness　　　　　　　C.　Actual scan time

    B.　Speed of computer　　　　　　D.　Size of the pixel

12. Air would have a _____ (higher or lower) differential absorption as compared to soft tissue.

13. The purpose of the detector collimator is to:

    A.　Reduce patient dose

    B.　Minimize amount of scatter radiation that strikes detector

    C.　Only allow high attenuation values to reach the detector

    D.　Minimize patient motion artifact

14. List the two primary components of a computed tomographic system:

    A.　_____　　　B.　_____

15. Which aspect of the CT system houses the x-ray tube and detector array? _____

16. What is another term for image storage? _____

17. The central opening in the CT support structure where the patient is scanned is called the: _____.

18. CT numbers is a numerical scale that represents tissue _____

19. List the correct CT number range for the following tissue types:

    A.　Cortical bone　　　_____

    B.　White brain matter　_____

    C.　Blood　　　　　　　_____

    D.　Fat　　　　　　　　_____

    E.　Lung tissue　　　　_____

    F.　Air　　　　　　　　_____

20. Which medium serves as the baseline for CT numbers? _____

21. Window width (WW) controls:

    A. Image density   C. Slice thickness

    B. Image contrast   D. Total number of slices

22. Window level (WL) controls:

    A. Image density   C. Slice thickness

    B. Image control   D. Total number of slices

23. Match the appearance of the following tissue types as seen on a CT image:

    _____ A. Bone   1. White

    _____ B. Gray brain matter   2. Gray

    _____ C. CSF   3. Black

    _____ D. Positive contrast media

24. Pitch is defined as _____ .

25. Calculate the pitch ratio using following parameters: Couch movement at a rate of 20 mm per second with a slice

    collimation of 10 mm. _____

26. The pitch ratio calculated in question 25 is an example of:

    A. Undersampling   C. Perfect pitch

    B. Oversampling   D. Intermittent pitch

27. Which of the following parameters would produce a 0.5:1.0 pitch ratio?

    A. 10 mm couch movement and 10 mm slice thickness

    B. 15 mm couch movement and 10 mm slice thickness

    C. 10 mm couch movement and 20 mm slice thickness

    D. 30 mm couch movement and 10 mm slice thickness

REVIEW EXERCISE B: Radiographic Anatomy of the Central Nervous System (see textbook pp. 705-713)

1. The central nervous system can be divided into two main divisions:

    A. _____

    B. _____

2. A. The solid spinal cord terminates at the level of the lower border of which vertebra? _____

    B. This tapered terminal area of the spinal cord is called the _____ .

3. A. The specialized cells of the nervous system that conduct electrical impulses are called _____ .

    B. The parts of these cells that receive the electrical impulse and conduct them toward the cell body are called

    _____ .

4. Three membranes or layers of coverings called *meninges* enclose both the brain and the spinal cord. Certain important spaces or potential spaces are associated with these meninges. List these three meninges and three associated spaces as follows:

MENINGES   *SPACES*

Skull or cranium

A. _____   D. _____
   (Outer "hard" or "tough" layer)   (Space or potential space)

B. _____   E. _____
   (Spider-like avascular membrane)   (Narrow space containing thin layer of fluid)

C. _____   F. _____
   (Inner "tender" layer)   (Wider space filled with cerebral spinal fluid)

5. The outer "hard" or "tough" membrane described above has an inner and outer layer tightly fused except for certain

   larger spaces between folds or creases of the brain and the skull, which provide for large venous blood channels

   called _____

6. The large cerebrum is divided into right and left hemispheres. Each hemisphere of the cerebrum is further divided into five lobes, with four of the lobes lying under the cranial bone of the same name. List these five lobes:

A. _____   D. _____

B. _____   E. _____

C. _____

7. The brain (encephalon) can be divided into three general divisions: the (1) forebrain, (2) midbrain, and (3) hindbrain. The forebrain and hindbrain are both divided into three divisions. List the three divisions of the forebrain and the hindbrain as labeled on Fig. 22-1. (Secondary terms for these divisions as found in the textbook are included in brackets.)

1. Forebrain   A. _____
   (Prosencephalon)   (Telencephalon) -Largest division

   (Diencephalon) {   B. _____

                           C. _____

2. Midbrain
   (Mesencephalon)

3. Hindbrain   D. _____

   (Rhombencephalon)   E. _____

                           F. _____

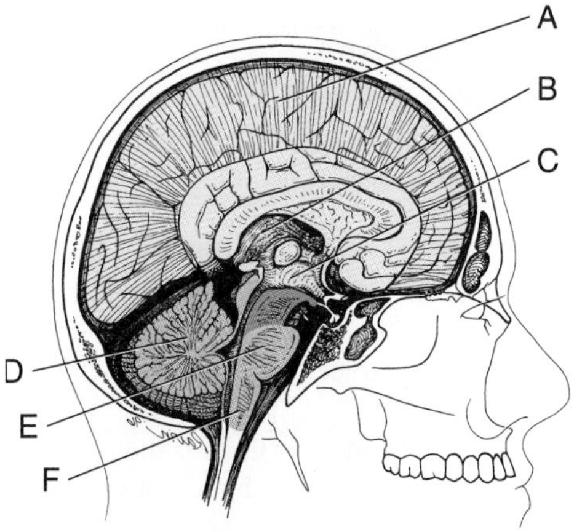

Fig. 22-1 Divisions of the forebrain and hindbrain, midsagittal view.

8. Identify the three lobes of the right cerebral hemisphere as labeled *A-C* in Fig. 22-2. The deep fissure separating the two cerebral hemispheres is labeled D. (Note: there is a fold of dura mater, called the *falx cerebri,* that extends deep within this fissure, separating the two hemispheres that is visualized on CT scans.)

   A. _____ lobe

   B. _____ lobe

   C. _____ lobe

   D. _____ fissure

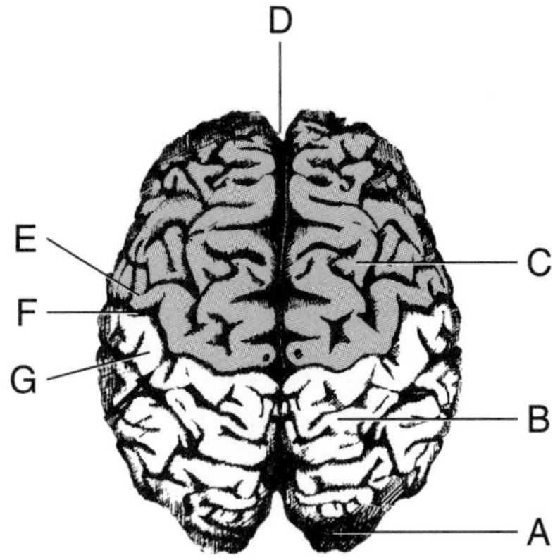

Fig. 22-2 Structures of the cerebral hemispheres.

9. The surface of each cerebral hemisphere contains numerous grooves and convolutions or raised areas. Identify labeled parts *E-G* in Fig. 22-2. Two of these raised areas, *E* and *G,* have specific names and are frequently demonstrated and identified on cranial CT scans. Part *F* is a shallow groove with a specific name.

   E. _____

   F. _____

   G. _____

10. What is the name of the arched mass of white matter that connects the two cerebral hemispheres?

    A. Falx cerebri   C. Central sulcus

    B. Anterior central gyrus   D. Corpus callosum

11. What is the name of the large groove that separates the cerebral hemispheres?

    A. Anterior central gyrus   C. Central sulcus

    B. Longitudinal fissure   D. Posterior central gyrus

12. The fluid manufactured and stored in the ventricular system is called (A) _____ , abbreviated as (B) _____ . This fluid completely surrounds the brain and spinal cord by filling the space called the (C) _____ space. A blockage within this system may result in excessive accumulation of this fluid within the ventricles, creating a condition known as (D) _____ .

13. The cerebrospinal fluid-filled subarachnoid space and ventricular system are important in computed tomography because these areas can be differentiated from tissue structures by their density differences.

    A. The larger spaces or areas within the subarachnoid space are called _____ .

    B. The largest of these is the _____ , located just posterior and inferior to the fourth ventricle.

14. The central midline portion of the brain connecting the midbrain, pons, and medulla to the spinal cord is called the

    _____ .

15. The optic chiasma, the site where some of the optic nerves cross to the opposite side, is located in the:

    A. _____ , a division of the forebrain.

    B. An important gland, which is located just inferior to this division of the forebrain is the

    _____ .

16. A second important midline structure gland is the (A) _____ , which is located just superior

    to the (B) _____ , a division of the hindbrain.

17. The central nervous system (CNS) can be divided by appearance into white matter and gray matter, which can be differentiated by CT. The difference in appearance between these two results from their makeup. Describe this difference by indicating what each consists of:

    A. White matter _____

    B. Gray matter _____

18. In general, the outer cerebral cortex is (A) _____ matter, while the more centrally located

    brain tissue is (B) _____ matter.

19. List the three structures associated with the hypothalamus:

    A. _____   B. _____   C. _____

20. List the three aspects of the brain stem:

    A. _____   B. _____   C. _____

21. Which aspect of the brain serves as an interpretation center for sensory impulses?
    A. Midbrain   C. Thalamus
    B. Pituitary gland   D. Hypothalamus

22. Which aspect of the brain coordinates important motor functions such as coordination, posture, and balance?
    A. Pons   C. Midbrain
    B. Cerebellum   D. Cerebrum

23. Which aspect of the brain controls important body activities related to homeostasis?
    A. Pons   C. Thalamus
    B. Cerebellum   D. Hypothalamus

24. Which aspect or structure of the brain controls a wide range of body functions including growth and reproductive functions?
    A. Pineal gland   C. Thalamus
    B. Pituitary gland   D. Hypothalamus

25. List the four cerebral nuclei or basal ganglia:

    A. _____   C. _____

    B. _____   D. _____

26. Ventricles: There are four cavities in the ventricular system. These are labeled in Fig. 22-3 and demonstrate the four ventricles in relationship to other brain structures. Two of the ventricles are located within the right and left cerebral hemispheres (A); the remaining two are midline structures (B and C).

    The larger two ventricles (A) have four significant parts labeled (1), (2), (3), and (6) in Fig. 22-4. The small duct-like structure (4) provides communication between ventricles, and (5) indicates a connection between the third and fourth ventricles. An important gland (8) is also shown. Number 7 represents an important communication with the sub-arachnoid space on each side of the fourth ventricle.

    Identify the ventricles and their parts as labeled on these two drawings.

    Fig.   22-3

    A.   Right and left _____ ventricles

    B.   _____ ventricle

    C.   _____ ventricle

    Fig.   22-4

    1.   _____ (occipital)

    2.   _____

    3.   _____ (frontal)

    4.   _____ (foramen)

    5.   _____

    6.   _____ (temporal)

    7.   _____

    8.   _____ (gland)

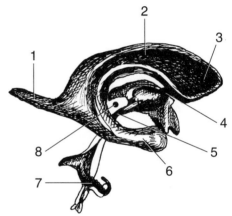

Fig. 22-3 Cavities in the ventricular system.

Fig. 22-4 Anatomy of the ventricles.

27. There are 12 pairs of cranial nerves, most of which originate from the brainstem and travel to various parts of the brain, controlling both sensory and motor functions. List these 12 pairs of cranial nerves:

    A. _____   E. _____   I. _____

    B. _____   F. _____   J. _____

    C. _____   G. _____   K. _____

    D. _____   H. _____   L. _____

REVIEW EXERCISE C: Cranial Computed Tomography and Sectional Anatomy of the Brain (see textbook pp. 714-716)

1. Which one of the following is not a common pathologic indicator for cranial computed tomography?

    A.   Brain atrophy   C.   Intracranial hemorrhage

    B.   Multiple sclerosis   D.   Aneurysm

2. Approximately _____ to _____% of all cranial CTs require contrast media.

3. True/False: Oxygen deprivation of 2 minutes will lead to permanent brain cell injury.

4. True/False: Contrast media are able to pass through the blood-brain barrier in the normal individual.

5. True/False: Contrast media are necessary for cranial CT for visualizing neoplasms.

6. Which one of the following substances will not pass through the blood-brain barrier?

   A. Proteins   C. Oxygen

   B. Glucose   D. Select ions found in the blood

7. Trauma to the skull may lead to a collection of blood accumulating under the dura mater called: _____

8. With routine cranial CT positioning, the neck is flexed to create a _____ angle of the IOML vertical and parallel to the x-ray beam.

   A. 10°   C. 25°

   B. 20°   D. 30°

9. On the average, it takes _____ to _____ axial scans to cover the entire brain.

10. The most important aspect of positioning the head for cranial CT is to ensure there is no

    _____ and no _____ of the head.

11. Identify the labeled parts on this axial section through the region of the mid-ventricular level (Figs. 22-5 and 22-6)

    A. _____   E. _____

    B. _____   F. _____

    C. _____   G. _____

    D. _____

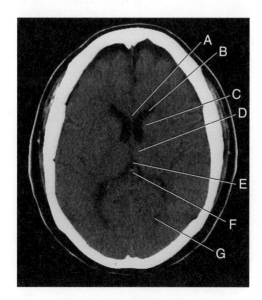

Fig. 22-5 Structure identification on an axial CT scan at mid-ventricular level.

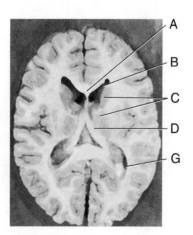

Fig. 22-6 Brain tissue specimen, mid-ventricular level.

12. Identify the labeled parts on this axial section through the level of the middle third ventricle (Figs. 22-7 and 22-8):

A. _____

B. _____

C. _____

D. _____

E. _____

13. Axial section at the level of the mid orbits (Figs. 22-9 and 22-10):

A. _____

B. _____

C. _____

D. _____

E. _____

F. _____

G. _____

H. _____

I. _____

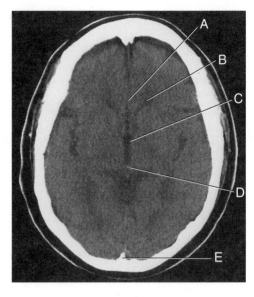

Fig. 22-7 Structure identification on an axial CT scan at mid-third ventricle level.

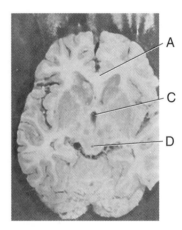

Fig. 22-8 Brain tissue specimen, mid-third ventricle level.

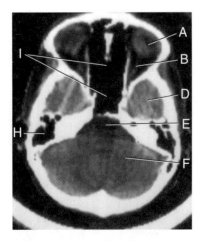

Fig. 22-9 Structure identification on an axial CT scan at the level of the mid orbits.

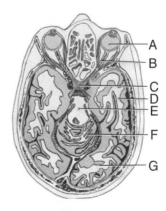

Fig. 22-10 Drawing of tissue in the axial section at the orbital plane level.

REVIEW EXERCISE D: Thoracic Computed Tomography Anatomy, Positioning, and Procedures (see textbook pp. 718-719)

Sectional Anatomy of the Thorax Identify the anatomy on these axial sections of the thorax at 10 mm-slice thickness obtained after bolus injections of contrast media. The patient's right is to your left as with conventional radiography.

1. Axial section through upper thorax at level of approximately T3 (Fig. 22-11). Parts *A, B, D,* and *E* represent veins and arteries of the lower neck and upper thorax just superior to the arch of the aorta. Parts *F* and *G* are well-known portions of the upper digestive tract and respiratory system that you should be able to identify by their relative locations

A. _____ vein

B. _____ artery

C. _____

D. _____ artery

E. _____ artery

F. _____

G. _____

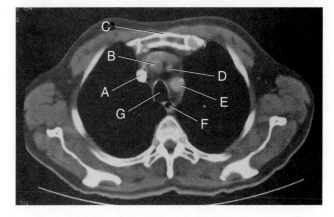

Fig. 22-11 Axial section through upper thorax at level of about T3.

2. Which one of the following structures is considered to be most posterior (as seen in Fig. 22-11)?

A. Esophagus   C. Left brachiocephalic vein

B. Trachea   D. Left common carotid artery

3. Axial section through level of carina (Fig. 22-12). Identify labeled structures *A-H,* which represent major vessels and bony structures of the chest.

A. _____

B. _____

C. _____

D. _____

E. _____

F. _____

G. _____

H. _____

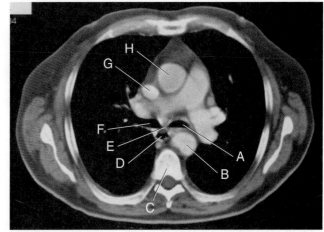

Fig. 22-12 Axial section through level of carina.

4. Which one of the following structures is located most anterior (as seen in Fig. 22-12)?

A. Superior vena cava   C. Descending aorta

B. Carina   D. Ascending aorta

5. Axial section through four chambers of the heart (Fig. 22-13). Identify labeled structures *A-H*, which represent the four chambers of the heart and other thoracic vessels and structures seen at this level.

A. _____

B. _____

C. _____

D. _____

E. _____

F. _____

G. _____

H. _____

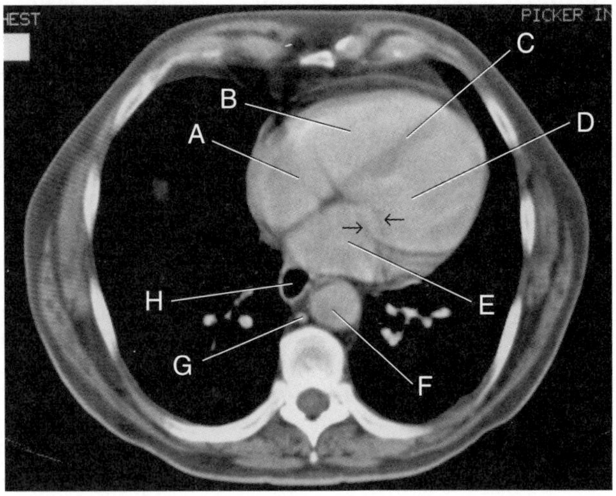

Fig. 22-13 Axial section through four chambers of the heart.

6. How can you determine whether structure *H* is the esophagus or the trachea?

_____

7. The valve between heart chambers D and E is the _____ valve (see arrows).

8. Which chamber of the heart is located closest to the spine? _____

Positioning and Procedures for Thoracic CT:

9. Describe the projection of the chest taken as a localizing radiograph or pilot scan for CT of the chest.

_____

10. What is the most common slice thickness for a CT study of the chest? _____

11. If a small pulmonary lesion is suspected, slice thickness will often be reduced to _____ .

12. Which of the following are not pathologic indicators for thoracic CT?

    A. Hilar lesions   E. Pericardial diseases

    B. Aneurysms   F. Evaluation of pulmonary nodules

    C. Abscess of thorax   G. All of the above are common indicators

    D. Cardiac disease

13. A mass seen on a thoracic CT study reveals a mass in the lungs. The attenuation of this mass is slightly above water (O). Which one of the following pathologic indicators would be most likely?

    A. Solid pulmonary nodule   C. Bronchogenic cyst

    B. Lung carcinoma   D. Pulmonary calcification

14. **Situation:** A patient with a clinical history of carcinoma of the lung comes to the radiology department for a CT of the thorax. Which one of the following scan ranges would be performed for this patient?

    A. From apex of lung to diaphragm   C. From apex of lung to left colic flexure

    B. From apex of lung to liver   D. From apex of lung to adrenal glands

15. Helical CT scanning uses a _____ breathing technique during CT of the thorax.

16. Describe the patient position for a routine CT examination of the thorax: _____

17. What is the name of the region located between the ascending aorta and the pulmonary artery? _____

_____ .

REVIEW EXERCISE E: Abdominal and Pelvic Computed Tomography Anatomy, Positioning, and Procedures (see textbook pp. 720-724)

The following CT images are 10 mm slice thickness. An intravenous contrast medium was given to enhance vascular structures as well as oral contrast for the GI tract.

1. Axial section through level of the pancreatic tail (Fig. 22-14). Identify labeled structures *A-K*, which represent major vessels and soft-tissue structures of the abdomen:

    A. _____

    B. _____

    C. _____

    D. _____

    E. _____

    F. _____

    G. _____

    H. _____

    I. _____

    J. _____

    K. _____

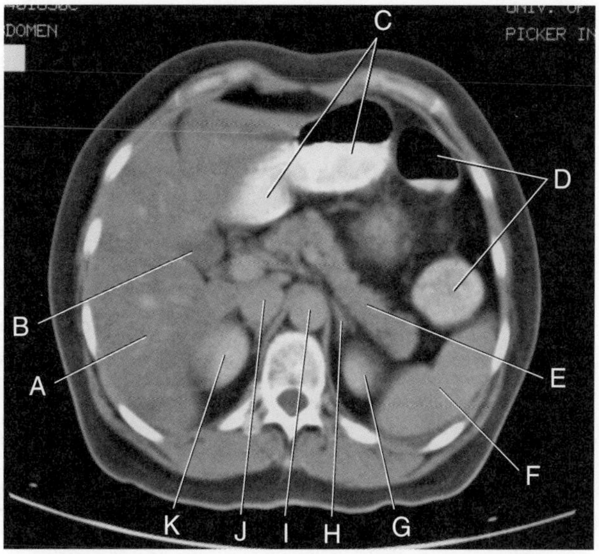

Fig. 22-14 Axial section through level of pancreatic tail.

Questions 2 and 3 relate to structures seen in Fig. 22-14.

2. Which two parts of the stomach are indicated by the two lead lines for label C? (Circle two of the four choices.)

    A. Pylorus   C. Fundus

    B. Body   D. Cardiac antrum

3. The adrenal glands often appear as an inverted _____ shape seen in sectional images of the abdomen.

4. Axial section through level of the second portion of duodenum (Fig. 22-15). Identify labeled structures *A-J*, which represent major vessels and soft-tissue structures of the abdomen:

A. _____

B. _____

C. _____

D. _____

E. _____

F. _____

G. _____

H. _____

I. _____

J. _____

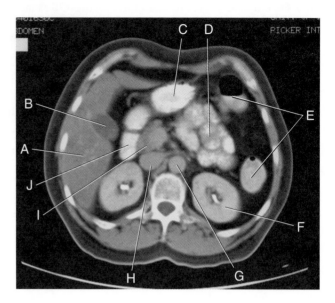

Fig. 22-15 Axial section through level of second portion of duodenum.

5. How can the second portion of the duodenum be distinguished from a tumor in the head of the pancreas as shown in Fig. 22-15?

_____

6. Axial section through level 2 cm caudad to the renal pelvis (Fig. 22-16). Identify labeled structures *A-I,* which represent major vessels and segments of both the large and small bowel, kidneys, and ureters.

A. _____

B. _____

C. _____

D. _____

E. _____

F. _____

G. _____

H. _____

I. _____

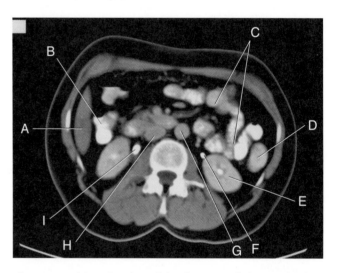

Fig. 22-16 Axial section through level 2 cm caudad to renal pelvis.

7. How can it be determined that the section in Fig. 22-16 is at a level just caudad to renal pelvis? (Hint: Look at the relationship of the kidneys and ureters.)

_____

8. How can it be determined which is the ascending colon and which is the descending colon on this section (Fig. 22-16)?

_____

9. Axial section through level of the ilium and the rectum (Fig. 22-17). Identify labeled structures *A-G,* which represent major vessels, soft tissues, and bony structures of the pelvis:

A. _____

B. _____

C. _____

D. _____

E. _____

F. _____

G. _____

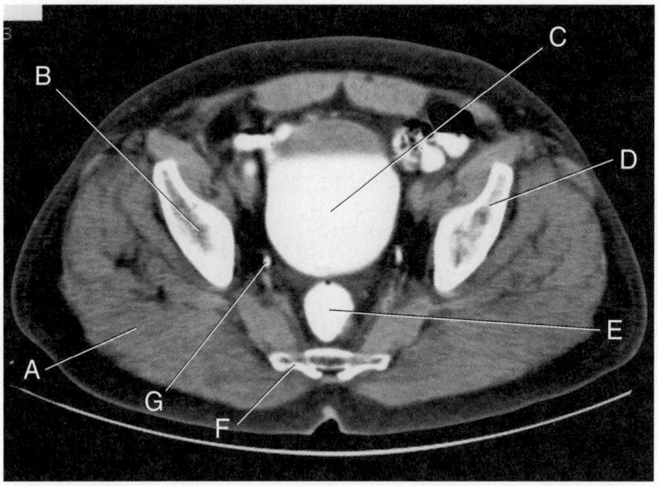

Fig. 22-17 Axial section through level of ilium and rectum.

Positioning and Procedures for Abdominal and Pelvic CT

10. True/False: The number of ERCP procedures performed has been greatly reduced due to the effectiveness of CT examinations of the abdomen.

11. True/False: Pregnancy is not a contraindication for CT of the abdomen.

12. True/False: CT has replaced (for the most part) lymphangiography in detecting lymph-node malignancies.

13. Pelvic CT is an excellent imaging modality for diagnosing occult disease. Occult disease is defined as:

_____

14. For most routine CT studies of the abdomen or pelvis, a slice thickness of _____ mm is often employed.

A. 10 to 15   C. 5 to 8

B. 20   D. 25 to 30

15. During a helical CT of the abdomen, a 15-mm couch movement per second with a slice collimation of 10 mm is used. Calculate the pitch ratio for this study.

_____

16. **Situation:** A patient with a clinical history of pancreatic cancer comes to CT for a study of the abdomen. What slice thickness should be used for this study at the level of the pancreas?

A. 5 to 8 mm   C. 10 mm

B. 2 to 3 mm   D. 1 to 1.5 mm

17. A. What percent of concentration of barium sulfate should be used for CT procedures of the abdomen and pelvis?

_____

B. How does this compare with regular "thin" barium as used in conventional upper GI studies as described in

Chapter 14? _____

18. Why is such a low concentration of barium used for CT studies?

   _____

19. Describe the appearance of beam-hardening artifacts.

   _____

20. When should the patient be given oral contrast media before a CT study of the small bowel?

   A. Night before the exam   C. Immediately before the exam

   B. 1 hour before the exam   D. 24 hours before the exam

21. What is the purpose of the insertion of a tampon for CT scans of the female pelvis and lower abdomen?

   _____

22. If the upper abdomen is the area of interest, scanning generally begins at the level of the

   (A) _____ , and continues inferiorly to the level of the (B) _____ .

23. If the pelvis is the area of interest, scanning begins at the level of the (A) _____ , and con-

   tinues to the (B) _____ .

24. To prevent respiratory and peristaltic artifacts on CT scans of the abdomen, maximum exposure times of

   _____ are needed.

25. A. What breathing instructions, if any, are required to obtain high-quality serial CT scans of the abdomen with

      non-spiral scanning? _____

   B. What are breathing requirements for volume (spiral) type scanning of the abdomen?

      _____

Laboratory Exercises (see textbook pp. 714-724)

Part A of this learning activity needs to be carried out in a special procedures room equipped for whole-body CT. A supervising technologist or instructor should be present for this activity. Part B can be carried out in a classroom or any room where illuminators and other CT viewing facilities are available.

LABORATORY EXERCISE A: Positioning

Complete the following and place a check by each when completed.

_____   1.   Review the equipment in the room, noting the location of patient support equipment such as oxygen, suction, the IV pole, and the emergency cart.

_____   2.   Role play using another student as the patient.   Prepare the patient by explaining the procedure, the breathing instructions they will be given, the sounds they will experience, and what they will see and experience as they are placed into the gantry aperture for the examination.

_____   3.   Place your patient on the table (couch) in a supine position with the arms above the head.   Raise the patient and table to the correct height and slowly move into the gantry aperture until the x-ray beam trajectory coincides with the starting scan position for the part being examined. Using the intercom device, talk to the patient from the control console. Finally, remove your patient when the procedure is completed.

_____   4.   Review the controls and monitors at the operator console.   Have someone demonstrate the image parameters and the other variables controlled by the technologist and explain how whole body scanning is different from cranial CT scanning.

LABORATORY EXERCISE B: Anatomy Review Using CT Scans

Use CT scans of the thorax (chest), abdomen, and pelvis as provided by your instructor. These may be "hard copies" as recorded on paper or film or they may be from disks or magnetic tape as displayed on monitors. They should include normal and abnormal sections displaying obvious pathology.

Locate and identify each of the organs and structures as labeled and identified on similar scans in the workbook and the textbook. (Pay particular attention to those parts you identified on similar scans in your workbook in the preceding Review Exercises A and B.)

_____   1.   Axial sections of the chest

_____   2.   Axial sections of the abdomen

_____   3.   Axial sections of the pelvis

Answers to Review Exercises

Review Exercise A: Basic Principles of Computed Tomography

1. A. Anatomy is presented in a series of slices that provides a more complete survey of a specific tissue.
   B. Better contrast resolution between various types of soft tissue.
   C. Ability to manipulate and adjust image after scanning is completed.
2. 1. B, 2. A, 3. E, 4. C, 5. C and D, 6. C, D and E, 7. C, 8. A, 9. D, 10. C and D 11. D, 12. E 13. C
3. True
4. False (multiple rotations possible)
5. D. Low cost system to maintain
6. B 0.5 mm or more
7. D source collimator
8. Volume element
9. Attenuation of radiation by a given tissue
10. Three, two
11. A. Slice thickness
12. Lower
13. B. Minimize amount of scatter radiation striking the detector
14. A. Scan unit
    B. Operator control console
15. Gantry
16. Image archiving
17. Aperture
18. Attenuation
19. A. Cortical bone: + 1000
    B. White brain matter: + 45
    C. Blood: + 20
    D. Fat: − 100
    E. Lung tissue: − 200
    F. Air: − 1000
20. Water
21. B. Image contrast
22. A. Image density
23. A. Bone - 1. white
    B. Gray brain matter - 2. gray
    C. CSF - 3. black
    D. Positive contrast media - 1. white
24. The ratio reflecting the relationship between patient couch movement and x-ray beam collimation or slice thickness
25. 2: 1 pitch
26. A. Undersampling
27. C. 10 mm couch movement and 20 mm slice thickness

Review Exercise B: Radiographic Anatomy of the Central Nervous System

1. A. Brain (encephalon)
   B. Spinal cord (medulla spinalis)
2. A. L1
   B. Conus medullaris
3. A. Neurons
   B. Dendrites
4. A. Dura mater
   B. Arachnoid
   C. Pia mater
   D. Epidural space
   E. Subdural space
   F. Subarachnoid space
5. Venous sinuses
6. A. Frontal lobe
   B. Parietal lobe
   C. Occipital lobe
   D. Temporal lobe
   E. Insula or central lobe
7. A. Cerebrum
   B. Thalamus
   C. Hypothalamus
   D. Cerebellum
   E. Pons
   F. Medulla (medulla oblongata)
8. A. Occipital lobe
   B. Parietal lobe
   C. Frontal lobe
   D. Longitudinal fissure
9. E. Anterior (precentral) central gyrus
   F. Central sulcus
   G. Posterior (post central) central gyrus
10. D corpus callosum
11. B longitudinal fissure
12. A. Cerebrospinal fluid
    B. CSF
    C. Subarachnoid
    D. Hydrocephalus
13. A. Cisterns
    B. Cistern cerebellomedullaris (Cisterna magna)
14. Brain stem
15. A. Hypothalamus
    B. Pituitary (hypophysis) gland
16. A. Pineal gland
    B. Cerebellum
17. A. Tracts of myelinated axons of nerve cells
    B. Primarily dendrites and cell bodies
18. A. Gray
    B. White
19. A. Infundibulum
    B. Posterior pituitary gland
    C. Optic chiasma
20. A. Midbrain
    B. Pons
    C. Medulla
21. C Thalamus
22. B Cerebellum
23. D Hypothalamus
24. B Pituitary gland
25. A. Caudate nucleus
    B. Lentiform nucleus
    C. Claustrum
    D. Amygdaloid nucleus
26. A. Right and left lateral ventricles
    B. Third ventricle
    C. Fourth ventricle
    1. Posterior horn
    2. Body
    3. Anterior horn
    4. Interventricular foramen
    5. Cerebral aqueduct
    6. Inferior horn
    7. Lateral recess
    8. Pineal gland
27. A. Olfactory
    B. Optic
    C. Oculomotor
    D. Trochlear
    E. Trigeminal
    F. Abducens
    G. Facial
    H. Acoustic
    I. Glossopharyngeal
    J. Vagus
    K. Spinal accessory
    L. Hypoglossal

Review Exercise C: Cranial Computed Tomography and Sectional Anatomy of the Brain

1. B. Multiple sclerosis
2. 50% to 90%
3. False. (4 minutes)
4. False (are not able to pass through)
5. True
6. A. proteins
7. Subdural hematoma
8. C. 25°
9. Six to ten
10. Rotation and no tilt
11. A. Anterior corpus callosum-genu
    B. Anterior horn of left lateral ventricle
    C. Region of caudate nuclei
    D. Region of thalamus
    E. Third ventricle
    F. Pineal gland or body
    G. Posterior horn of left lateral ventricle
12. A. Anterior corpus callosum-genu
    B. Anterior horn of left lateral ventricle (CT only)
    C. Third ventricle
    D. Region of pineal gland
    E. Internal occipital protuberance (CT only)
13. A. Orbital bulb or eyeball
    B. Left optic nerve
    C. Optic chiasma (drawing only)
    D. Temporal lobe of cerebrum

E. Pons
F. Cerebellum
G. Occipital lobe (drawing only)
H. Mastoid air cells (CT only)
I. Sphenoid and ethmoid sinuses-CT only

Review Exercise D: Thoracic Computed Tomography Anatomy, Positioning, and Procedures

1. A. Right brachiocephalic vein
   B. Brachiocephalic artery
   C. Sternum (manubrium)
   D. Left common carotid artery
   E. Left subclavian artery
   F. Esophagus
   G. Trachea
2. A esophagus
3. A. Left main stem bronchus
   B. Descending aorta
   C. T5 vertebra
   D. Esophagus
   E. Carina
   F. Right main stem bronchus
   G. Superior vena cava
   H. Ascending aorta
4. D ascending aorta
5. A. Right atrium
   B. Right ventricle
   C. Interventricular septum
   D. Left ventricle
   E. Left atrium
   F. Descending aorta
   G. Azygos vein
   H. Esophagus
6. This level (through the four chambers of the heart) is below or inferior to the carina, so *H* couldn't be the trachea.
7. Mitral
8. Left atrium
9. PA, tube and detectors stationary; patient and couch are moved at intervals through the aperture.
10. 10 mm
11. Scale 3 to 5 mm
12. G all are common indications
13. C. Bronchogenic cyst

14. D. From apex of lung to adrenal glands
15. Breath hold or single breath
16. Supine position with arms above head
17. Aortopulmonary window

Review Exercise E: Abdominal and Pelvic Computed Tomography Anatomy, Positioning, and Procedures

1. A. Right lobe of the liver (posterior segment)
   B. Gallbladder
   C. Stomach
   D. Colon
   E. Tail of pancreas
   F. Spleen
   G. Upper lobe of left kidney
   H. Left adrenal gland
   I. Aorta
   J. Inferior vena cava
   K. Upper lobe of right kidney
2. A and B (pylorus and body)
3. "V"
4. A. Right lobe of liver
   B. Gallbladder
   C. Stomach
   D. Jejunum
   E. Colon
   F. Left kidney
   G. Abdominal aorta
   H. Inferior vena cava
   I. Head of pancreas
   J. Second portion of duodenum
5. Give the patient oral contrast media to opacify the duodenum
6. A. Lower portion of right lobe of liver
   B. Ascending colon
   C. Jejunum
   D. Descending colon
   E. Left kidney
   F. Left ureter
   G. Abdominal aorta
   H. Inferior vena cava
   I. Right ureter

7. The ureters are seen in cross-section totally separate from the kidneys. (Above the renal pelvis ureters would not be visible, and at level of the renal pelvis ureters and kidneys would appear connected.)
8. Ascending would be on patient's right (side of liver) and descending would be on left.
9. A. Gluteus maximus muscle
   B. Right ilium
   C. Urinary bladder
   D. Left ilium
   E. Rectum
   F. Sacrum
   G. Right ureter
10. True
11. False (is a contraindication). Although the radiologist may still order CT if no other imaging modality will produce the needed diagnosis.
12. True
13. A hidden or concealed disease difficult to diagnose
14. A. 10 to 15
15. 1.5:1.0
16. A. 5 to 8 mm
17. A. 1% to 3%
    B. Much thinner, thin barium is about a 50% concentration for conventional upper GI studies
18. Higher concentrations of barium sulfate will produce beam-hardening artifacts.
19. Linear streaks arising from the high density structures
20. B. 1 hour before exam
21. To aid in localization of the vagina by entrapment of air
22. (A) Xiphoid process
    (B) Iliac crest
23. (A) Iliac crest
    (B) Symphysis pubis
24. 1 to 3 seconds
25. A. Ask patient to suspend respiration at same phase of respiration for all exposures for consistency
    B. With volume or spiral scanning a single breath hold of 20 to 30 seconds is needed.

SELF-TEST

My Score = _____ %

This self-test should be taken only after completing all of the readings, review exercises, and laboratory activities for a particular section. The purpose of this test is not only to provide a good learning exercise but also to serve as a good indicator of what your final evaluation grade will be. It is strongly suggested that if you do not get at least a 90% to 95% grade on this self-test, you should review those areas in which you missed questions before going to your instructor for the final evaluation exam for this chapter. (There are 87 questions or blanks—each is worth 1.2 points.)

1. Which generation of CT scanner used a pencil-thin x-ray beam and a single detector?

    A. First-generation   C. Third-generation

    B. Second-generation   D. Fourth-generation

2. Which generation of CT scanner allows helical or continuous volume-type scanning (may be more than one correct answer)?

    A. First-generation   C. Third-generation

    B. Second-generation   D. Fourth-generation

3. Which devices in the helical CT scanners allow continual tube rotation in the same direction?

    _____

4. CT can detect tissue density (contrast) differences as low as:

    A. 1%   C. 10%

    B. 5%   D. 20%

5. Which device controls slice thickness in a CT image? _____

6. What must be done to the numerical data to create the actual CT image or picture?

    _____

7. The two major components of the scan unit are:

    A. _____   B. _____

8. Each tiny picture element in the display matrix is called a (an) _____ .

9. Which of the following parameters *cannot* be varied by appropriate manipulation at the operator console?

    A. kVp   D. Vertical adjustment of table height

    B. Scan time   E. Thickness of slice

    C. Pitch selections

10. Contrast media will not ordinarily cross the _____ .

11. Which one of the following pathologic indications does *not* apply to cranial CT?

    A. Brain neoplasm   D. Trauma

    B. Brain atrophy   E. All of the above apply

    C. Multiple sclerosis

12. Considering the blood-brain phenomenon, which of the following would require the use of contrast media? (There may be more than one correct answer.)

   A. Hydrocephalus   D. Epidural hematoma

   B. Possible neoplasia   E. Brain tumor

   C. Subdural hematoma

13. In what year did the first successful clinical demonstration of computed tomography (CT) take place?

   A. 1895   B. 1966   C. 1972   D. 1981

14. A. The parts of the neuron that conduct impulses toward the cell body are called _____.

   B. The part that conducts impulses away from the cell body is the _____.

15. Three protective membranes that cover or enclose the entire central nervous system are called

   _____

16. The three membranes from question 2 are called (starting externally):

   A. _____   B. _____   C. _____

17. The various layers of the membranes just discussed have specific spaces of various sizes between these layers. Each has a specific name. Identify these various membrane layers and their associated spaces on Fig. 22-18.

   Membranes and associated spaces:

   A. _____

   B. _____

   C. _____

   D. _____

   E. _____

   F. _____

   G. _____

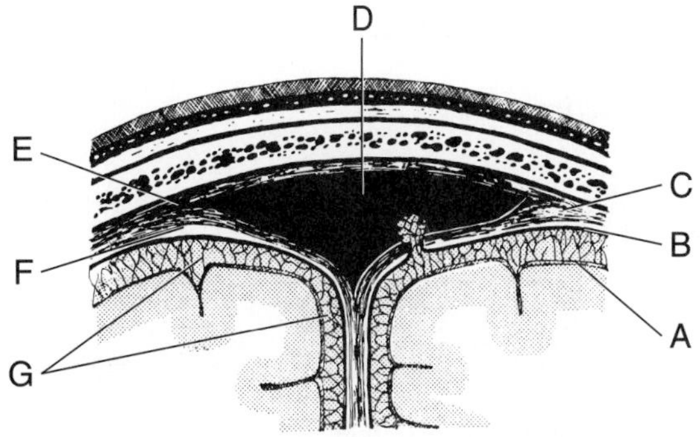

Fig. 22-18 Meninges and meningeal spaces.

18. Which of the spaces in Question 17 is normally filled with cerebrospinal fluid? _____

19. Match the following areas and divisions of the brain.

   _____ 1. Pons   A. Forebrain

   _____ 2. Cerebellum   B. Midbrain

   _____ 3. Cerebrum   C. Hindbrain

   _____ 4. Thalamus

   _____ 5. Medulla

20. The largest division of the brain is the _____.

21. The right and left cerebral hemispheres are separated by a deep fissure called the _____.

22. The fibrous band of white tissue deep within this fissure connecting the right and left hemispheres is called the

     _____.

23. What is the name of the tissue found within the fissure mentioned in question 22? _____

24. Which of the following ventricles are located within the cerebral hemispheres

     A. Lateral ventricles   C. Third ventricle

     B. Fourth ventricle   D. Cisterna magna

25. The diamond-shaped fourth ventricle connects inferiorly with a wide portion of subarachnoid space called the:

     A. Interventricular foramen   C. Cisterna cerebellomedullaris

     B. Lateral recesses   D. Cisterna pontis

26. Identify the ventricles, their parts, and their associated structures as labeled on both the lateral and top-view drawings (Figs. 22-19 and 22-20).

Ventricles:

A. _____

B. _____

C. _____

Connecting ducts:

a. _____

b. _____

c. _____

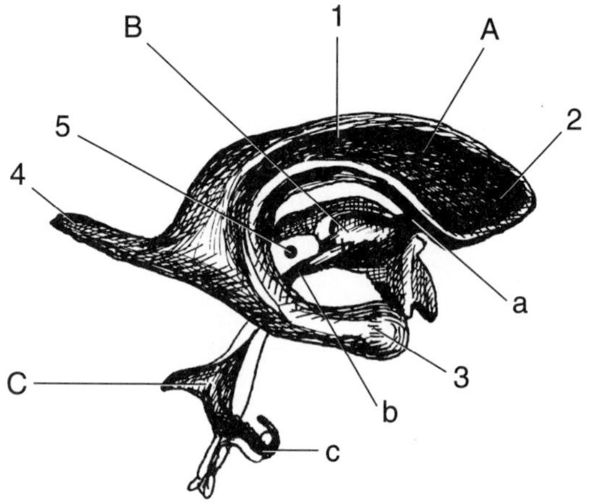

Fig. 22-19 Ventricles, lateral view.

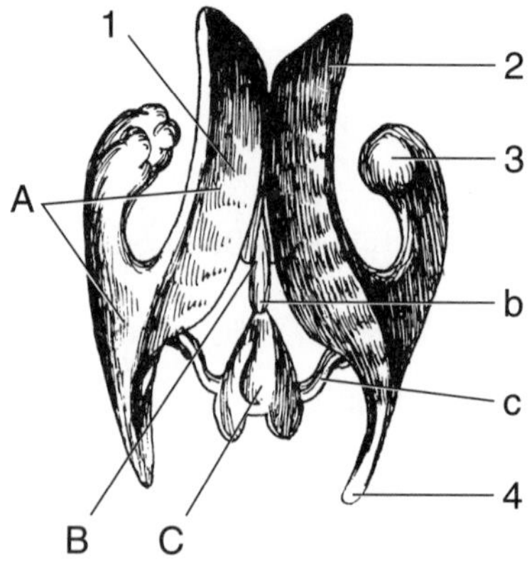

Parts of lateral ventricles:

1. _____

2. _____

3. _____

4. _____

Associated structure: (only in Fig. 22-19)

5. _____

Fig. 22-20 Ventricles, superior view.

27. The condition known as _____ results from abnormal accumulation of cerebrospinal fluid

     within the _____.

28. Enlarged regions of the subarachnoid space are called _____.

29. Identify the four lobes of the cerebrum as labeled on

    Fig. 22-21.

    A. _____

    B. _____

    C. _____

    D. _____

    E. The fifth lobe, which is more centrally located and not
       shown on this drawing, is called the

    _____.

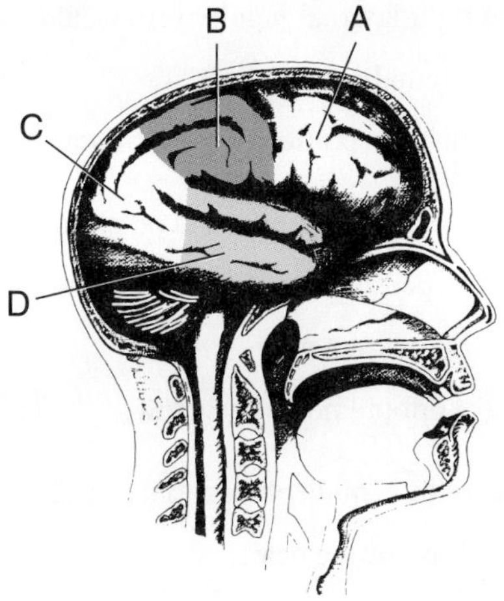

Fig. 22-21 Four lobes of the cerebrum.

30. Identify each of the following terms as either gray matter or white matter:

    _____ 1. Cerebral cortex   A. Gray matter

    _____ 2. Axons (fibrous parts of neuron) B. White matter

    _____ 3. Corpus callosum

    _____ 4. Thalamus

    _____ 5. Centrum semiovale

    _____ 6. Cerebral nuclei

Questions 31 through 35 refer to anatomy as seen on the axial CT brain sections (see textbook pp.715- 716)

31. Select the structure that would *not* lie in the same axial section as the others (section through the orbital plane):

    A. Temporal lobe   C. Longitudinal fissure

    B. Cerebellum   D. Optic nerve

32. Select the structure that would not lie in the same axial section as the others (section through mid third ventricle):

    A. Pons   D. Genu

    B. Parietal lobe of cerebrum E. Anterior horn of lateral ventricle

    C. Internal occipital protuberance

33. Select the structure that would *not* lie in the same axial section as the others (section through mid ventricular level):

    A. Frontal bone   D. Mid brain

    B. Third ventricle E. Caudate nucleus

    C. Genu

Questions 34 through 37 refer to anatomy as seen on axial thoracic CT sections (see textbook pp. 718 - 719)

34. The brachiocephalic artery would be best demonstrated on an axial section at the level of the:

    A. Sternal notch   C. Body portion of manubrium

    B. Inferior portion of manubrium D. Carina

35. The right internal jugular vein would only be clearly seen on axial sections at the level of the:

    A. Sternal notch   C. Carina

    B. Inferior portion of manubrium   D. Base of the heart

36. The ascending aorta would be clearly seen on axial sections at the level of the:

    A. Superior portion of manubrium   D. Carina

    B. Sternal notch   E. All of the above

    C. Aortopulmonary window

37. The right hemidiaphragm only would generally be seen on axial sections at the level of the:

    A. Base of the heart   D. Aortopulmonary window

    B. 2 cm below the base of the heart E. None of the above

    C. Carina

38. The space between the ascending and descending aorta is called _____.

39. Which one of the following structures is considered to be most anterior at the level of the carina?

    A. Ascending aorta   D. Left main stem bronchus

    B. Descending aorta   E. Azygos vein

    C. Carina

40. Which chamber of the heart is considered to be most posterior at the level of the base of the heart?

    A. Right atrium   C. Left atrium

    B. Right ventricle   D. Left ventricle

41. Which of the following is not a pathologic indication for CT of the thorax?

    A. Evaluation of pulmonary nodules   C. Hilar lesions

    B. Aneurysms   D. Mitral valve prolapse

42. A _____ slice thickness is commonly used for routine scans of the thorax.

    A. 10 mm   B. 5 mm   C. 2 mm   D. 10 cm

Questions 43 through 47 refer to anatomy as seen on the axial abdomen and pelvic CT sections (see textbook pp. 722-724)

43. The uncinate process refers to:

    A. A section of the liver located posteriorly and inferiorly

    B. A hooklike process of the spleen as seen lying next to the duodenum

    C. A process of the gallbladder seen only in the appropriate axial section

    D. The hooklike extension of the head of the pancreas

44. The right lobe of the liver is demonstrated on axial sections at the same level(s) of the:

    A. Pancreatic tail   C. Uncinate process of pancreas

    B. Mid portion of the kidneys D. All of the above

45. The gallbladder is visualized on the same axial level as the:

    A. Renal pelves of kidneys   C. Right lobe of the liver

    B. Uncinate process of the pancreas   D. All of the above

46. The prostate gland is best visualized at the same axial section level as the:

    A. Ischial rami   C. Urinary bladder

    B. Acetabular roof   D. Symphysis pubis

47. Which one of the following structures is considered to be most anterior (at the level of the femoral heads)?

    A. Rectum   C. Urinary bladder

    B. Seminal vesicles   D. Coccyx

48. A common couch incrementation for abdominal scanning is:

    A. 10 cm   B. 10 mm   C. 1 cm   D. 5 mm

49. Beam hardening artifacts for CT of the abdomen are most likely to occur when:

    A. Patient has metallic parts such as a hip prosthesis

    B. High concentration of a large bolus of barium is present with a low concentration of water

    C. Low concentration of barium (too diluted with water) is present

    D. Peristalsis occurs in GI tract

50. The first slice for an upper abdomen CT scan is commonly taken at the level of:

    A. First lumbar vertebrae   C. Xiphoid process

    B. Inferior rib margin   D. Iliac crest

51. True/False: The use of CT has greatly reduced the ERCP as a common standard diagnostic procedure for evaluating the biliary ducts.

52. True/False:The use of water-soluble contrast agents rather than barium sulfate suspensions for GI tract radiography is desirable because they tend to slow peristaltic action.

53. True/False: Because of the relatively short exposure times, patients are not required to hold their breath during CT exposures of the abdomen.

54. True/False: The use of both oral and/or rectal contrast media is essential for CT abdominal and pelvic exams.

55. True/False: Contrast media are injected intravenously in a similar manner to excretory urography to visualize structures within the mediastinum for thoracic CT.

CHAPTER 23

Additional Imaging Procedures

This chapter discusses additional imaging procedures less common in most radiology departments. Arthrograms, sialograms, myelograms, and conventional tomograms are being replaced with other new imaging modalities such as computerized tomography (CT) or magnetic resonance imaging (MRI). However, in some departments, these procedures are still being performed in sufficient numbers that technologists need to be familiar with them so that they can perform them when requested.

The anatomy for these procedures has been studied in previous chapters; this chapter therefore covers only the procedures themselves and the related positioning. The exception to this is the anatomy of the female reproductive organs as described in the section on hysterosalpingography.

CHAPTER OBJECTIVES

After you have completed **all** the activities of this chapter, you will be able to:

ARTHROGRAPHY

_____ 1. Identify the purpose, indications, patient preparation, equipment, general procedure, and the positioning routines related to knee arthrography.

_____ 2. Identify the purpose, indications, patient preparation, equipment, general procedure, and the positioning and filming sequence related to shoulder arthrography.

HYSTEROSALPINOGRAPHY

_____ 1. Identify specific aspects of the female reproductive system.

_____ 2. Identify the purpose, indications, patient preparation, equipment, general procedure, and the positioning routines related to hysterosalpingography.

ORTHOROENTGENOGRAPHY

_____ 1. Define *orthoroentgenography* and the purpose of this procedure.

_____ 2. Identify the specific positioning and procedure for lower and upper limb orthoroentgenography.

MYELOGRAPHY

_____ 1. Identify the purpose, indications, contraindications, equipment, and general procedure related to myelography.

_____ 2. Identify positioning routines performed for lumbar, thoracic, and cervical myelography.

SIALOGRAPHY

_____ 1. Identify major aspects of the salivary glands

_____ 2. Identify the purpose, indications, patient preparation, equipment, general procedure, and the positioning routines related to sialography.

BONE DENSITOMETRY

_____   1.   Define and list the risk factors for osteoporosis.

_____   2.   Identify the types of bone densitometry methods available, and the advantages and disadvantages for each method.

_____   3.   Identify the purpose, indications, patient preparation, equipment, general procedure, and the positioning routines related to bone densitometry.

CONVENTIONAL TOMOGRAPHY

_____   1.   Define the specific terms associated with conventional tomography.

_____   2.   Identify the five basic types of trajectories for tube movement in conventional tomography.

_____   3.   Identify the controls and variables that are common features on conventional tomographic units.

_____   4.   Define the difference between a variable and a fixed fulcrum.

_____   5.   Identify the four controlling factors related to tomographic blur.

_____   6.   Describe briefly the two variations of conventional tomography, including autotomography (breathing technique) and pantomography (Panorex).

_____   7.   Demonstrate the principles and controlling factors of conventional tomography in laboratory exercises.

Learning Exercises

Complete the following review exercises after reading the associated pages in the textbook as indicated by each exercise. Answers to each review exercise are given at the end of the review exercises.

REVIEW EXERCISE A: Arthrography (see textbook pp. 726-730)

1.   What classifications of joints are studied with arthrography? _____

2.   Other than conventional radiography of synovial joints (e.g., arthrography), what other imaging procedure is preferred by physicians for studying synovial joints? _____

3.   List the three common forms of knee injury that require arthrography:

   A.   _____

   B.   _____

   C.   _____

4.   Give an example of nontraumatic pathology of the knee joint indicating arthrography. _____

5.   What are the contraindications for arthrography of any joint? _____

6.   True/False: An arthrogram must be approached as a sterile procedure; proper skin prep and sterility must be maintained.

7.   True/False: Once the contrast medium is introduced into the knee joint, the knee must *not* be flexed or exercised.

8. A. For a knee arthrogram, a _____ cc syringe is used with a _____ gauge needle to draw up _____ cc of positive contrast medial for injection.

    B. If dual contrast media is used, a _____ cc syringe is used to inject the negative contrast media.

9. List the two types of contrast media used for a knee arthrogram:

    A. _____

    B. _____

10. List the two projections for conventional "overhead" projections used for knee arthrography?

    A. _____

    B. _____

11. A. How much is the limb rotated between fluoroscopic spot films of the knee joint? _____

    B. How many exposures of each meniscus are generally taken with this method? _____

12. A. How many exposures are taken of each meniscus during horizontal beam arthrography of the knee?

        _____

    B. How many degrees of rotation of the leg between exposures? _____

13. What four aspects of shoulder anatomy are demonstrated with shoulder arthrography?

    A. _____   C. _____

    B. _____   D. _____

14. What is the general name for the conjoined tendons of the four major shoulder muscles? _____

15. What type of needle is commonly used for shoulder arthrograms? _____

16. A. For a single contrast study of the shoulder, how much positive contrast medium is commonly used?

        _____

    B. For a dual contrast study, _____ cc of positive contrast media and _____ cc of negative medium is used (e.g., room air).

17. List the five or six projections frequently taken during a shoulder arthrogram:

    A. _____   D. _____

    B. _____   E. _____

    C. _____   or F. _____

REVIEW EXERCISE B: Hysterosalpingography (see textbook pp. 731-733)

1. The hysterosalpingogram is a radiographic study of the _____ and _____ .

2. The uterus is situated between the _____ posteriorly and the

    _____ anteriorly.

3. List the four divisions of the uterus:

   A. _____

   B. _____

   C. _____

   D. _____

4. The largest division of the uterus is the _____ .

5. The distal aspect of the uterus extending to the vagina is the _____

6. List the three layers of tissue that form the uterus (from the innermost to the outermost layer):

   A. _____

   B. _____

   C. _____

7. Which of the following terms is not an aspect of the uterine tube?

   A. Cornu   C. Isthmus

   B. Ampulla   D. Infundibulum

8. True/False: Fertilization of the ovum occurs in the uterine tube.

9. True/False: The distal portion of the uterine tube opens into the peritoneal cavity.

10. Which of the following terms is used to describe the "degree of openness" of the uterine tube?

    A. Stenosis   C. Atresia

    B. Patency   D. Gauge

11. The most common indication for the hysterosalpingogram (HSG) is:

    _____

12. In addition to the answer for question 11, what are two additional pathologic indications for HSG?

    A. _____

    B. _____

13. List the three common types of lesions that can be demonstrated during a hysterosalpingogram:

    A. _____

    B. _____

    C. _____

14. The contrast medium preferred by most radiologists for a hysterosalpingogram is:

    A. Water-soluble, iodinated   C. Oxygen

    B. Oil-based, iodinated   D. Nitrogen

15. What device may be needed to aid the insertion and fixation of the cannula or catheter during the hysterosalpin-

    gogram? _____

16. To help facilitate the flow of contrast media into the uterine cavity, which position is the patient placed into follow-

    ing the injection of contrast media? _____

17. In addition to the supine position, what two other positions may be imaged to adequately visualize pertinent
    anatomy for an HSG?:

    A. _____

    B. _____

18. Where is the CR centered for overhead projections taken during a HSG using a 24 × 30 (10 × 12 in.) image receptor?

    A. At level of ASIS   C. Iliac crest

    B. Symphysis pubis   D. 2 in. (5 cm) superior to symphysis pubis

REVIEW EXERCISE C: Myelography (see textbook pp. 734-738)

1. Myelography is a radiographic study of the:

    A. _____

    B. _____

2. List the four common lesions or abnormalities (indications) demonstrated during myelography:

    A. _____   C. _____

    B. _____   D. _____

3. Of the four indications just mentioned, which is the most common for myelography?_____.

4. True/False: Myelography of the cervical and thoracic spine regions is most common.

5. List the four common contraindications for myelography:

    A. _____   C. _____

    B. _____   D. _____

6. What type of radiographic table must be used for myelography? _____

7. To reduce patient anxiety, a sedative is usually administered _____ hour(s) before the procedure.

8. Into what space is the contrast medium introduced with myelography? _____

9. List the two common puncture sites for contrast media injection during myelography:

    A. _____

    B. _____

10. Which one of the puncture sites from question 9 is preferred? _____

11. What is the patient's general body position(s) for the following punctures?

    A. Lumbar _____

    B. Cervical _____

12. Why is a large positioning block placed under the abdomen for a lumbar puncture in the prone position?

    _____

13. Which type of contrast medium is commonly used for myelography? _____

14. The contrast medium in question 13 will provide good radiopacity up to _____ after injection.

    A. 20 minutes   C. 1 hour

    B. 30 minutes   D. 8 hours

15. What dosage range of contrast medium is ideal for myelography?

    A. 8 to 10 cc   C. 6 to 17 cc

    B. 20 to 30 cc   D. Approximately 1 ml

16. Indicate the correct sequence of events for a myelogram by listing the following in order (1 through 8):

    _____ A. Introduce needle into subarachnoid space

    _____ B. Collect CSF and send to laboratory

    _____ C. Take conventional radiographic images

    _____ D. Explain the procedure to the patient

    _____ E. Introduce the contrast medium

    _____ F. Have patient sign informed consent form

    _____ G. Take fluoroscopic spot images

    _____ H. Prepare patient's skin for puncture

17. Which position is performed to demonstrate the region of C7 to T4 during a cervical myelogram?

    _____

18. Why should the patient's head and neck remain hyperextended during cervical myelography?

    _____

19. True/False: Generally, AP supine, PA prone, or horizontal beam lateral projections are not taken during thoracic spine myelography.

20. Complete the following for suggested basic routine projections (following fluoroscopy and spot-filming) for the different levels of the spine:

                                                      PROJECTION/POSITION   *LEVEL OF CR*

    1. Cervical region   A. _____

                                B. _____

    2. Thoracic region   A. _____

                                B. _____

                                C. _____

    3. Lumbar region   A. _____

21. True/False: Myelography is largely being replaced by MRI and CT.

REVIEW EXERCISE D: Sialography (see textbook pp. 739-741)

1. List the three pairs of salivary glands:

    A. _____

    B. _____

    C. _____

2. Which is the largest of the salivary glands? _____

3. Which is the smallest of the salivary glands? _____

4. List the two terms for the duct that carries saliva from the parotid gland to the oral cavity:

    A. _____

    B. _____

5. Which one of the following is not a correct term for the duct leading from the submandibular gland to the oral cavity?

    A. Wharton's duct   C. Submandibular duct

    B. Submaxillary duct   D. Bartholin's duct

6. The 12 small ducts leading form the sublingual glands to the oral cavity is/are called:

    A. Wharton's duct   C. Stenson's duct

    B. Duct of Rivinus   D. Accessory salivary ducts

7. What is the term for the center, vertical fold membrane located under the tongue? _____

8. Identify the salivary glands and associated structures labeled on Fig. 23-1:

   A. _____

   B. _____

   C. _____

   D. _____

   E. _____

   F. _____

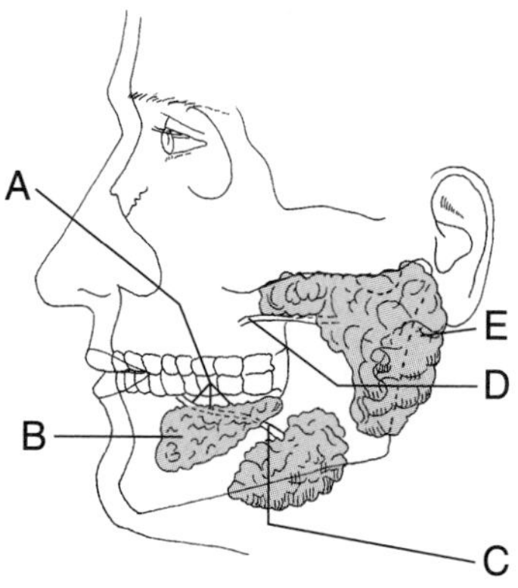

Fig. 23-1 Salivary glands and associated structures.

9. List the three most common pathologic indications that can lead to an obstruction of the salivary ductal system:

   A. _____

   B. _____

   C. _____

10. Sialectasia is:

    A. Dilation of the salivary duct   C. Inflammation of the salivary gland

    B. Stricture of the salivary duct   D. Inability to produce saliva

11. Why is the patient given a lemon slice to suck at the onset of the sialogram?

    _____

12. List the two devices used to cannulate a salivary duct once the duct is located.

    A. _____

    B. _____

13. If conventional tomography is used during a sialogram, _____ (oil-based or water-soluble) contrast media should be used.

14. If calculi in one of the salivary ducts are suspected, _____ contrast media should be used (oil-based or water-soluble).

15. On the average, how much contrast medium is injected to fill a salivary duct? _____

16. Which one of the following imaging modalities is not used during a sialogram?

    A. Conventional radiography   C. CT

    B. Sonography   D. Digital fluoroscopy

17. Which one of the following imaging positions is not performed during a sialogram?

    A. Superoinferior projection   C. AP/PA projection

    B. Lateral position   D. Lateral oblique position

REVIEW EXERCISE E: Orthoroentgenography (see textbook pp. 742-744)

1. Why is orthoroentgenography more commonly used in long bone measurements rather than CT?

    _____

2. What is the literal definition or meaning of the term *orthoroentgenogram*?

    _____

3. Why should separate projections be taken of limb joints rather than including the entire extremity on a single projection?

    _____

4. When performing an orthoroentgenographic procedure, what device needs to be placed on top of the table next to

    the affected limb? _____

5. What is the name of the surgical procedure that shortens a limb by fusing the epiphyses? _____

6. Which three joints are included on one image receptor for a long bone study of the lower limb?

    _____

7. True/False: Both right and left lower limbs can be placed on the same radiograph for a long bone study.

8. True/False: For a bilateral study, all three joints of both lower limbs can be placed on the same 35 × 43 cm (14 × 17 inch) IR.

9. If both lower limbs are radiographed together on one image receptor, why should two rulers be used with one under each limb rather than placing one midway between the two limbs?

    _____

10. True/False: For a long bone study of the upper limb, all three projections must be taken with the Bucky grid.

11. True/False: The wrist is examined in the pronated position (PA) for a long bone study of the upper limb.

12. True/False: The proximal humerus must be rotated internally for the shoulder projection taken during upper limb orthoroentgenography.

REVIEW EXERCISE F: Bone Densitometry (see textbook pp. 745-748)

1. Each year in the United States, approximately _____ million people have, or are at risk of developing, osteoporosis.

2. For osteoporosis to be visible radiographically, a loss of _____% to _____% of the trabecular bone must occur.

3. Cells responsible for new bone formation are called _____, and cells that help to break

    down old bone are _____ .

4. The purpose of bone densitometry is to _____ .

5. Central or axial analysis includes bone density measurements of the:

    A. _____

    B. _____

6. Peripheral site analysis includes bone density measurements of the fingers, wrist, _____ ,

    _____ , or _____ .

7. True/False: Osteoporosis leads to an increased risk of fractures

8. True/False: Loss of magnesium and phosphorus from the bony cortex is the primary cause of osteoporosis

9. True/False: Osteoporosis affects primarily pre-menopausal women.

10. True/False: Hormone therapy may retard the effects of osteoporosis

11. Place a check by each of the following that are **not** risk factors for osteoporosis as listed in the texbook:

    _____ A. Family history of osteoporosis

    _____ B. Excessive physical activity

    _____ C. Low sodium and niacin intake

    _____ D. Smoking

    _____ E. Low body weight

    _____ F. Alcohol consumption

    _____ G. High fat diet

    _____ H. Low calcium intake

    _____ I. Height greater than 6 feet (180 cm)

    _____ J. Previous fractures

12. True/False: Severe scoliosis or kyphosis may result in less accurate results for bone densitometry procedures.

13. True/False: Bone densitometry needs to be scheduled at least 1 week following an iodinated contrast media or radionuclide procedure.

14. List the three most common types of bone densitometry equipment, methods, and techniques in current use:

    A. _____

    B. _____

    C. _____

15. Which one of the following bone densitometry techniques and equipment methods uses a dual-energy, fan-beam x-ray source?

    A. Radioabsorptiometry (RA)   C. (Dual-energy x-ray absorptiometry (DXA)

    B. Dual-energy photon absorptiometry   D. Quantitative computed (DPA) tomography (QCT)

16. Z-score obtained with the DXA system compares the patient to:

    A. Young, healthy individual with peak bone mass   C. Patient with moderate osteoporosis

    B. Patient with severe osteoporosis   D. Average individual of the same age and gender

17. True/False: Patient dose with the DXA system ranges between 1 to 30 microSieverts.

18. Quantitative computed tomography (QCT) provides bone mineral density measurements of

    _____ and _____ bone.

19. The anatomical site most commonly evaluated with quantitative ultrasound (QUS) is _____ .

20. True/False: DXA of the hip requires the lower limb to be rotated 15 to 20° internally.

21. The "T" score compares the patient's bone density to: _____ .

22. Which of the following is the method of choice for evaluating both trabecular and cortical bone?

    A. Quantitative computed tomography (QCT)

    B. Dual-energy x-ray absorptiometry (DXA)

    C. Quantitative ultrasound (QUS)

    D. Dual-energy photon absorptiometry

23. Which of the methods from question 22 provides a true three-dimensional or volumetric analysis?

    _____

REVIEW EXERCISE G: Conventional Tomography (see textbook pp. 749-754)

1. Define each of the following terms. (Give short, concise answers.)

    A. Tomograph _____

    B. Fulcrum _____

    C. Fulcrum level _____

    D. Objective (focal) plane _____

    E. Sectional thickness _____

    F. Exposure angle _____

    G. Tube movement (shift) _____

    H. Amplitude _____

    I. Tube trajectory _____

    J. Blur _____

    K. Blur margin _____

2. Identify the correct term for the five tube movement trajectories in Fig. 23-2:

   A. _____

   B. _____

   C. _____

   D. _____

   E. _____

3. Which of the tube trajectories from the previous question are multidirectional? Which are unidirectional? (indicate by letter)

   1. Multidirectional _____

   2. Unidirectional _____

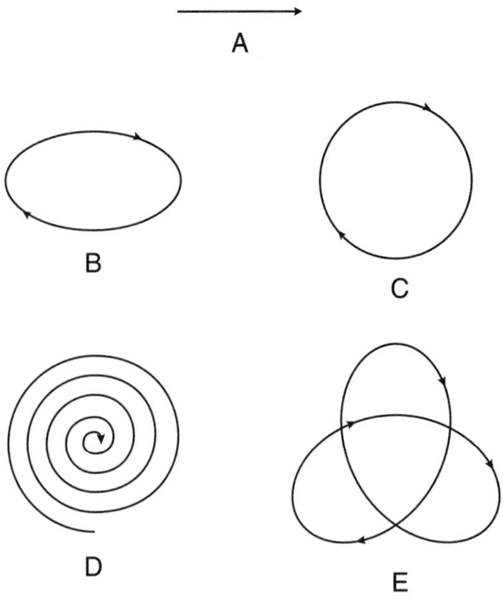

Fig. 23-2 Tube movement trajectories.

4. Which two of these tube trajectories are considered the most complex?

   _____

5. List the five common adjustments or settings found on the tomographic control panel:

   A. _____

   B. _____

   C. _____

   D. _____

   E. _____

6. True/False: Objects closer to the objective plane will experience maximum blurring.

7. True/False: The fixed-type fulcrum (rather than the variable type) is most commonly used with multidirectional specialized tomographic equipment.

8. Which one of the methods from the previous question (fixed or variable type) will alter the fulcrum by moving the

   patient and tabletop up or down? _____

9. Briefly describe the tomographic blurring principle. (Why, or how, does blurring of some objects occur while others remain in sharp focus?)

   _____

   _____

10. Describe the method of determining focal level settings and centering when beginning a tomographic procedure:

   _____

   _____

11. List the four factors that determine the amount of blurring:

    A. _____

    B. _____

    C. _____

    D. _____

12. True/False: As the exposure angle decreases, slice thickness also decreases (becomes thinner).

13. True/False: As the distance from the image receptor increases, object blurring will increase.

14. To explain how variations in tube trajectories or movement patterns influence the amount of blurring, complete the following (study the various tube trajectories of Fig. 23-2 as you answer these questions):

    A. Maximum blurring occurs when objects are _____ (parallel or perpendicular) to the direction of tube movement.

    B. A circular movement pattern will create _____ (more or less) blurring than an elliptical pattern.

    C. The elliptical pattern has more objects nearer _____ (parallel or perpendicular) to the line of tube travel than the circular pattern.

    D. Maximum blurring occurs with spiral and hypocycloidal tube patterns because they include a

       _____ dimension as part of their movement.

15. Multidirectional tube trajectories are needed for visualizing small anatomical structures of _____ or less.

16. Which type of tomographic equipment demonstrates the following satisfactorily:

    _____ 1. Lung tumor   A. Linear tomogram only

    _____ 2. Nephrotomogram   B. Multidirectional or multitiered capabilities

    _____ 3. Sella turcica

    _____ 4. TMJs

    _____ 5. Middle ear structures

    _____ 6. Biliary ducts (ERCP)

17. True/False: The human eye accepts a certain degree of blurring as normal, making the actual amount of blurring somewhat subjective.

18. A tomographic principle in which the anatomical structure moves but the image receptor/tube remain stationary is

    called _____. (Hint: It is used in certain lateral spine and sternum projections to blur out

    overlying structures)

19. What is the most common application for pantotomography? _____

20. What device minimizes penumbra blurring during a pantotomographic procedure? _____

Laboratory Exercises

The following exercises are for two procedures for which supplies and equipment are most commonly available to students.

EXERCISE A.   ORTHOROENTGENOGRAPHY-LONG BONE MEASUREMENT (see textbook pp. 742-744)

1.   Using an upper and lower limb radiographic phantom (if available), produce long bone measurement radiographs of the following:

_____   Unilateral lower limb (AP projection of hip, knee, and ankle on one image receptor with a correctly placed Bell-Thompson ruler)

_____   Bilateral lower limbs (AP projections of hips, knees, and ankles on one image receptor with correctly placed Bell-Thompson rulers)

_____   Unilateral upper limb (AP projections of shoulder, elbow, and wrist on one image receptor with correctly placed ruler)

EXERCISE B.   CONVENTIONAL TOMOGRAPHY (see textbook pp. 749-754)

This part of the learning exercise needs to be carried out in an energized radiographic room equipped with at least a linear type tomographic unit. The use of multidirectional and/or multitiered tomographic units is optional. Check the following steps when they are completed:

_____   **Step 1**   **Equipment setup:** Set up the necessary tomographic equipment, including the adjustable fulcrum level attachment connected to the tube and to the Bucky.   Ensure that the Bucky tray locks are released (as well as the tube angle and tube distance locks), allowing the tube and Bucky tray to move freely.

_____   **Step 2**   **Preparation of "phantom" for experiments:** Design a series of experiments to demonstrate the tomographic blurring principle and the effect of the four controlling and influencing factors on blurring.

   Commercial tomographic phantoms are available with various lead numbers or other metallic devices placed at specific levels within the phantom.   If these are not readily available, one can easily be made with paper clips in combination with a wire mesh or other flat metallic objects placed in horizontal layers in three different books, or in three different layers within the same book. The shape or the configuration of the metallic objects can be varied in each layer so that the various levels can be differentiated on the radiograph.

_____   **Step 3**   **Determine exposure factors:** Determine approximate exposure factors to visualize the metallic objects as placed in the books and stacked on the x-ray table.   Start with an approximate upper limb exposure technique. Make a test exposure. Set the factors on the control panel of the tomographic unit as needed.

OPTIONAL EXPERIMENTS TO DEMONSTRATE TOMOGRAPHIC PRINCIPLES AND VARIABLES:

Using your knowledge and understanding of tomographic blurring principles as studied in this chapter, design and carry out exercises as needed to demonstrate the following:

Experiment A: Orientation of Body Part to Tube Travel Demonstrate that those objects parallel to the direction of tube movement create "streaks" and are not as effectively blurred as when they are perpendicular to the tube movement.   This can be readily shown by changing the longitudinal direction of the metallic objects (e.g., paper clips) so the levels above and below the focal plane will be at some angle or completely perpendicular to the direction of the tube travel. This should demonstrate increased blurring of the objects above and below the focal plane.

Experiment B: Influencing and Controlling Factors for Tomographic Blurring Design experiments to demonstrate how each of the following four factors or variables influence or control the amount of blurring. On these types of experiments, remember to change only one factor at a time, keeping all other factors constant.

_____   **Factor 1   Object-focal plane distance**

   Demonstrate that those objects farther from the focal plane have greater movement on the image receptor and therefore increased blurring as compared with those closer to the focal plane.

This can be done by first taking tomographs with the objects above and below those in the focal plane. Compare these with tomographs taken when the objects above and below are placed at increased distances from the focal plane. You should be able to demonstrate markedly increased blurring on the second set of tomographs.

_____ **Factor 2   Exposure angle**

By changing the exposure angle, demonstrate that an increase in exposure angle with greater tube travel will increase the blurring, resulting in a thinner focal plane. Likewise, a decrease in exposure angle with less tube travel will decrease the movement of the objects above and below the focal plane, creating less blurring and a thicker section remaining in focus.

Remember that the amplitude or speed of tube movement must also increase as the exposure angle is increased so that the exposure continues throughout the full arc of tube travel.

_____ **Factor 3   Object-image receptor (IR) distance**

Demonstrate that as the distance of the objects from the IR is increased, greater blurring will occur.

Sponge blocks can be placed between objects (e.g., books or phantom) and the table to increase the object-IR distance. (This will demonstrate why the upside or side away from the IR on a tomogram of a lateral TMJ or of a lateral of inner ear structures should be examined rather than the downside.)

Optional

_____ **Factor 4   Tube trajectory** (if equipment is available)

This can be done only if equipment is available that has multidirectional and/or multitiered trajectory possibilities.

By changing to a circular or elliptical movement, demonstrate that increased blurring and a thinner focal plane can be achieved as compared with only linear tube movement.

Demonstrate that maximum blurring occurs with the multidirectional, multitiered (spiral and hypocycloidal) trajectories, even when the distance between the objects above and below the focal plane is very small. This should demonstrate that blurring of objects even as close as 1 mm to the focal plane can be achieved.

Answers to Review Exercises

Review Exercise A: Arthrography

1. Synovial joints
2. Magnetic resonance imaging (MRI)
3. A. Tears of the joint capsule
   B. Tears of the menisci
   C. Tears of ligaments
4. Baker's cyst
5. Allergic reactions to iodine-based contrast media, or to local anesthetics
6. True
7. False (needs to be flexed to distribute contrast media)
8. A. 10, 20, 5
   B. 50
9. A. Positive or radiopaque media such as iodinated, water-soluble contrast agent
   B. Negative or radiolucent contrast agents such as room air, oxygen, or carbon dioxide
10. A. AP
    B. Lateral
11. A. 20°
    B. 9
12. A. 6 (six views per meniscus)
    B. 30°
13. A. Joint capsule
    B. Rotator cuff
    C. Long tendon of biceps muscle
    D. Articular cartilage
14. Rotator cuff
15. 2½ to 3½ in. spinal needle
16. A. 10 to 12 cc
    B. 3 to 4, 10 to 12
17. A. AP scout
    B. AP internal rotation
    C. AP external rotation
    D. Glenoid fossa (Grashey) projection
    E. Transaxillary (inferosuperior axial) projection
    F. Bicipital (intertubercular) groove projection

Review Exercise B: Hysterosalpingography

1. Uterus
   Uterine tubes
2. Rectosigmoid colon
   Urinary bladder
3. A. Fundus
   B. Corpus (body)
   C. Isthmus
   D. Cervix
4. Corpus or body
5. Cervix
6. A. Endometrium
   B. Myometrium
   C. Serosa

7. A. Cornu
8. True
9. True
10. B. Patency
11. Assessment of female infertility
12. A. Demonstrate intrauterine pathology
    B. Evaluation of the uterine tubes following tubal ligation in reconstructive surgery
13. A. Endometrial polyps
    B. Uterine fibroids
    C. Intrauterine adhesions
14. A. Water-soluble, iodinated
15. Tenaculum
16. Slight Trendelenburg
17. A. LPO
    B. RPO
18. D. 2 in. (5 cm) superior to symphysis pubis

Review Exercise C: Myelography

1. A. Spinal cord
   B. Nerve root branches
2. A. Herniated nucleus pulposus (HNP)
   B. Cancerous or benign tumors
   C. Cysts
   D. Possible bone fragments
3. Herniated nucleus pulposus (HNP)
4. False (most common are cervical and lumbar regions)
5. A. Blood in the cerebrospinal fluid
   B. Arachnoiditis
   C. Increased intracranial pressure
   D. Recent lumbar puncture (within 2 weeks)
6. 90/15° tilting table
7. One (1)
8. Into the subarachnoid space (of spinal canal)
9. A. Lumbar (L3-4)
   B. Cervical (C1-2)
10. Lumbar (L3-4)
11. A. Prone or left lateral
    B. Erect or prone
12. For spinal flexion to widen the interspinous spaces to facilitate needle placement
13. Nonionic water-soluble iodine based
14. C. 1 hour
15. C. 6 to 17 cc
16. A. 4, B. 5, C. 8, D. 1, E. 6, F. 2, G. 7, H. 3
17. Swimmer's lateral using a horizontal x-ray beam
18. To keep the contrast media from entering the cranial subarachnoid space
19. True (right and left lateral decubitus positions are taken)

20. 1. A. Horizontal beam lateral (prone), C5
       B. Horizontal beam lateral (swimmers), C7
    2. A. R lateral decubitus (AP or PA), T7
       B. L lateral decubitus (AP or PA), T7
       C. R or L lateral, vertical beam, T7
    3. A. Semi-erect horizontal beam lateral (prone), L3

20. True

Review Exercise D: Sialography

1. A. Parotid glands
   B. Submandibular glands
   C. Sublingual glands
2. Parotid gland
3. Sublingual glands
4. A. Parotid duct
   B. Stensen's duct
5. D. Bartholin's duct
6. B. Ducts of Rivinus
7. Frenulum
8. A. Ducts of Rivinus (Bartholin's ducts)
   B. Sublingual gland
   C. Submandibular duct (Wharton's duct)
   D. Submandibular gland (submaxillary gland)
   E. Parotid duct (Stenson's duct)
   F. Parotid gland
9. A. Calculi
   B. Strictures
   C. Tumors
10. A. Dilation of the salivary duct
11. To cause the patient to express saliva and help locate the opening of a particular duct
12. A. Butterfly needle
    B. Sialography catheter
13. Oil-based
14. Water-soluble
15. 1 to 2 ml
16. B. Sonography
17. A. Superoinferior projection

Review Exercise E: Orthoroetgenography

1. CT is more costly and requires specialized equipment.
2. A straight or right angle radiograph
3. To prevent elongation of the limb due to the divergence of the x-ray beam
4. A special metallic (Bell-Thompson) ruler to measure bone length from one joint to another
5. Epiphysiodeses
6. Hip, knee, and ankle

7. True
8. True
9. A single center-placed ruler makes it difficult or impossible to shield the gonads without obscuring the upper part of the ruler.
10. True
11. False (PA would cross radius and ulna)
12. False (The proximal humerus is rotated into an external rotation position)

13. Review Exercise F: Bone Densitometry

1. 28
2. 30% to 50%
3. Osteoblasts, osteoclasts
4. Evaluate bone mineral density
5. A. Lumbar spine
   B. Proximal femur
6. Forearm, heel, or lower leg
7. True
8. False (loss of calcium and collagen)
9. False (post-menopausal)
10. True
11. B, C, G, I
12. True
13. True
14. A. Dual-energy x-ray absorptiometry (DXA)
    B. Quantitative computed tomography (QCT)
    C. Quantitative ultrasound (QUS)
15. C. Dual-energy x-ray absorptiometry (DXA)
16. D. Average individual of the same age and gender
17. True
18. Trabecular, cortical
19. Os calcis (heel)
20. True

21. An average healthy individual with peak bone mass
22. A. Quantitative computed tomography (QCT)
23. A. QCT

Review Exercise G: Conventional Tomography

1. A. The radiograph produced during a tomographic procedure
   B. The pivot point of the connecting rod between tube and film holder
   C. The distance from table top to fulcrum
   D. The plane or section of the object that is clear and in focus
   E. The thickness of the objective plane
   F. The angle resulting from the x-ray tube beam movement
   G. The distance the tube travels
   H. The speed the tube travels in inches per second or cm per second
   I. The geometric configuration or pattern of tube travel
   J. The area of distortion of objects outside the objective plane
   K. The outer edges of the blurred object
2. A. Linear
   B. Elliptical
   C. Circular
   D. Spiral
   E. Hypocycloidal
3. 1. B, C, D, E
   2. A
   4. D (spiral) and E (hypocycloidal)
   5. A. Tube travel speed
      B. Objective plane

C. Direction or type of tube trajectory (for units that are multidirectional)
D. Tube center
E. Fulcrum level
6. False (objects away from objective plane have greatest blurring)
7. True
8. Fixed fulcrum type
9. Objects farther from the fulcrum level or objective plane will be blurred by the movement of the tube and film. Objects closer to this fulcrum level and those that are parallel to tube travel will remain almost stationary and experience little or no blurring.
10. Two 90° conventional radiographs are generally taken to determine depth and centering of the object of interest
11. A. Distance the object is from the objective plane
    B. Exposure angle
    C. Distance the object is from the film
    D. Tube trajectory
12. False (increases)
13. True
14. A. Perpendicular
    B. More
    C. Parallel
    D. Vertical or multitiered
15. 1 mm
16. 1. A, 2. A, 3. B, 4. B, 5. B, 6. A
17. True
18. Autotomography or breathing technique
19. Mandible studies
20. Slit beam restrictor or diaphragm

SELF-TEST

This self-test should be taken only after completing **all** the readings, review exercises, and laboratory activities for a particular section. The purpose of this test is not only to provide a good learning exercise but also to serve as a good indicator of what your final evaluation grade will be. It is strongly suggested that if you do not get at least a 90% to 95% grade on this self-test, you should review those areas in which you missed questions **before** going to your instructor for the final evaluation exam for this chapter. (There are 83 questions or blanks—each is worth 1.2 points.)

1. The formal term for a radiographic long bone measurement study is _____ .

2. True/False: To properly measure the length of a long bone, the entire lower limb should be included on a single projection.

3. True/False: Epiphysiodeses is an operation to lengthen bone by widening the epiphyseal plate.

4. True/False: Movement of the body part between exposures will compromise the long bone study.

5. True/False: If a long bone study of both lower limbs is ordered, the use of two metal rulers is recommended with both limbs exposed at the same time on the same image receptor.

6. What is the proper name for the special metal ruler used for long bone measurement? _____

7. What size of image receptor and how may exposures are recommended for a long bone study of the upper limbs for

   an adult? _____

8. List the two synovial-type joints most commonly examined with an arthrogram.

   A. _____   B. _____

9. List the two contraindications for an arthrogram:

   A. _____   B. _____

10. An indication of a possible "Baker's cyst" would suggest the need for an arthrogram procedure for the

    _____ .

11. List the two types and the amounts of contrast media commonly used for a knee arthrogram:

	TYPE	*AMOUNT*
A.	_____	_____
B.	_____	_____

12. What size needle is used to introduce the contrast media during a knee arthrogram? _____

13. What is the purpose of flexing the knee gently after the contrast media has been injected for an arthrogram procedure?

    _____

14. What size image receptor is recommended for horizontal beam arthrogram projections?

    _____

15. How many exposures are made, and how much is the leg rotated, between each exposure for horizontal beam knee arthrograms?

    A. Number of exposures: _____

    B. Degrees of rotation between exposures: _____

16. The term *rotator cuff* refers to what structures of the shoulder? _____

17. List the overhead projections that may be requested for a shoulder arthrogram:

Scout

    A. _____

Post Injection

    B. _____

    C. _____

    D. _____

    E. _____

    F. _____

18. List the three common lesions or conditions diagnosed through a myelogram:

    A. _____   C. _____

    B. _____

19. List the four common contraindications for a myelogram:

    A. _____   C. _____

    B. _____   D. _____

20. The most common clinical indication for a myelogram is:

    A. Benign tumors   C. HNP

    B. Spinal cysts   D. Bony injury to the spine

21. Which position will move the contrast media column from the lumbar to the cervical region during a myelogram?

    A. Fowler's   C. Trendelenburg

    B. Left lateral decubitus   D. Prone

22. What is the most common spinal puncture site for a lumbar myelogram?

    A. L3-4   C. L4-5

    B. L1-2   D. L5 -S1

24. A cervical puncture is indicated for an upper spinal region myelogram if:

    A. The patient has severe lordosis   C. The patient has HNP of the L4-5 level

    B. The patient has mild scoliosis   D. The patient has complete blockage at T-spine level

25. The absorption of the water-soluble contrast media into the vascular system of the body begins approximately _____ minutes after injection and is totally undetectable radiographically after _____ hours.

26. Which position is performed during a cervical myelogram to demonstrate the C7-T1 region?

    _____

27. Another term for tomography is _____ .

28. Match the following tomographic terms with the correct definition:

    _____ 1. Objective plane   A. The area of distortion

    _____ 2. Exposure angle   B. The speed of tube travel

    _____ 3. Tomograph   C. Radiograph produced by a tomographic unit

    _____ 4. Blur   D. The plane where the object is clear

    _____ 5. Fulcrum   E. The pivot point between tube and image receptor

    _____ 6. Amplitude   F. The factor that determines slice thickness

29. Match the following tube trajectories: (Fig. 23-3)

    _____ 1. Spiral

    _____ 2. Elliptical

    _____ 3. Circular

    _____ 4. Hypocycloidal

    _____ 5. Linear

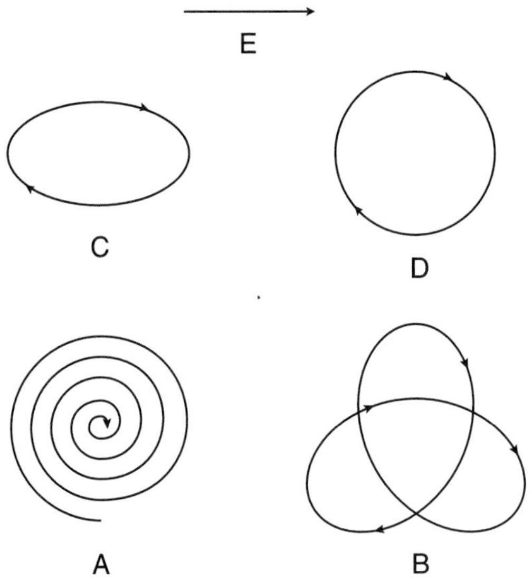

Fig. 23-3 Tube movement trajectories.

30. List the two methods of adjusting the fulcrum level:

    A. _____   B. _____

31. True/False: Maximum blurring of an object will be achieved when it is perpendicular to tube travel.

32. True/False: The primary factor affecting the sectional thickness as controlled by the operator is the type of tube trajectory.

33. True/False: Increased blurring occurs when the object is farther from the image receptor.

34. True/False: In pantomography, the image receptor and tube move with the patient stationary similar to conventional tomography.

35. True/False: Amplitude does not influence or control the amount of blurring.

36. Which one of the following exposure times would be suitable for breathing technique (autotomography)?

    A. 2 to 3 seconds   C. ½ second

    B. 1 second   D. 10 milliseconds

37. List the four divisions of the uterus:

    A. _____

    B. _____

    C. _____

    D. _____

38. Which of the following is *not* a tissue layer of the uterus?

    A. Osseometrium   C. Endometrium

    B. Myometrium   D. Serosa

39. True/False: The uterine tubes are connected directly to the ovaries.

40. List the two contraindications for a hysterosalpingogram:

    A. _____

    B. _____

41. True/False: Oil-based contrast medium is preferred for the majority of hysterosalpingograms.

42. True/False: Hysterosalpingography can be a therapeutic tool in correcting certain obstructions in the uterine tube.

43. Match the following salivary ducts to the correct salivary gland:

    _____ A. Parotid gland   1. Ducts of Rivinus

    _____ B. Submandibular gland   2. Stenson's duct

    _____ C. Sublingual gland   3. Wharton's duct

44. Sialography is contraindicated for:

    A. Possible obstruction of the salivary duct   C. Salivary duct fistula

    B. Severe inflammation of the salivary gland or duct D. Calculi lodged in salivary duct

45. What type of contrast media should be used for the majority of sialograms? _____

46. Which of the following is *not* a risk factor for osteoporosis:

    A. Excessive physical activity   C. Low body weight

    B. Alcohol consumption   D. Low calcium intake

47. Newer dual-energy x-ray absorptiometry (DXA) uses:

    A. Fan-beam x-ray source   C. Pencil-thin x-ray source

    B. Positron-emission source   D. Super voltage x-ray source

48. A T-score obtained with the DXA system compares the patient to a(n):

    A. Average patient of the same age and gender   C. Patient with moderate osteoporosis

    B. Healthy individual with peak bone mass   D. Patient with severe osteoporosis

49. The two negatives with quantitative computed tomography (QCT) are:

    A. _____

    B. _____

50. The area that is most commonly scanned with quantitative ultrasound (QUS) is the _____ .

CHAPTER 24

Additional Diagnostic and Therapeutic Modalities

This chapter introduces select alternative diagnostic and therapeutic imaging modalities, including nuclear medicine, radiation oncology, diagnostic ultrasound, and resonance imaging. The information and review exercises contained in Chapter 24 are intended to introduce students to basic concepts related to each of these modalities. Basic definitions, physical principles, clinical applications, and technologist responsibilities will be covered.

A more extensive presentation is provided in the magnetic resonance imaging (MRI) section, which introduces MRI terminology and the basics of MRI physics and instrumentation. The important clinical aspects related to personnel and patient safety are discussed. An introduction to the imaging parameters that affect the quality of the images and clinical applications of MRI is included. Although portions of the chapter may appear complex and will require careful study, the authors have provided a thorough introduction to understanding this exciting and rapidly developing field.

CHAPTER OBJECTIVES

After you have completed **all** the activities of this chapter, you will be able to:

_____ 1. Identify basic operating principles related to nuclear medicine imaging.

_____ 2. List the purpose, radionuclide used, and pathologic indications demonstrated with select nuclear medicine procedures.

_____ 3. List specific responsibilities for members of the nuclear medicine team.

_____ 4. Distinguish between internal and external types of radiation therapy.

_____ 5. Identify the energy level, characteristics, and advantages of the major types of radiation therapy units.

_____ 6. List the specific responsibilities of radiation oncology team members.

_____ 7. Identify basic operating principles related to ultrasound.

_____ 8. List the characteristics, advantages, and disadvantages of specific types of ultrasound systems.

_____ 7. List the purpose, transducer used, and pathologic indications demonstrated with select ultrasound procedures.

_____ 8. Explain how MRI produces an image.

_____ 9. Compare the process of MRI image production with that of other imaging modalities.

_____ 10. Explain how a signal is generated and received from body tissues.

_____ 11. Explain how contrast is produced in the MR image.

_____ 12. Identify specific MRI system components.

_____ 13. Identify basic MRI safety considerations.

_____ 14. Identify information to be included when preparing a patient for an MRI exam.

_____ 15. Identify the type of contrast agent used in MRI.

_____ 16. Identify the different types of RF coils.

_____ 17. State the appearance of specific tissue types on both T1- and T2-weighted images.

_____ 18. Define the terms and pathologic indications related to MRI.

Learning Exercises

Complete the following review exercises after reading the associated pages in the textbook as indicated by each exercise. Answers to each review exercise are given at the end of the review exercises.

REVIEW EXERCISE A: Nuclear Medicine (see textbook pp. 756-757)

1. Nuclear medicine uses radioactive materials called _____ in the study and treatment of various medical conditions.

2. Radioactive materials that are introduced into the body and concentrate in specific organs are called

    _____

3. How are the materials identified in question 2 introduced into the body?

    A. Inhalation   C. Injection

    B. Orally   D. All of the above

4. One of the most common radioactive materials used in nuclear medicine procedures is:

    A. Sulfur colloid   C. Technetium 99m

    B. Iodine 131   D. Thallium

5. The term *SPECT* is an abbreviation for _____.

6. The SPECT camera provides a _____ -dimensional view of the anatomy.

7. A study of the skeletal system using radioactive materials is called: _____.

8. A common genitourinary nuclear medicine study is performed for:

    A. Kidney transplants   C. Pyelonephritis

    B. Renal cyst   D. All of the above

9. Nuclear medicine is considered the ideal modality for diagnosing _____ of the gastrointestinal tract.

    A. Peptic ulcers   C. Gastroesophageal reflux

    B. Meckel's diverticulum   D. Colitis

10. Which one of the following radiopharmaceutical is used during myocardial perfusion studies?

    A. Technetium 99m   C. Iodine 131

    B. Thallium   D. Neo Tect

11. Which one of the following radiopharmaceuticals is used to determine if a pulmonary lesion is benign or malignant?

    A. Technetium 99m   C. Iodine 131

    B. Thallium   D. Neo Tect

12. Match the following responsibilities to the correct nuclear medicine team member:

_____ A. Properly disposes contaminated materials   1. Nuclear medicine technologist

_____ B. Calibrates nuclear medicine imaging equipment   2. Nuclear medicine physician

_____ C. Performs statistical analysis of study data   3. Medical nuclear physicist

_____ D. Administers radionuclide to patient

_____ E. Interprets procedure

_____ F. Often serves as department radiation safety officer

_____ G. Licensed to acquire and use radioactive materials

_____ H. Prepares radioactive materials

_____ I. Digitally processes the images

REVIEW EXERCISE B: Radiation Oncology (see textbook p. 758)

1. Cancer is second only to _____ as the leading cause of death in the United States and Canada.

2. Identify the two types of radiation therapy treatment:

    A. _____

    B. _____

3. Prostate cancer is a common candidate for which of the two types of radiation therapy treatment from question 2?

    _____

4. List the three sources of external beam radiation:

    A. _____

    B. _____

    C. _____

5. Cobalt-60 units emit gamma rays at the intensity of _____ MeV.
    A. 1.25   C. 10.4
    B. 5.25   D. 15.25

6. What is the source of the high energy x-rays produced with a linear accelerator therapy unit?
    A. Cobalt-60   C. Uranium 235
    B. High-speed neutrons striking an anode   D. High-speed electrons striking an anode

7. Which of the following is most effective for the treatment of shallow or superficial cancerous tissue?
    A. Cobalt-60   C. High voltage x-ray type unit
    B. Linear accelerator   D. Internal, brachytherapy type

8. Linear accelerators produce energy levels between _____ and _____ MeV.

    A. 1 to 2   C. 4 to 30

    B. 3 to 5   D. 30 to 50

9. What is the purpose of radiation therapy simulation?

    _____

10. Match the following responsibilities to the correct radiation oncology team member:

    _____ A. Outlines plan to deliver the desired dosage   1. Radiation therapist

    _____ B. Administers radiation treatments   2. Radiation oncologist

    _____ C. May use fluoroscopy to determine treatment fields   3. Medical dosimetrist

    _____ D. Calibrates equipment   4. Medical health physicist

    _____ E. Prescribes treatment plan

    _____ F. Advises oncologists on dosage calculations

    _____ G. Maintains treatment records

REVIEW EXERCISE C: Ultrasound (see textbook pp 759-762)

1. List three additional terms for ultrasound:

    A. _____

    B. _____

    C. _____

2. Medical ultrasound uses high frequency sound waves in the range between _____ to _____ MHz .

3. True/False: Ultrasound is an ideal imaging modality for diagnosing an ileus.

4. True/False: Ultrasound is often used to locate a bone cyst in the femur.

5. True/False: Research studies conclude that there are no adverse biologic effects associated with the use of medical ultrasound.

6. True/False: The first A-mode ultrasound unit was built in Germany in the late 1950s.

7. Which generation of ultrasound unit introduced two-dimensional gray scale?

    A. A-mode   C. Real time dynamic

    B. B-mode   D. Doppler

8. Which type of ultrasound unit is used to examine the structure and behavior of flowing blood?

    A. A-mode   C. Real time dynamic

    B. B-mode   D. Doppler

9. What major improvement is offered by the new high-definition digital ultrasound systems?

   A. Smaller size unit   C. Increase in dynamic range

   B. Can alter between A-mode and B-mode   D. Introduction of gray scale

10. What is the fundamental purpose or function of the transducer?

    _____

11. What type of material comprises the functional aspect of the transducer, which creates the high-frequency sound waves?

    A. Tungsten alloy   C. Silver/chromium alloy

    B. Ceramic   D. Ferrous alloy

12. What physical principle is applied when the transducer produces a sound wave?

    A. Piezoelectric effect   C. Thermionic emission

    B. Modulation transfer   D. Larmor effect

13. Match the correct frequency transducer to the following procedures and/or situations:

    _____ A. For an average or small abdomen   1. 3.5 MHz

    _____ B. For a larger abdomen   2. 5.0 to 7.0 MHz

    _____ C. For a study of a superficial structure   3. 17 MHz

14. True/False: A transducer serves as both a transmitter and receiver of echoes.

15. True/False: A sonographer must provide initial interpretation of the ultrasound images.

16. Ultrasound is the "gold standard" for studies of the following structures except the:

    A. Liver   C. Gallbladder

    B. Stomach   D. Uterus

17. What is the name of the ultrasound procedure in which amniotic fluid is withdrawn from the uterus for genetic analysis?

    _____

18. Ultrasound is very effective in evaluating the fetus before birth for early indications of:

    A. Heart defects   C. Spina bifida

    B. Hydrocephaly   D. All of the above

19. What is the advantage of using ultrasound for studies of the musculoskeletal system over MRI?

    A. Less expensive   C. Provides a functional study of joint movement

    B. Noninvasive   D. All of the above

20. Match the following sonographic terms to the correct definition:

_____ A. An image that possesses both width and height

1. Anechoic

_____ B. Alteration in frequency or wavelength reflected by moving objects

2. Backscatter

_____ C. Acoustic energy that travels through a medium

3. Doppler effect

_____ D. An anatomical object that does not produce any echoes

4. Echogenic

_____ E. Ultrasound images that demonstrate dynamic motion

5. Hyperechoic

_____ F. An anatomical object that produces more echoes than normal

6. Hypoechoic

_____ G. Acoustic energy reflected from a structure that interferes with the expected path of the acoustic wave

7. Real time imaging

_____ H. An anatomical structure that possesses echo-producing structures

8. Two-dimensional image

_____ I. An aspect of acoustic energy reflected back toward the source or origin

9. Wave

_____ J. An anatomical object that produces fewer echoes than normal

10. Reflection

REVIEW EXERCISE D: Physical Principles of MRI (see textbook pp. 763-768)

1. MRI uses _____ and _____ to obtain a mathematically reconstructed image.

2. The MRI image represents differences in the tissues of the patient in the number of _____ and the rate at which they recover from radiofrequency stimulation.

3. To compare the energy of x-rays and MRI radio waves and the relative effect on irradiated tissue, complete the following:

		WAVELENGTH	FREQUENCY	ENERGY
1.	Typical x-rays	A. 10^{-9}cm	B. 10^{19} cycles/sec.	C. 60,000 electron volts
2.	MRI radio waves	A. _____	B. _____	C. _____

4. A. Which nucleus is most suitable for MR? _____

   B. Why? _____

5. Which component of the nucleus is affected by radio waves and static magnetic fields?

_____

6. A typical cubic centimeter of the human body may contain approximately how many _____ hydrogen atoms?

   A. 1000   C. 10^{10}

   B. 10,000   D. 10^{20}

7. Define and briefly describe the term *precession*. (Compare this with some well-known phenomenon.)

_____

8. The rate of precession of a proton in a magnetic field _____ (increases or decreases) as the strength of the magnetic field increases.

9. Precession occurs due to _____ acting on a spinning nuclei.

10. The angle of precession of protons can be altered by the introduction of _____ .

11. How does an increase in the length of applicaton time of the radio wave affect the angle of precession?

   _____

12. Timing of the radio wave to the rate of the precessing nuclei is an example of the concept of

   _____ .

13. The signal that is received by the antenna or the receiving coil comes from which part of the atoms in the body tissues?

   _____

14. The nucleus emits _____ waves because it is a tiny magnet that is also

   _____ .

15. Relaxation of the nuclei as soon as the radiofrequency pulse is turned off can be divided into two categories:

   _____ and _____ .

16. T1 relaxation is known as _____ or *spin-lattice relaxation.* (Hint: Transverse or longitudinal)

17. T2 relaxation is known as _____ or spin-spin relaxation.   (Hint: Transverse or longitudinal)

18. The quantity of hydrogen nuclei per given volume of tissue is referred to as the _____ ,

   which is a _____ (major or minor) contributor to the appearance of the MR image.

19. Describe the main purpose of the gradient magnetic fields (the magnetic field strengths through only specific regions or slices of body tissue).

   _____

20. What are three primary factors that determine the signal strength and therefore the brightness of an image?

   _____

   _____

   _____

REVIEW EXERCISE E: Equipment Components (see textbook pp.769-772)

1. List the five main components of the MRI system.

   A. _____   D. _____

   B. _____   E. _____

   C. _____

2.   The two units of measurement pertaining to magnetic fields are _____ and _____.

3.   List the three types of MRI magnet systems and their approximate field strengths.   (The earth's magnetic field strength is provided as a comparison.)

Type of Magnet   *Field Strength*

Earth _____   __.00005_____ Tesla

A.   _____   _____ Tesla

B.   _____   _____ Tesla

C.   _____   _____ Tesla

4.   MRI systems generally include gradient coils in _____ directions.

5.   What is the major advantage of the new 3.0 Tesla ultra-fast MRI imaging systems?

     _____

6.   What is the major advantage of the flared or short bore design MRI imaging systems?

     _____

7.   The radiofrequency coils act as _____ to both produce and detect the radio waves, which are referred to as the MRI "signal."

8.   A.   A circumferential whole-volume coil is one which _____.

     B.   Two examples of this type of coil are the _____ and _____.

9.   An example of a surface coil is the _____.

10. The display or workstation allows the technologist to control the operation of the system and view the images. List at least three variables that can be controlled or set at this workstation.

     A.   _____

     B.   _____

     C.   _____

Summary of MRI Imaging Process and System Components Used

Following is a five-step summary of the entire MR imaging process. It identifies the component used and the results of each step:

STEP	COMPONENT	RESULT
1. Apply static magnetic field	_____	Nuclei align and precess
2. Select slice by applying gradient magnetic field (variation of magnetic field strength over patient)	_____	Nuclei precess at a particular frequency
3. Apply RF pulses	_____	Nuclei in the slice area precess in phase at a greater angle
4. Receive RF signal	RF receiving coil or antenna	_____
5. Convert signal to image	_____	Reconstructed image is displayed

Fig. 24-1 Summary of MRI process and system components used.

11. Complete the omitted parts by filling in the blanks of the steps, components, and results as listed in the following summary of MRI imaging process and system components used (Fig. 24-1).

REVIEW EXERCISE F: Clinical Applications, Safety Considerations, and Appearance of Anatomy (see textbook pp. 773-777)

1. Complete the following list of MRI safety concerns.

   A. _____

   B. _____

   C. _____

   D. Local heating of tissues and metallic objects

   E. Electrical interference with normal functions of nerve cells and muscle fibers.

2. The danger of projectiles becomes _____ (greater/lesser) as ferromagnetic objects are moved toward the scanner because the field strength is _____ (directly/inversely) proportional to the cube of the distance from the bore of the magnet.

3. In a code blue situation, the patient is removed from the scan room due to the danger of _____ .

4. Pacemakers are not allowed inside the _____ gauss line.

5. As a general rule, O_2 tanks, IV pumps, and wheelchairs are not allowed inside the _____ gauss line.

6. Magnetic tapes, credit cards, and cochlear implants are not allowed inside the _____ gauss line.

7. Identify the most important contraindication to MRI involving torquing of metallic objects.

    _____

8. The unit for measuring local heating of tissues is: _____ (Hint: Initials are SAR)

    _____

9. MRI has the ability to show anatomy in _____, _____, and

    _____ planes.

10. MRI has excellent _____, which allows visualization of soft tissue structures.

11. Diagnosis of diseases such as those involving the CNS can be made with MRI by comparing the signals produced

    in _____ tissues with those produced in _____ tissues (normal or

    abnormal).

12. List three types of histories that should be obtained from patients before an MRI exam.

    A. _____   C. _____

    B. _____

13. Name the IV contrast agent commonly used in MRI: _____.

14. Describe how this contrast agent affects T1 and T2 relaxation rates: _____

    _____

15. The average amount of contrast media given during an MRI examination is _____ ml/kg; the injection rate should

    not exceed _____ ml/min.

16. List eight absolute contraindications to patient MRI scanning.

    A. _____

    B. _____

    C. _____

    D. _____

    E. _____

    F. _____

    G. _____

    H. _____

17. Match the following pulse sequence description with the correct designation.

    _____ 1. Pulse sequences using a combination of short TR and short TE   A. T1 relaxation

    _____ 2. Pulse sequences using a combination of long TR and long TE   B. T2 relaxation

18. List the T1- and T2-weighted appearances for the following tissues: dark, bright, light gray, or dark gray

		_T1_	_T2_
A.	Cortical bone	Dark	Dark
B.	Red bone marrow	_____	_____
C.	Fat	_____	_____
D.	White brain matter	_____	_____
E.	CSF	_____	_____
F.	Muscle	_____	_____
G.	Vessels	_____	_____

19. True/False: Flowing blood is not visualized with a conventional spin-echo pulse sequence.

20. True/False: Tissues filled with air do not produce a T1 or T2 signal and therefore appear as bright.

REVIEW EXERCISE G: MRI Examinations (see textbook: pp. 778-781)

1. Complete the list of six structures or tissue types best demonstrated by MRI of the brain.

    A. Gray matter   D. _____

    B. _____   E. Basal ganglia

    C. _____   F. Brain stem

2. Complete the list of six possible pathologies demonstrated by MRI of the brain.

    A. _____   E. Hemorrhagic disorders

    B. _____   F. CVA

    C. _____

    D. _____

3. MRI of the brain is considered superior to the CT in visualizing the following three regions of the body or tissue types.

    A. _____

    B. _____

    C. _____

4. Which of the following technical factors may be used in spine imaging?

   A. T1-weighted sequence   C. Cardiac gating

   B. T2-weighted sequence   D. All of the above

5. Complete the list of seven structures best demonstrated by MRI of the spine.

   A. _____   E. Facet joint spaces

   B. _____   F. Basivertebral vein

   C. _____   G. Ligamentus flavum

   D. _____

6. List two major advantages of MR over CT imaging of the spine.

   A. _____

   B. _____

7. True/False: CT is superior to MRI for evaluation of spinal trauma.

8. Complete the list of structures best demonstrated by MRI of the limb or joints.

   A. _____   C. _____   E. Blood vessels

   B. _____   D. _____   F. Marrow

                                                G. Fat

9. Complete the list of structures (organs) best demonstrated by MRI of the abdomen and pelvis.

   A. _____   E. _____

   B. _____   F. Kidneys

   C. _____   G. Vessels

   D. _____   H. Reproductive organs

10. True/False: Sonography and CT are the modalities of choice for demonstrating renal cysts.

11. True/False: Transrectal coils may be used to demonstrate prostate and other reproductive organs.

12.   Match the following terms with the correct definition (refer to textbook [pp. 782-783] for questions 12 and 13):

_____   1.   MR technique to minimize motion artifacts   A.   T2

_____   2.   False features on an image caused by patient instability or   B.   Tesla
                equipment deficiencies

_____   3.   Slow gyration of an axis of a spinning body caused by an   C.   Signal averaging
                application of torque

_____   4.   Method of improving SNR by averaging several FIDs or spin   D.   Acoustic neuroma
                echos

_____   5.   Spin lattice or longitudinal relaxation time   E.   Fringe field

_____   6.   SI unit of magnetic field intensity   F.   Schwannoma

_____   7.   Stray magnetic field that exists outside the imager   G.   Artifacts

_____   8.   A new growth of the white substance of the nerve sheath   H.   Gating

_____   9.   A tumor growing from nerve cells affecting the sense of hearing   I.   Precession

_____   10.   Spin-spin or transverse relaxation time   J.   T1

13.   Match the following terms with the correct definition:

_____   1.   Measure of the geometric relationship between the RF coil and the body.   A.   Contrast resolution

_____   2.   Atmospheric gases such as nitrogen and helium used for cooling   B.   Chordoma

_____   3.   Reappearance of an NMR signal after the FID has disappeared   C.   Turbulence

_____   4.   Amount of rotation of the net magnetization vector produced by an RF   D.   Spin echo
                pulse.

_____   5.   Force that causes or tends to cause a body to rotate   E.   Filling factor

_____   6.   Repetition time   F.   Meningioma

_____   7.   In flowing fluid, velocity component that fluctuates randomly   G.   Cryogen

_____   8.   A malignant tumor arising form the embryonic remains of the notocord   H.   Torque

_____   9.   A hard, slow growing vascular tumor   I.   TR

_____   10.   Ability of an imaging process to distinguish adjacent soft tissue structures J.   Flip angle
                from one another

Answers to Review Exercises

Review Exercise A: Nuclear Medicine

1. Radiopharmaceuticals
2. Tracers
3. D. All of the above
4. C. Technetium 99m
5. Single photon emission computed tomography
6. Three
7. Bone scintigraphy
8. A. Kidney transplants
9. B. Meckel's diverticulum
10. B. Thallium
11. D. Neo Tect
12. A. 1
    B. 3
    C. 1
    D. 1
    E. 2
    F. 3
    G. 2
    H. 3
    I. 1

Review Exercise B: Radiation Oncology

1. Heart-related diseases
2. A. Internal, brachytherapy
   B. External beam, teletherapy
3. Internal, brachytherapy
4. A. X-ray units
   B. Cobalt-60 gamma rays units
   C. Linear accelerator or betatron units
5. A. 1.25
6. D. High-speed electrons striking an anode
7. B. Linear accelerator
8. C. 4 to 30
9. Determine the area and volume of tissue to be treated
10. A. 3
    B. 1
    C. 1
    D. 4
    E. 2
    F. 4
    G. 1

Review Exercise C: Ultrasound

1. A. Sonography
   B. Ultrasonography
   C. Echosonography
2. 1 to 17
3. False (is not ideal for ileus)
4. False (not used for bone cyst)
5. True
6. False (in the early 1950s)
7. B. B-mode
8. D. Doppler

9. C. Increase in dynamic range
10. Converts electrical energy to ultrasonic energy
11. B. Ceramic
12. A. Piezoelectric effect
13. A. 2
    B. 1
    C. 3
14. True
15. True
16. B. Stomach
17. Amniocentesis
18. D. All of the above
19. D. All of the above
20. A. 8
    B. 3
    C. 9
    D. 1
    E. 7
    F. 5
    G. 10
    H. 4
    I. 2
    J. 6

Review Exercise D: Physical Principles of MRI

1. Magnetic fields and radio waves
2. Nuclei
3. 2. A. 10^3 to 10^{-2} meters
      B. 10^5 to 10^{10} hertz
      C. 10^{-7} electron volts
4. A. Hydrogen (single proton nucleus)
   B. The large amount of hydrogen present in any organism.
5. Proton
6. A. 1000
7. Is similar to the wobble of a slowly spinning top
8. Increases
9. An outside force (the magnetic field)
10. Radio waves
11. Increase in time increases the angle of precession
12. Resonance
13. Nucleus, or proton
14. Radio, precessing or rotating
15. T1 relaxation and T2 relaxation
16. Longitudinal
17. Transverse
18. Spin density, minor
19. So that the returning signal can be located (because only the precessing nuclei within these regions or slice transmit signals).
20. A. Spin density
    B. T1 relaxation rate
    C. T2 relaxation rate

Review Exercise E: Equipment Components

1. A. Magnet
   B. Gradient coils
   C. Radiofrequency coils
   D. Electronic support system
   E. Computer and display
2. Tesla and Gauss
3. A. Resistive, 0.3
   B. Permanent, 0.3
   C. Superconducting, 2.0 to 3.0
4. Three (3)
5. Improved signal-to-noise ratio for brain mapping and real-time brain acquisitions
6. Helps to alleviate claustrophobia
7. Antennas
8. A. Encircles the part being imaged
   B. Any two of the following: body coil, limb (extremity) coil, head coil, or volume neck coil
9. Shoulder coil or planar coil
10. Any three of the following:
    A. Select pulse sequences
    B. Adjust parameters such as signal averages and pulse repetition time (TR)
    C. Initiate scan, or alter brightness and contrast of image
11. 1. Magnet
    2. Gradient coils
    3. RF sending coil or antenna
    4. Electric signal is received from nuclei and sent to computer
    5. Computer

Review Exercise F: Clinical Application, Safety Considerations, and Appearance of Anatomy

1. A. Potential hazards of projectiles
   B. Electrical interference with implants
   C. Torquing of metallic objects
2. Greater, directly
3. Metallic objects used in blue code situations becoming projectiles
4. 5
5. 50
6. 10
7. Presence of intracranial aneurysm clips
8. Specific absorption ratio
9. Transverse, sagittal, and coronal
10. Contrast resolution
11. Normal, abnormal
12. A. Surgical history
    B. Occupational history
    C. Accidental history
13. Gd - DTPA (Gadolinium - DTPA)
14. Shortens T1 and T2 relaxation rates

15. 0.2, 10
16. A. Cardiac pacemakers
    B. Electronic implant
    C. Aneurysm clip in the brain
    D. Inner ear surgery
    E. Metallic fragments in the body
    F. Metal in and/or removed from
       the eye
    G. Eye prostheses
    H. Pregnancy
17. 1. A. (T1 relaxation)
    2. B. (T2 relaxation)
18.

	T1	T2
B. Red bone marrow	Light gray	Dark gray
C. Fat	Bright	Dark
D. White brain matter	Light gray	Dark gray
E. CSF	Dark	Bright
F. Muscle	Dark gray	Dark gray
G. Vessels	Dark	Dark

19. True
20. False (appears black)

Review Exercise G: MRI Examinations

1. B. White matter
   C. Nerve tissue
   D. Ventricles
2. A. White matter disease (multiple sclerosis or demyelinating disease)
   B. Ischemic disorders
   C. Neoplasm
   D. Infectious diseases (such as AIDS and herpes)
3. A. Posterior fossa
   B. Brainstem
   C. Detecting small changes in tissue water content
4. D. All of the above
5. A. Spinal cord
   B. Nerve tissue
   C. Intervertebral disks
   D. Bone marrow

6. A. MR does not require the use of intrathecal (within a sheath) contrast media
   B. It covers a large area of the spine in a single sagittal view
7. True
8. A. Fat and Muscle
   B. Ligaments
   C. Tendons
   D. Nerves
9. A. Liver
   B. Pancreas
   C. Spleen
   D. Adrenals
   E. Gallbladder
10. True
11. True
12. 1. H, 2. G, 3. I, 4. C, 5. J,
    6. B, 7. E, 8. F, 9. D, 10. A
13. 1. E, 2. G, 3. D, 4. J, 5. H,
    6. I, 7. C, 8. B, 9. F, 10. A

SELF-TEST

My Score = _____ %

This self-test should be taken only after completing all of the readings, review exercises, and laboratory activities for a particular section. The purpose of this test is not only to provide a good learning exercise but also to serve as a good indicator of what your final evaluation grade will be. It is strongly suggested that if you do not get at least a 90% to 95% grade on this self-test, you should review those areas where you missed questions before going to your instructor for the final evaluation exam for this chapter. (There are 75 questions or blanks—each is worth 1.3 points.)

1. One of the most common radionuclides used in nuclear medicine is:

    A. Thallium   C. Cardiolyte

    B. Techetium 99m   D. Sulfur colloid

2. What type of imaging device used in nuclear medicine provides a three-dimensional image of anatomical structures?

    A. SPECT camera   C. Linear accelerator

    B. B-mode unit   D. Real-time scanner

3. An abnormal region detected during a nuclear medicine skeletal scan is described as a/an:

    A. Signal void   C. Acoustic shadow

    B. Hot spot   D. Region of high attenuation

4. Which one of the following is a common pathologic indicator for a nuclear medicine gastrointestinal study?

    A. Duodenal ulcer   C. Meckel's diverticulum

    B. Bezoar   D. Ileus

5   If a treadmill is not available for a nuclear medicine cardiac study, the patient is given:

    A. Glucagon   C. Lasix

    B. Valium   D. Vasodilator

6. True/False: The perfusion phase of a nuclear medicine lung ventilation/perfusion study is performed **before** the ventilation phase.

7. Which one of the following duties is *not* a typical responsibility of the nuclear medicine technologist?

    A. Calibrate instrumentation   C. Administer radionuclides

    B. Process images   D. Decontaminate area due to spills

8. Which one of the following is *not* an example of a teletherapy unit?

    A. Linear accelerator   C. X-ray units

    B. Neutron accelerator   D. Cobalt-60 unit

9. Linear accelerators deliver energy levels to target tissues between:

    A. 50 to 100 kVp   C. 100 to 300 kVp

    B. 1.25 to 5.0 MeV   D. 4 to 30 MeV

10. True/False: The patient is often skin-tattooed during radiation therapy simulations.

11. Which one of the following is *not* a responsibility of the radiation therapist?

    A. Uses fluoroscopy for treatment planning   C. Prescribes the treatment

    B. Interacts directly with patient   D. Maintains therapy records

12. Which of the following is *not* an alternative term for medical ultrasound?

    A. Echosonography   C. Piezosonography

    B. Sonography   D. Ultrasonography

13. Medical ultrasound operates at a frequency range between:

    A. 1 to 5 KHz   C. 1 to 17 KHz

    B. 25 to 50 KHz   D. 1 to 17 MHz

14. Which generation of ultrasound equipment first introduced gray scale imaging?

    A. A-mode   C. Real time dynamic

    B. B-mode   D. Doppler

15. An ultrasound transducer converts _____ energy to ultrasonic energy.

    A. Electrical   C. Light

    B. Heat   D. Magnetic

16. Which one of the following transducers would be used on a large abdomen?

    A. 3.5 MHz   C. 10 MHz

    B. 5.0 to 7.0 MHz   D. 17 MHz

17. True/False: A higher frequency transducer will increase penetration through the anatomy but will produce lower image resolution.

18. True/False: A normal gallbladder is an example of a *hyperechoic* structure.

19. True/False: Breast ultrasound is used primarily to distinguish between solid and cystic masses.

20. With color-flow Doppler, blood flowing away from the transducer is:

    A. Red   C. Blue

    B. Gray   D. Black

21. The MR image represents differences in the number of:

    A. X-rays attenuated   C. Frequencies of nuclei

    B. Nuclei and the rate of their recovery   D. Radio waves

22. MRI technique makes use of:

    A. X-rays   C. Sound waves

    B. Radio waves   D. Visible light

23. The nuclei in the body used to receive and re-emit radio waves are:

    A. Hydrogen   C. Oxygen

    B. Carbon   D. Phosphorus

24. The nuclei that receive and re-emit radio waves are under the influence of:

    A. Gravitational force   C. X-ray energy

    B. The sun and the planets   D. A static magnetic field

25. Which of the following properties results in a nucleus becoming a small magnet?

    A. An even number of neutrons and protons   C. An even number of electrons

    B. An odd number of neutrons or protons   D. The presence of a magnet

26. Precession occurs because spinning magnetic nuclei:

    A. Oscillate in the presence of other atoms   C. Are acted on by a static magnetic field

    B. Regress under the face of a magnet   D. Ionize atoms

27. A precessing nucleus causes _____ to occur in a nearby loop of wire.

    A. An alternating current   C. A direct current

    B. A dipole   D. Magnetic regression

28. Precession can be altered by the application of:

    A. X-rays   C. Microwaves

    B. Radio frequency waves   D. Visible light

29. Resonance occurs when radio waves are:

    A. Of the same frequency as the precessing nuclei   C. At the same rate as T2 relaxation

    B. At the same rate as T1 relaxation   D. Received by an antenna

30. The angle of precession of the nuclei is altered because the:

    A. Nuclei must be vertical   C. Electrostatic properties of the nuclei dominate

    B. The magnetic force dominates   D. MR signal is strongest when nuclei are horizontal

31. Emitted waves from the nuclei are _____ and sent to the computer.

    A. Evaluated   C. In resonance

    B. Received by an antenna   D. Precessing

32. The _____ among T1, T2, and spin density of tissues produces image contrast.

    A. Similarities   C. Differences

    B. Phase   D. Frequency

33. In T2 relaxation, the spins:

    A. Are vertical in orientation   C. Are reduced in density

    B. Move to the north   D. Become out of phase with one another

34. In T1 relaxation, the spins:

    A. Are relaxing to a vertical orientation   C. Are reduced in density

    B. Stay in a horizontal position   D. Become out of phase with one another

35. Spin density refers to the _____ of hydrogen nuclei.

    A. Quality   C. Phase D

    B. Quantity   D. Wavelength

36. The signal strength and thus the brightness of points in the image is primarily determined by:

    A.   Differences in T1 and T2 relaxation rates of tissues
    C.   The longitudinal component of nuclei
    B.   Differences in spin density of tissues
    D.   Exposure of the nuclei to the static magnetic field

37. Gradient magnetic fields are useful because:

    A.   The strength is consistent along the patient
    B.   The strength determines the frequency of the MR signal
    C.   They allow the location of the signal to be moved
    D.   The precessional rate of the nuclei must be constant

38. Gradient magnetic fields allow:

    A.   Slice selection and locating the signal
    C.   Slice selection and spin echo
    B.   Locating the signal and relaxation of nuclei
    D.   Spin echo and relaxation of nuclei

39. TR can be defined as:

    A.   Time reversal
    C.   Timing range
    B.   Repetition time
    D.   Time of resonance

40. TE can be defined as:

    A.   Echo phase
    C.   Temporary echo
    B.   Time net
    D.   Echo time

41. TR and TE have a profound influence upon:

    A.   Image noise deletion
    C.   Signal averaging
    B.   Image contrast
    D.   Image density

42. One Tesla equals:

    A.   10,000 times the earth's magnetic field
    C.   10 Gauss
    B.   0.00005 Gauss
    D.   10,000 Gauss

43. Superconducting magnet systems produce magnetic field strengths of up to:

    A.   2.0 or 3.0 Tesla
    C.   0.3 Tesla
    B.   1.0 Tesla
    D.   0.1 Tesla

44. Which one of the following diagrams (Fig. 24-2) is correctly labeled according to the x, y, and z gradient coils (A, B, or C)? _____

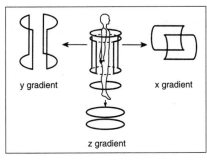

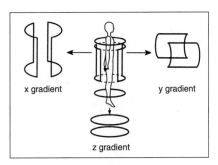

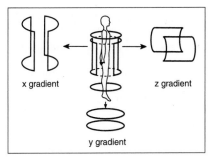

Fig. 24-2 Labeling of gradient coils.

45. Typical permanent magnet systems produce magnetic field strengths of up to:

    A. 2.0 Tesla   C. 0.3 Tesla

    B. 1.0 Tesla   D. 0.1 Tesla

46. Superconducting magnets require _____ to allow the low temperatures necessary for the property of superconductivity.

    A. Cryogens   C. Alternating electrical current

    B. Liquid hydrogen   D. Friction

47. The RF coils act as:

    A. The antennas to produce and receive radio waves   C. A shield from extraneous RF pulses

    B. A means of producing a gradient magnetic field   D. A superconducting magnet

48. Coils that are smaller than the body coil and that do not surround the anatomy are generally referred to as:

    A. Circumferential coils   C. Surface coils

    B. Whole-volume coils   D. Head coils

49. Which one of the following is not a similarity between MRI and CT?

    A. The outward appearance of the unit   C. The use of ionizing radiation

    B. The use of a computer to analyze information   D. Images viewed as a slice of tissue

50. Primary safety concerns for the technologist, patient, and medical personnel are due to:

    A. Fringe field strengths less than 1 Gauss

    B. Gravitational pull on metallic objects

    C. Magnetic fields and heat production

    D. Interaction of magnetic fields with metallic objects and tissues

51. Projectiles are a concern due to:

    A. Force of metallic objects being pulled to the magnet   C. Nerve cell function

    B. Fringe fields less than 10 Gauss   D. Local heating of tissues and metallic objects

52. Pacemakers are not allowed inside the:

    A. 5 Gauss line   C. 1.0 Gauss line

    B. 2.5 Gauss line   D. 0.5 Gauss line

53. IV pumps, wheelchairs, and O_2 tanks are not allowed inside the:

    A. 150 Gauss line   C. 5 Gauss line

    B. 50 Gauss line   D. 1 Gauss line

54. The most important contraindication in regard to torquing of metallic objects is:

    A. Intraabdominal surgical staples   C. Intracranial aneurysm clips

    B. Shrapnel   D. Hip prosthesis

55. Local heating of tissues (referred to as *SAR* or *specific absorption ratio*) is measured in:

    A. W/kg   C. RF frequency

    B. C°   D. F°

56. The contrast agent commonly used for MR examinations is:

   A. Iodine 131   C. Gadolinium oxysulfide

   B. Lanthanum oxybromide   D. Gadolinium-diethylene triamine pentaacetic acid

57. Contrast agents are generally used with:

   A. T1-weighted pulse sequences   C. Spin-density weighted pulse sequences

   B. T2-weighted pulse sequences   D. All of the above

58. Which of the following is considered a circumferential whole volume coil:

   A. Shoulder coil   C. Head coil

   B. C-spine coil   D. Planar coil

59. The three sets of gradient coils are typically:

   A. Visible on the external surface of the magnet

   B.   Situated in two different directions

   C. Located within the bore of the magnet or gantry

   D. All of the above

60. Surface coils improve:

   A. SNR   C. Safety

   B. Anatomical magnification   D. Heat dissipation

61. Proton (spin) density images use a pulse sequence that has a combination of:

   A. Long TR, short TE   C. Short TR, long TE

   B. Long TR, long TE   D. Short TR, short TE

62. T1-weighted images use a pulse sequence that has a combination of:

   A. Long TR, short TE   C. Short TR, long TE

   B. Long TR, long TE   D. Short TR, short TE

63. T2-weighted images use a pulse sequence that has a combination of:

   A. Long TR, short TE   C. Short TR, long TE

   B. Long TR, long TE   D. Short TR, short TE

64. On T1-weighted images, CSF will be:

   A. Dark   C. Same as white matter

   B. Bright   D. Same as gray matter

65. On T2-weighted images, CSF will be:

   A. Dark   C. Same as white matter

   B. Bright   D. Same as gray matter

66. MRI of the brain allows visualization of:

   A. White matter disease   C. Small calcifications

   B. Acute blood   D. Fractures

67. MRI of the brain includes the use of a standard head coil and:

    A. Prone position   C. Sedation

    B. Cardiac gating   D. T1- and T2-weighted pulse sequences

68. Which of the following is not best evaluated by MRI of the spine:

    A. Bone marrow changes   C. Disk herniation

    B. Cord abnormalities   D. Scoliosis

69. MRI of the lumbar spine requires the patient to be positioned:

    A. Feet first, prone   C. Head first, prone

    B. Feet first, supine   D. Head first, supine

70. MRI of the joints or limbs demonstrates all of the following except:

    A. Ligaments   C. Muscle

    B. Tendons   D. Skin

71. During MRI of the joints, the patient must lie so that the anatomy of interest is:

    A. Centered to the coil, coil then moved to magnet center   C. Prone and centered to the magnet

    B. Supine and centered to the magnet   D. None of the above

72. The patient is positioned for abdominopelvic MRI by placing the patient:

    A. Prone, head first   C. Prone, feet first

    B. Supine, feet first   D. Supine, head first

73. The largest drawback for MRI of the abdomen is:

    A. Motion artifacts   C. Coil selection

    B. Metallic implants   D. Sequence times

74. A RF pulse sequence for MRI in which the net magnetization is inverted is called:

    A. Inversion recovery   C. Flip angle

    B. Spin-echo   D. Saturation recovery

75. A mathematical procedure to separate frequency components of a signal from its amplitudes is called:

    A. Gradient moment nulling   C. Fourier transformation

    B. Signal averaging   D. Free induction decay

SELF-TEST ANSWERS

Chapter 14 Upper Gastrointestinal System

1. C. Production of hormones
2. C. Pineal
3. Barium swallow
4. Mumps
5. A. Mastication
6. B. Epiglottis
7. D. T11
8. A. Trachea
9. Peristalsis
10. Stomach
11. D. Incisura angularis
12. A. Fundus
13. False (in the stomach)
14. False (the greater curvature)
15. Fundus
16. Head of pancreas and C-loop of duodenum
17. 1. E, 2. F, 3. I, 4. H, 5. C, 6. A, 7 D, 8. G, 9. B
18. A. Distal esophagus
    B. Region of esophagogastric junction
    C. Fundus
    D. Greater curvature
    E. Body
    F. Pyloric antrum
    E. Pyloric canal
    H. Pyloric orifice (sphincter)
    I. Descending portion of duodenum
    J. Duodenal bulb
    K. Lesser curvature
19. A. Prone
    B. Air in fundus
20. Lateral
21. A. Supine
    B. Barium-filled fundus (air in pylorus)
22. A. Posterior
    B. Air in pylorus indicated semi-supine position
    C. (p. 440) RAO
    D. Air in fundus indicated a semi-prone position and duodenal bulb and C-loop in profile indicated an RAO and not an LAO.
23. Chyme
24. A. Vitamins
25. C. Rhythmic segmentation
26. Hyposthenic or asthenic, L3-4
27. Hypersthenic, T11-12
28. Barium sulfate
29. Carbon dioxide
30. A. Three or four parts of barium to one part of water
    B. One part barium to one part water

31. When there is a possibility that the contrast media may spill into the peritoneum (such as pre-surgery or a perforated bowel)
32. Output
33. C. 1000 to 6000 times
34. True
35. Lower
36. B. 0.50
37. A. Zenker's diverticulum
38. B. Nuclear medicine
39. D. Trapped vegetable fiber in the stomach
40. To detect signs of esophageal reflux (also see question 49 and answer)
41. 35 to 40°
42. The RAO visualizes the esophagus between the heart and vertebra better than an LAO.
43. Majority of esophagus is superimposed over the spine and thus is not well visualized
44. Shredded cotton or marshmallows
45. Right lateral
46. Reduce patient oblique to less than 40 degrees for asthenic patient.
47. Supine position for an AP projection
48. To rule-out esophageal varices (a condition of dilation of the veins, which in advanced stages may lead to internal bleeding)
49. The Valsalva maneuver, to rule out esophageal reflux (a condition wherein gastric contents return back through the gastric orifice into the esophagus causing irritation of esophageal lining).
50. An ulcer

Chapter 15 Lower Gastrointestinal System

1. A. 15 to 18 ft (4.5 to 5.5 m)
2. C. Ileum
3. D. Suspensory ligament of the duodenum
4. A. Ileum
5. C. Jejunum
6. A. Cecum
   B. Rectum
7. Veniform appendix
8. True
9. False (these are in large intestine)
10. Left
11. A. Jejunum
    B. Ileum
    C. Region of ileocecal valve
    D. Duodenum
    E. Pyloric portion of stomach
    F. Left colic (splenic) flexure

G. Descending colon
H. Sigmoid colon
I. Rectum
J. Cecum
K. Ascending colon
L. Right colic (hepatic)flexure
M. Transverse colon

12. C. Transverse colon
13. B. Large intestine
14. B. Rhythmic segmentation
15. 1. F, 2. D, 3. I, 4. L, 5. B, 6. G, 7. J, 8. C, 9. A, 10. E, 11. M, 12. K, 13. H
16. 1. D, 2. G, 3. E, 4. H, 5. A, 6. C, 7. B, 8. F
17. A. Barium enema
18. False
19. Hold breath on expiration
20. Produces compression of the abdomen that leads to separation of the loops of small intestine
21. 8 hours
22. Cathartic
23. Rectal retention enema tip
24. Glucagon
25. Lidocaine
26. D. Prolapse of rectum
27. B. Anorectal angle
28. True
29. RAO
30. Two hours
31. D. Anatrast
32. C. Center chamber only
33. 35 to 45 degrees
34. 2 inches (5 cm)
35. Defecography
36. LPO
37. Right lateral decubitus will drain excess barium from the descending colon allowing for detection of small polyp
38. Evacuative proctography
39. False
40. False
41. True
42. D. 2000 to 3000 mrad
43. A. Right. Iliac crest
    B. Left. 1 to 2 inches (2.5 to 5 cm) above the iliac crest

Chapter 16 Gallbladder and Biliary Ducts

1. A. Anterior inferior
2. C. Inferior
4. Falciform ligament
5. To break down or emulsify fats
6. Common hepatic duct
7. 30 to 40 cc
8. Hydrolysis

9. Cholecystokinin (CCK)
10. Common bile duct
11. 1. H, 2. F, 3. G, 4. A, 5. I, 6. B, 7. D, 8. E, 9. C
12. Supine, because the body and fundus of the gallbladder are anterior and the neck and cystic duct posterior
13. A. Fundus
    B. Body
    C. Neck
    D. Cystic duct
    E. Duodenum
    F. Common bile duct
    G. Common hepatic duct
    H. Right hepatic duct
    I. Left hepatic duct
14. 1. H, 2. I, 3. A, 4. B, 5. C, 6. F, 7. E, 8. G, 9. D
15. True
16. True
17. 1. C, 2. D, 3. E, 4. G, 5. B, 6. A, 7. F
18. At least 8 hours
19. 10 to 12 hours before the procedure
20. 70 to 76 kVp
21. Allow for better drainage of the gallbladder and free superimposition of biliary ducts and gallbladder from spine
22. 5 to 10 minutes
23. False (the patient needs to be NPO only 4 hours before the ultrasound procedure)
24. True
25. Through a small catheter placed into the remnant portion of the cystic duct after the gallbladder has been surgically removed
26. 6 to 8 cc
27. The grid must be turned crosswise to prevent grid cutoff.
28. A much smaller incision is required with the laparoscopic technique.
29. To detect postoperatively in the radiology department any residual stones in the biliary ducts that may have gone undetected during the cholecystectomy
30. B. Obstructive jaundice
31. D. Skinny needle
32. A. R, B. S, C. R
33. True
34. True
35. True
36. False
37. True
38. Center chamber
39. Operative cholangiogram is "immediate," performed during surgery, and the T-tube cholangiogram is "delayed," or done in radiology following surgery.

40. Increase the obliquity of the LAO position
41. Because of the more anterior location of the gallbladder
42. Either the erect, PA, or a right lateral decubitus positions will stratify or "layer" any possible stones in the gallbladder.
43. RPO
44. Keep the patient NPO for 4 hours then perform an ultrasound study of the gallbladder.
45. D. PTC

Chapter 17 Urinary System

1. A. Retroperitoneal
2. C. Posterolateral
3. Anterior
4. 30 degree
5. A. Uteropelvic junction
   B. Near brim of pelvis
   C. Ureterovesical (UV) junction
6. 2 inches, 5 cm
7. Uremia
8. D. 1.5 liter
9. D. Inferior vena cava
10. Renal pyramids
11. Renal pelvis
12. Nephron
13. True
14. False (99% is reabsorbed)
15. Trigone
16. A. Urinary bladder
    B. Ureter
    C. Ureteropelvic junction
    D. Renal pelvis
    E. Major calyces
    F. Minor calyces
17. Retrograde pyelogram (Note catheter in right ureter)
18. When the benefit of the procedure outweighs the risks of the radiation exposure
19. Ionic and nonionic
20. 1. I, 2. N, 3. I, 4. I, 5. I, 6. N, 7. I, 8. N, 9. I, 10. N
21. B. 0.6 to 1.5 mg/dl
22. A. 48 hours
23. C. Diabetes mellitus
24. A. Observe and reassure patient
25. B. Mild reaction
26. B. Mild reaction
27. D. Severe reaction
28. C. Moderate reaction
29. C. Axillary vein
30. 20 to 45 degrees
31. Anuria or anuresis
32. Lithotripsy
33. D. Vesicourethral reflux
34. A. Renal obstruction
35. A. Ectopic kidney
36. True
37. True
38. B. Ureteric calculi
39. 20 minutes following injection

40. Nephrogram or nephrotomography; immediately after completion of injection
41. Retrograde urethrogram on a male patient
42. Left posterior oblique (LPO)
43. False (higher for female)
44. False (primarily the ureter)
45. Angle the CR more caudally to project the symphysis pubis inferior to the bladder.

Chapter 18 Mammography

1. Mammography Quality Standards Act, 1994
2. Only VA facilities
3. 40
4. 8
5. Inframammary crease
6. Upper, outer quadrant (UOQ)
7. 11 o'clock
8. Pectoralis major muscle
9. Lactation or production of milk
10. Cooper's ligaments
11. Adipose (fatty)
12. Trabeculae
13. Base
14. A. Fibro-glandular
15. B. Fibro-fatty
16. C. Fatty
17. A. Fibro-fatty
18. A. Glandular tissue
    B. Nipple
    C. Adipose (fatty) tissue
    D. Pectoral muscle
    E. Mediolateral oblique (MLO)
    F. Axillary
19. Molybdenum
20. Apex
21. True (only not for implants)
22. True
23. False (grid is used due to the large amount of scatter and secondary)
24. O.1 mm
25. 2x the original size of the object
26. B. 200 to 300 mrad (130 to 150 per projection)
27. Sonography (ultrasound)
28. Magnetic resonance imaging (MRI)
29. True
30. False (patient dose reduced by minimizing repeats)
31. True
32. A. Sulphur colloid
33. Noninvasive and invasive
34. D. XCCL
35. MLO
36. A. Craniocaudal (CC)
    B. Mediolateral oblique (MLO)
37. Mediolateral oblique projection
38. 25 to 28 kVp
39. Laterally exaggerated craniocaudal (XCCL) projection
40. LMO

41. Over
42. A. Eklund
    B. Implant displaced (ID)
43. Axillary tail view (AT); sometimes called the *Cleopatra view*
44. Axillary side
45. Have patient hold the breast back with her opposite hand
46. MLO (mediolateral oblique)
47. XXCL (laterally exaggerated cranio-caudad)
48. Inframammary crease at its upper limits
49. B. Mediolateral oblique
50. C. Use manual exposure factors

Chapter 19 Trauma and Mobile Radiography

1. A. Spiral fracture
   B. Compound fracture
   C. Comminuted fracture
   D. Greenstick fracture
   E. Colles' fracture
   F. Impacted fracture
   G. Compression fracture
   H. Stellate fracture
   I. Pott's fracture
2. A. Dislocation or luxation
   B. Subluxation
3. Spine (although, it can occur in the elbow as well)
4. B. lack of apposition
5. A. valgus angulation
6. 1. E, 2. I, 3. D, 4. H, 5. A, 6. B, 7. C, 8. G, 9. F
7. True
8. True
9. D AP shoulder
10. B 6:1 to 8:1
11. A. Grid frequency
    B. Grid ratio
12. True
13. Battery-operated, battery driven
14. Standard power source
15. False (mobile fluoroscopy units)
16. True
17. False (PA is recommended due to less exposure to operator and less OID)
18. True
19. Roadmapping
20. Reducing patient dose
21. A. Time
    B. Distance
    C. Shielding
22. Distance
23. A. less than 10 mR/hr
24. 4 mR (30 ÷ 60 × 8 = 4)
25. False (greater on tube side)
26. False (by a factor of four)
27. A right lateral decubitus
28. 3 to 4 in (7 to 10 cm) below the jugular notch

29. 15 to 20° mediolateral angle and horizontal beam lateral projections
30. C left lateral decubitus
31. Two
32. Parallel to the interepicondylar plane
33. A horizontal beam lateromedial projection
34. 25 to 30°, or until the CR can be projected parallel to the scapular blade (wing)
35. 10° posteriorly from perpendicular to the plantar surface of the foot
36. Perform a cross-angle CR projection of the ankle, with CR 15 to 20° lateromedial from the long axis of the foot
37. C affected leg is rotated 10 to 20° internally if possible
38. A 35 to 40° cephalad AP axial projection
39. C double angle oblique with IR perpendicular to CR
40. A. it reduces distortion
    B. the long OID produces an air gap effect, which improves image quality without the use of a grid thus allowing a double CR angle (which would cause grid cutoff if a grid were used)
41. B trauma, horizontal beam lateral
42. A. Crosswise
    B. 2 in. (5 cm) superior to EAM
43. C. Lateral
44. A. AP or PA and lateral wrist
45. D. Epiphyseal

Chapter 20 Pediatric Radiography

1. B. 2 years
2. D. Describe the . . .
3. D. Do none of the abovex
4. D. Hold-em Tiger
5. C. Pigg-O-Stat
6. A. Proper immobilization
   B. Short exposure times
   C. Accurate technique charts
7. Is she pregnant?
8. C. Pigg-O-Stat
9. D. 3-D ultrasound
10. B. Functional MRI
11. A. 4, B. 9, C. 7, D. 2, E. 13, F. 3, G. 12, H. 11, I. 1, J. 6, K. 10, L. 8, M. 5
12. A. (+), B. (+), C. (−), D. (+), E. (−), F. (+), G. (−)
13. C. Extend arms upward
14. 55 to 65 kVp
15. True
16. True
17. Kite method
18. Between the umbilicus and just above the pubis

19. 1. D, 2. E, 3. EP, 4. D, 5. E and EP
20. 1. B, 2. B, 3. E, 4. A, 5. E, 6. D, 7. A, 8. B, 9. D, 10. A, 11. E, 12. A, 13. A
21. D. 30°
22. B. Midway between glabella and inion
23. A. 4 hours
24. Diminish the risk of aspiration from vomiting
25 C. Appendicitis
26. A. Level of iliac crest
    B. 1 in. (2.5 cm) above umbilicus
27. Mammillary (nipple) level
28. 6 to 12 ounces
29. Manually, very slowly, using a 60 ml syringe and a #10 French flexible silicone catheter
30. No bowel prep is required
31. When the bladder is full and when voiding
32. One
33. A. Vesicoureteral reflux
    B. Before
34. False (shielding should be used in all positions using tape when necessary)
35. True

Chapter 21 Angiography and Interventional Procedures

1. D. Right and left coronary arteries
2. D. Right common carotid
3. C. Upper margin of thyroid cartilage
4. A. Pulmonary veins
5. C. Right common carotid
6. A. Anterior portion of brain
7. B. Anterior and middle cerebral arteries
8. D. Basilar artery
9. D. Sphenoid
10. C. Internal and external cerebral veins
11. B. Internal jugular vein
12. C. Azygos vein
13. 1. E, 2. J, 3. D, 4. I, 5. K, 6. B, 7. F, 8. H, 9. G, 10. A, 11. L, 12. C
14. False (from brachiocephalic)
15. False (median cubital vein)
16. True
17. True
18. B. Synthesize simple carbohydrates
19. C. 8
20. 1. O, 2. Q, 3. P, 4. N, 5. L, 6. D, 7 A, 8. K, 9. R, 10. M, 11. G, 12. C, 13. F, 14. B, 15. H
21. C. Body temperature
22. B. Color duplex ultrasound
23. False (Does not need to be used)
24. True

25. C. Coarctation
26. C. 8 to 10 seconds
27. B. Pulmonary emboli
28. A. Femoral vein
29. A. 45 RPO
30. C. Left ventricle
31. D. 15 to 30 frames per second
32. D. Malabsorption syndrome
33. C. 30 to 40 ml
34. False (unilateral for upper limb but bilateral for lower limb)
35. True
36. A. Helps to visualize the lymph vessels
37. True
38. False (oil-based is used. Water-soluble is too quickly absorbed)
39. D. Hepatic malignancies
40. 1. C, 2. D, 3. F, 4. A, 5. G, 6. B, 7. E
41. False (placed inferior to renal veins)
42. True

Chapter 22 Computed Tomography

1. A. First generation
2. C and D, third and fourth generation
3. Slip rings
4. A. 1%
5. Source collimator
6. Assign various shades of gray to the numerical values
7. A. Scan unit
   B. Operator control console
8. Pixel
9. D. Vertical adjustment of table height
10. Blood-brain barrier
11. C. Multiple sclerosis
12. B and E Possible neoplasia and brain tumor
13. C. 1972
14. A. Dendrites
    B. Axon
15. Meninges
16. A. Dura mater
    B. Arachnoid
    C. Pia mater
17. A. Pia mater
    B. Arachnoid mater
    C. Dura mater
    D. Venous sinus
    E. Epidural space
    F. Subdural space
    G. Subarachnoid spaces
18. Subarachnoid space
19. 1. C, 2. C, 3. A, 4. A, 5. C
20. Cerebrum
21. Longitudinal fissure
22. Corpus callosum
23. Falx cerebri

24. A. Lateral ventricles
25. C. Cisterna cerebellomedullaris
26. A. Lateral
    B. Third
    C. Fourth
    a. Interventricular foramen
    b. Cerebral aqueduct
    c. Lateral recess
    1. Body
    2. Anterior horn
    3. Inferior (temporal) horn
    4. Posterior horn
    5. Pineal gland
27. Hydrocephalus, ventricles
28. Cisterns
29. A. Frontal
    B. Parietal
    C. Occipital
    D. Temporal
    E. Insula or central lobe
30. 1. A, 2. B, 3. B, 4. B, 5. B, 6. A
31. C. Longitudinal fissure
32. A. Pons
33. D. Mid brain
34. B. Inferior portion of manubrium
35. A. Sternal notch
36. C. Aortopulmonary window
37. A. Base of heart
38. Aortopulmonary window
39. A. Ascending aorta
40. C. Left atrium
41. D. Mitral valve prolapse
42. A. 10 mm
43. D. The hooklike extension of the head of the pancreas
44. D. All of the above
45. D. All of the above
46. D. Symphysis pubis
47. C. Urinary bladder
48. B. 10 mm
49. B. High concentration of a large bolus of barium is present with a low concentration of water
50. C. Xiphoid process
51. True
52. False (They speed up peristaltic action)
53. False (Need to hold breath)
54. True
55. True

Chapter 23 Additional Imaging Procedures

1. Orthoroentgenography
2. False (Ends of bone must be on separate projections)
3. False (Is a premature fusion of the epiphysis to shorten a bone)
4. True
5. True
6. Bell-Thompson ruler

7. 24 x 39 cm (10 x 12 in.) or 30 x 35 cm (11 x 14 in.) with three exposures placed on the same IR
8. A. Knee
   B. Shoulder
9. A. Sensitivity to iodine
   B. Sensitivity to local anesthetics
10. Knee
11. A. Iodinated water soluble, 5 cc
    B. Room air, 80 to 100 cc
12. 20 gauge
13. To provide a thin, even coating of positive contrast media over the soft tissues of the knee joint
14. 18 x 43 cm (7 x 17 in.)
15. A. 6, B. 30°
16. The conjoined tendons of the four major shoulder muscles
17. A. AP internal and external rotation shoulder scout
    B. AP internal rotation
    C. AP external rotation
    D. Glenoid fossa projection (Grashey)
    E. Transaxillary (inferosuperior axial) projection
    F. Bicipital (intertubercular) groove projection
18. A. Herniated nucleus pulposus (HNP)
    B. Cancerous or benign tumors
    C. Cysts
19. A. Blood in the cerebrospinal fluid
    B. Arachnoiditis
    C. Increased intracranial pressure
    D. Recent lumbar puncture (2 weeks)
20. C HNP
21. C Trendelenburg
22. A L3-4
24. D blockage at T-spine level
25. 30, 24
26. Horizontal beam swimmer's lateral
27. Body section radiography
28. 1. D, 2. F, 3. C, 4. A, 5. E, 6. B
29. 1. A, 2. C, 3. D, 4. B, 5. E
30. A. Variable fulcrum
    B. Fixed fulcrum
31. True
32. False (is the exposure angle)
33. True
34. True
35. True
36. A 2 to 3 seconds
37. A. Fundus
    B. Corpus or body
    C. Isthmus
    D. Cervix
38. A. Osseometrium
39. False (connect to the uterus at the corna)

40. A. Acute pelvic inflammatory disease
    B. Active uterine bleeding
41. False (water-soluble is preferred)
42. True
43. A. 2
    B: 3
    C: 1
44. B. Severe inflammation of the salivary gland or duct
45. Water-soluble contrast media
46. A. Excessive physical activity
47. A. Fan-beam x-ray source
48. B. Healthy individual with peak bone mass
49. A. Higher patient dose
    B. More expensive as compared to other bone densitometry systems
50. Os calcis or calcaneus

Chapter 24 Additional Diagnostic and Therapeutic Modalities

1. B. Techetium 99m
2. A. SPECT camera
3. B. Hot spot
4. C. Meckel's diverticulum
5. D. Vasodilator
6. False (during the ventilation phase)
7. A. Calibrate instrumentation
8. B. Neutron accelerator
9. D. 4 to 30 MeV
10. True
11. C. Prescribes the treatment
12. C. Piezosonography
13. D. 1 to 17 MHz
14. B. B-mode
15. A. Electrical

16. A. 3.5 MHz
17. False (higher resolution)
18. False (gall bladder is anechoic)
19. True
20. C. Blue
21. B. Nuclei and the rate of their recovery
22. B. Radio waves
23. A. Hydrogen
24. D. A static magnetic field
25. B. An odd number of neutrons or protons
26. C. Are aced on by a static magnetic
27. A. An alternating current
28. B. Radio frequency waves
29. A. Of the same frequency as the precessing nuclei
30. D. MR signal is strongest when nuclei are horizontal
31. B. Received by an antenna
32. C. Differences
33. D. Become out of phase with one another
34. A. Are relaxing to a vertical orientation
35. B. Quantity
36. A. Differences in T1 and T2 relaxation rates of tissues nuclei
37. B. The strength determines the frequency of the MR signal
38. A. Slice selection and locating the signal
39. B. Repetition time
40. D. Echo time
41. B. Image contrast
42. D. 10,000 Gauss
43. A. 2.0 or 3.0 Tesla
44. B.

45. C. 0.3 tesla
46. A. Cryogens
47. A. The antennas to produce and receive radio waves
48. C. Surface coils
49. C. The use of ionizing radiation
50. D. Interaction of magnetic fields with metallic objects and tissues
51. A. Force of metallic objects being pulled to the magnet
52. A. 5 Gauss line
53. B. 50 Gauss line
54. C. Intracranial aneurysm clips
55. A. W/kg
56. D. Gadolinium-diethylene triamine pentaacetic acid
57. A. T1-weighted pulse sequences
58. C. Head coil
59. C. Located in bore of magnet
60. A. SNR
61. A. Long TR, short TE
62. D. Short TR, short TE
63. B. Long TR, long TE
64. A. Dark
65. B. Bright
66. A. White matter disease
67. D. T1- and T2-weighted pulse sequences
68. D. Scoliosis
69. B. Feet-first, supine
70. D. Skin
71. A. Centered to the coil, coil then moved to magnet center
72. B. Supine, feet first
73. A. Motion artifacts
74. A. Inversion recovery
75. C. Fourier transformation

A food web may also contain another level of **tertiary consumers** (carnivores that consume other carnivores). In a real community, these webs can be extremely complex, with species existing on multiple trophic levels. Communities also include **decomposers**, which are organisms that break down dead matter.

The collection of biotic (living) and abiotic (nonliving) features in a geographic area is called an **ecosystem**. For example, in a forest, the ecosystem consists of all the organisms (animals, plants, fungi, bacteria, etc.), in addition to the soil, groundwater, rocks, and other abiotic features.

Biomes are collections of plant and animal communities that exist within specific climates. They are similar to ecosystems, but they do not include abiotic components and can exist within and across continents. For example, the Amazon rainforest is a specific ecosystem, while tropical rainforests in general are considered a biome that includes a set of similar communities across the world. Together, all the living and nonliving parts of the earth are known as the **biosphere**.

Terrestrial biomes are usually defined by distinctive patterns in temperature and rainfall, and aquatic biomes are defined by the type of water and organisms found there. Examples of biomes include:

- **deserts**: extreme temperatures and very low rainfall with specialized vegetation and small mammals
- **tropical rainforests**: hot and wet with an extremely high diversity of species
- **temperate grasslands**: moderate precipitation and distinct seasons with grasses and shrubs dominating
- **temperate forests**: moderate precipitation and temperatures with deciduous trees dominating
- **tundra**: extremely low temperatures and short growing seasons with little or no tree growth
- **coral reefs**: a marine (saltwater) system with high levels of diversity
- **lake**: an enclosed body of fresh water

If the delicate balance of an ecosystem is disrupted, the system may not function properly. For example, if all the secondary consumers disappear, the population of primary consumers would increase, causing the primary consumers to overeat the producers and eventually starve. **Keystone species** are especially important in a particular community, and removing them decreases the overall diversity of the ecosystem.

PRACTICE QUESTIONS

11. An abiotic environmental factor that influences population size is
  a. food availability
  b. rate of precipitation
  c. mutualism
  d. competition
  e. predation

parts of the digestive tract, blood vessels, and the reproduction system. Finally, cardiac muscle is the involuntary muscle that contracts the heart, pumping blood throughout the body.

🔍 Some skeletal muscles, such as the diaphragm and those that control blinking, can be voluntarily controlled but usually operate involuntarily.

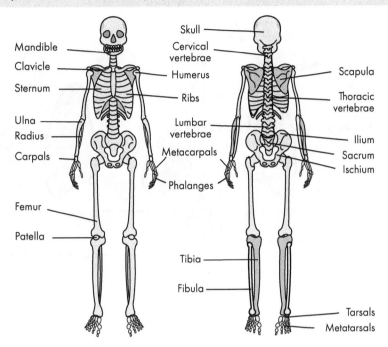

Figure 6.12. The Skeletal System

The **immune system** protects the body from infection by foreign particles and organisms. It includes the **skin** and mucous membranes, which act as physical barriers, and a number of specialized cells that destroy foreign substances in the body. The human body has an adaptive immune system, meaning it can recognize and respond to foreign substances once it has been exposed to them. This is the underlying mechanism behind vaccines.

The immune system is composed of **B cells**, or B lymphocytes, that produce special proteins called **antibodies** that bind to foreign substances, called **antigens**, and neutralize them. **T cells**, or T lymphocytes, remove body cells that have been infected by foreign invaders like bacteria or viruses. **Helper T cells** coordinate production of antibodies by B cells and removal of infected cells by T cells. **Killer T cells** destroy body cells that have been infected by invaders after they are identified and removed by T cells. Finally, **memory cells** remember antigens that have been removed so the immune system can respond more quickly if they enter the body again.

🔍 Memory B cells are the underlying mechanisms behind vaccines, which introduce a harmless version of a pathogen into the body to activate the body's adaptive immune response.

The **nervous system** processes external stimuli and sends signals throughout the body. It is made up of two parts. The central nervous system (CNS) includes the brain and spinal cord and is where information is processed and stored. The brain has three parts: the cerebrum,

b. is correct. Precipitation is a nonliving (abiotic) factor that influences population size.

12. The terrestrial biome characterized by moderate rainfall and the dominance of deciduous trees is called

a. desert
b. tropical rainforest
c. temperate forest
d. tundra
e. grasslands

Answer:

c. is corret. Temperate forests have moderate rainfall and are dominated by deciduous trees.

Human Anatomy and Physiology

In a multicellular organism, cells are grouped together into **tissues**, and these tissues are grouped into **organs**, which perform specific **functions**. The heart, for example, is the organ that pumps blood throughout the body. Organs are further grouped into **organ systems**, such as the digestive or respiratory systems.

Anatomy is the study of the structure of organisms, and **physiology** is the study of how these structures function. Both disciplines study the systems that allow organisms to perform a number of crucial functions, including the exchange of energy, nutrients, and waste products with the environment. This exchange allows organisms to maintain **homeostasis**, or the stabilization of internal conditions.

🔍 In science, a **system** is a collection of interconnected parts that make up a complex whole with defined boundaries. Systems may be closed, meaning nothing passes in or out of them, or open, meaning they have inputs and outputs.

The human body has a number of systems that perform vital functions, including the digestive, excretory, respiratory, circulatory, skeletal, muscular, immune, nervous, endocrine, and reproductive systems.

The **digestive system** breaks food down into nutrients for use by the body's cells. Food enters through the **mouth** and moves through the **esophagus** to the **stomach**, where it is physically and chemically broken down. The food particles then move into the **small intestine**, where the majority of nutrients are absorbed. Finally, the remaining particles enter the **large intestine**, which mostly absorbs water, and waste exits through the **rectum** and **anus**. This system also includes other organs, such as the **liver**, **gallbladder**, and **pancreas**, that manufacture substances needed for digestion.

The **genitourinary system** removes waste products from the body. Its organs include the liver, which breaks down harmful substances, and the **kidneys**, which filter waste from the bloodstream. The excretory system also includes the **bladder** and **urinary tract**, which expel the waste filtered by the kidneys; the lungs, which expel the carbon dioxide created by cellular metabolism; and the skin, which secretes salt in the form of perspiration.

The **respiratory system** takes in oxygen (which is needed for cellular functioning) and expels carbon dioxide. Humans take in air primarily through the nose but also through the mouth. This air travels down the **trachea** and **bronchi** into the **lungs**, which are composed of millions of small structures called alveoli that allow for the exchange of gases between the blood and the air.

The circulatory system carries oxygen, nutrients, and waste products in the blood to and from all the cells of the body. The **heart** is a four-chambered muscle that pumps blood throughout the body. The four chambers are the right atrium, right ventricle, left atrium, and left ventricle. Deoxygenated blood (blood

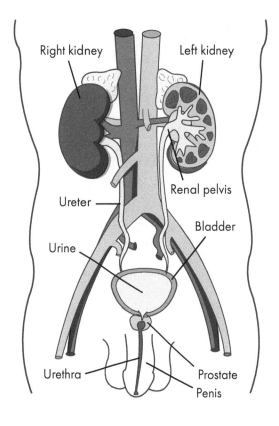

Figure 6.9. Genitourinary System

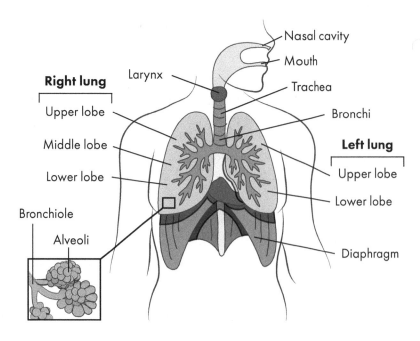

Figure 6.10. Respiratory System

from which all the oxygen has been extracted and used) enters the right atrium and then is sent from the right ventricle through the pulmonary artery to the lungs, where it collects oxygen. The oxygen-rich blood then returns to the left atrium of the heart and is pumped out the left ventricle to the rest of the body.

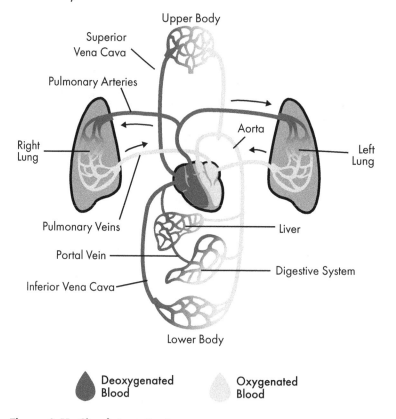

Figure 6.11. Circulatory System

Blood travels through a system of vessels. **Arteries** branch directly off the heart and carry blood away from it. The largest artery is the aorta, which carries blood from the heart to the rest of the body. **Veins** carry blood back to the heart from other parts of the body. Most veins carry deoxygenated blood, but the pulmonary veins carry oxygenated blood from the lungs back to the heart to then be pumped to the rest of the body. Arteries and veins branch into smaller and smaller vessels until they become **capillaries**, which are the smallest vessels and the site where gas exchange occurs.

The **skeletal system**, which is composed of the body's **bones** and **joints**, provides support for the body and helps with movement. Bones also store some of the body's nutrients and produce specific types of cells. Humans are born with 237 bones. However, many of these bones fuse during childhood, and adults have only 206 bones. Bones can have a rough or smooth texture and come in four basic shapes: long, flat, short, and irregular.

The **muscular system** allows the body to move and also moves blood and other substances through the body. The human body has three types of muscles. Skeletal muscles are voluntary muscles (meaning they can be controlled) that are attached to bones and move the body. Smooth muscles are involuntary muscles (meaning they cannot be controlled) that create movement in cerebellum, and medulla. The **cerebrum** is the biggest part of the brain, the wrinkly gray part at the front and top, and controls different functions like thinking, vision, hearing, touch, and smell. The **cerebellum** is located at the back and bottom of the brain and controls motor movements. The **medulla**, or brain stem, is where the brain connects to the spinal cord and controls automatic body functions like breathing and heartbeat.

The peripheral nervous system (PNS) includes small cells called **neurons** that transmit information throughout the body using electrical signals. Neurons are made up of three basic parts: the cell body, dendrites, and axons. The cell body is the main part of the cell where the organelles are located. Dendrites are long arms that extend from the main cell body and communicate with other cells' dendrites through chemical messages passed across a space called a synapse. Axons are extensions from the cell body and transmit messages to the muscles.

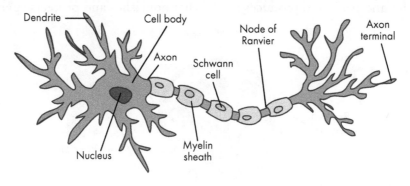

Figure 6.13. Neuron

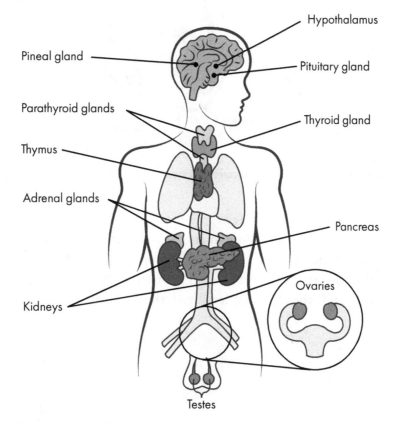

Figure 6.14. Endocrine System

The **endocrine system** is a collection of organs that produce **hormones**, which are chemicals that regulate bodily processes. These organs include the pituitary gland, hypothalamus, pineal gland, thyroid gland, parathyroid glands, adrenal glands, testes (in males), ovaries (in females), and the placenta (in pregnant females). Together, the hormones these organs produce regulate a wide variety of bodily functions, including hunger, sleep, mood, reproduction, and temperature. Some organs that are part of other systems can also act as endocrine organs, including the pancreas and liver.

The reproductive system includes the organs necessary for sexual reproduction. In males, sperm is produced in the **testes** (also known as **testicles**) and carried through a thin tube called the **vas deferens** to the **urethra**, which carries sperm through the **penis** and out of the body. The **prostate** is a muscular gland approximately the size of a walnut that is located between the male bladder and penis and produces a fluid that nourishes and protects sperm.

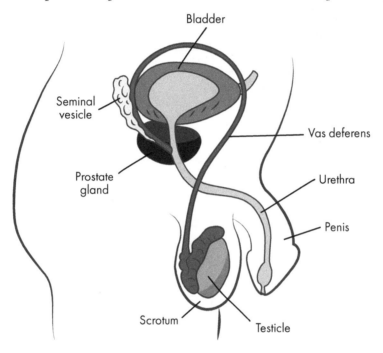

Figure 6.15. Male Reproductive System

In the female reproductive system, eggs are produced in the **ovaries** and released roughly once a month to move through the **fallopian tubes** to the **uterus**. If an egg is fertilized, the new embryo implants in the lining of the uterus and develops over the course of about nine months. At the end of **gestation**, the baby leaves the uterus through the cervix, and exits the body through the **vagina.** If the egg is not fertilized, the uterus will shed its lining.

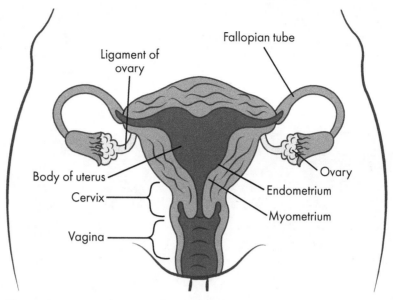

Figure 6.16. Female Reproductive System

PRACTICE QUESTIONS

13.   The small bones in the hands are known as the

      a.   tarsals

      b.   ribs

      c.   metatarsals

      d.   vertebrae

      e.   phalanges

Answer:

e. is correct. The small bones in the fingers of the hands are the phalanges.

14.   In the digestive tract, most of the nutrients are absorbed in the

      a.   small intestine

      b.   rectum

      c.   stomach

      d.   large intestine

      e.   esophagus

Answer:

a. is correct. Most nutrients are absorbed by the small intestine.

Test Your Knowledge

Read the question, and then choose the most correct answer.

1. Which of the following is NOT a nucleobase of DNA?

   a. adenine
   b. guanine
   c. thymine
   d. uracil

2. Which of the following is a monomer used to build carbohydrates?

   a. glucose
   b. thymine
   c. aspartic acid
   d. histone

3. Which of the following processes uses the information stored in RNA to produce a protein?

   a. replication
   b. translation
   c. transcription
   d. mutation

4. The information stored in DNA is used to make which of the following molecules?

   a. amino acids
   b. proteins
   c. fatty acids
   d. monosaccharides

5. Which of the following is NOT present in an animal cell?

   a. nucleus
   b. mitochondria
   c. cytoplasm
   d. cell wall

6. Which of the following cell organelles are the site of lipid synthesis?

   a. smooth endoplasmic reticulum
   b. ribosome
   c. rough endoplasmic reticulum
   d. Golgi apparatus

7. Which of the following cellular processes does NOT use ATP?

   a. facilitated diffusion
   b. DNA replication
   c. active transport through the cell membrane
   d. movement of the mot complex in a flagellum

8. Which of the following molecules can be found in abundance in a fatigued muscle?

   a. glucose
   b. lactic acid
   c. ATP
   d. myoglobin

9. Why do some photosynthetic structures, like leaves, appear green?

   a. The epidermis of the leaf absorbs red and blue light.
   b. The epidermis of the leaf absorbs green light.
   c. The chlorophyll of the leaf absorbs red and blue light.
   d. The chlorophyll of the leaf absorbs green light.

10. The Calvin cycle produces one molecule of glucose from which of the following three molecules?

    a. ATP, NADPH, and O_2
    b. ATP, NADPH, and CO_2
    c. CO_2, H_2O, and ATP
    d. CO_2, H_2O, and O_2

11. The result of meiosis and cytokinesis is

    a. two haploid (1n) cells.
    b. four haploid (1n) cells.
    c. two diploid (2n) cells.
    d. four diploid (2n) cells.

12. Alleles for brown eyes (B) are dominant over alleles for blue eyes (b). If two parents are both heterozygous for this gene, what is the percent chance that their offspring will have brown eyes?

    a. 25
    b. 50
    c. 75
    d. 100

13. If a plant that is homozygous dominant (T) for a trait is crossed with a plant that is homozygous recessive (t) for the same trait, what will be the phenotype of the offspring if the trait follows Mendelian patterns of inheritance?

    a. All offspring will show the dominant phenotype.
    b. All offspring will show the recessive phenotype.
    c. Half the offspring will show the dominant trait, and the other half will show the recessive phenotype.
    d. All the offspring will show a mix of the dominant and recessive phenotypes.

14. A female who carries the recessive color blindness gene mates with a color-blind male, resulting in a male child. Which of the following numbers represents the likelihood the offspring will also be color blind?

    a. 25 percent
    b. 50 percent
    c. 100 percent
    d. 0 percent

15. Type AB blood—the expression of both A and B antigens on a red blood cell surface—occurs as the result of which of the following?

    a. incomplete dominance
    b. recombination
    c. codominance
    d. independent assortment

16. Which of the following is NOT a condition of natural selection?

    a. differential reproduction
    b. competition between species
    c. overproduction of offspring
    d. inheritance of traits

17. Which of the following is the type of nonrandom mating that leads to changes in allele frequency?

    a. sexual selection
    b. genetic drift
    c. migration
    d. gene flow

18. Which of the following aquatic biomes are located where freshwater streams empty into the ocean?

    a. wetlands
    b. coral reef
    c. estuaries
    d. littoral

19. Which of the following scenarios accurately describes primary succession?

   a. The ground is scorched by a lava flow; later the establishment of lichens begins on the volcanic rock, leading to the eventual formation of soils.

   b. A meadow is destroyed by a flood; eventually small grasses begin to grow again to begin establishing a healthy meadow ecosystem.

   c. A fire destroys a section of a forest; once the ashes clear, small animals begin making their homes within the area.

   d. A farmer overuses the land causing all the minerals and nutrients in the soil to be used up. Some leftover grass seeds in the soil begin to sprout, repopulating the land.

20. A barnacle is attached to the outside of the whale to collect and consume particulate matter as the whale moves through the ocean. The barnacle benefits, while the whale is unaffected. The phenomenon described is an example of

   a. predation
   b. commensalism
   c. mutualism
   d. parasitism

21. Which of the following organisms generate their own food through photosynthesis and make up the first level of the energy pyramid?

   a. heterotrophs
   b. autotrophs
   c. producers
   d. consumers

22. Which of the following is composed only of members of the same species?

   a. ecosystem
   b. community
   c. biome
   d. population

23. Which of the following type of muscle is responsible for voluntary movement in the body?

   a. cardiac
   b. visceral
   c. smooth
   d. skeletal

24. Which of the following organs is an accessory organ that food does NOT pass through as part of digestion?

   a. pharynx
   b. mouth
   c. small intestine
   d. liver

25. Which of the following is NOT a function of the respiratory system in humans?

   a. to exchange gas
   b. to produce sound and speech
   c. to distribute oxygen to the rest of the body
   d. to remove particles from the air

ANSWER KEY

1. d.

Uracil (U) is a pyrimidine found in RNA, replacing the thymine (T) pyrimidine found in DNA.

2. a.

Glucose is a monosaccharide that can be used to build larger polysaccharides.

3. b.

Translation is a process of matching codons in RNA to the correct anti-codon to manufacture a protein.

4. b.

Proteins are the expressed products of a gene.

5. d.

The cell wall is the structure that gives plant cells their rigidity.

6. a.

The smooth endoplasmic reticulum is a series of membranes attached to the cell nucleus and plays an important role in the production and storage of lipids. It is called smooth because it lacks ribosomes on the membrane surface.

7. a.

Facilitated diffusion is a form of passive transport across the cell membrane and does not use energy.

8. b.

Lactic acid, a byproduct of anaerobic respiration, builds up in muscles and causes fatigue. This occurs when the energy exerted by the muscle exceeds the amount of oxygen available for aerobic respiration.

9. c.

Light passes through the epidermis and strikes the pigment chlorophyll, which absorbs the wavelengths of light that humans see as red and blue and reflects the wavelengths of light that the human eye perceives as green.

10. b.

Glucose is produced from CO_2 by the energy stored in ATP and the hydrogen atoms associated with NADPH.

11. b.

Four haploid (1n) cells are produced during meiosis.

12. c.

The Punnett square shows that there is a 75 percent chance the child will have the dominant B gene, and thus have brown eyes.

	B	b
B	BB	Bb
b	Bb	bb

13. a.

Because each offspring will inherit the dominant allele, all the offspring will show the dominant phenotype. The offspring would only show a mix of the two phenotypes if they did not follow Mendelian inheritance patterns.

14. b.

The offspring has a 50 percent chance of inheriting the dominant allele and a 50 percent chance of inheriting the recessive allele from his mother.

15. c.

Type AB blood occurs when two equally dominant alleles (A and B) are inherited. Since they are both dominant, one does not mask the other; instead, both are expressed.

16. b.

Competition between species is not necessary for natural selection to occur, although it can influence the traits that are selected for within a population.

17. a.

Sexual selection changes allele frequency because it leads to some members of the population reproducing more frequently than others.

18. c.

Estuaries are found at the boundary of ocean and stream biomes and are very ecologically productive areas.

19. a.

Primary succession can only occur on newly exposed earth that was not previously inhabited by living things. Often this new land is the result of lava flows or glacial movement.

20. b.

In a commensal relationship, one species benefits with no impact on the other.

21. c.

Producers are a kind of autotroph that are found on the energy pyramid and produce food via photosynthesis.

22. d.

A population is all the members of the same species in a given area.

23. d.

Skeletal muscles are attached to the skeletal system and are controlled voluntarily.

24. d.

The liver is an accessory organ that detoxifies ingested toxins and produces bile for fat digestion.

25. c.

The cardiovascular system distributes oxygen to the rest of the body.

SEVEN: PHYSICAL SCIENCE

The Structure of the Atom

All matter is composed of very small particles called **atoms**. Atoms can be further broken down into subatomic particles. **Protons**, which are positive, and **neutrons**, which are neutral, form the nucleus of the atom. Negative particles called **electrons** orbit the nucleus.

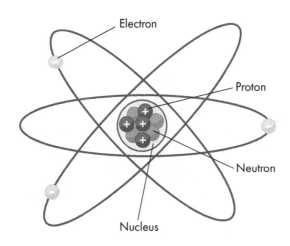

Figure 7.1. Structure of the Atom

While electrons are often depicted as orbiting the nucleus like a planet orbits the sun, they're actually arranged in cloud-like areas called **shells**. The shells closest to the nucleus have the lowest energy and are filled first. The high-energy shells farther from the nucleus only fill with electrons once lower-energy shells are full.

The outermost electron shell of an atom is its **valence shell**. The electrons in this shell are involved in chemical reactions. Atoms are most stable when their valence shell is full (usually with eight electrons), so the atom will lose, gain, or share electrons to fill its valence shell.

A neutral atom will have an equal number of protons and electrons. When a neutral atom loses or gains electrons, it gains or loses charge accordingly, forming an **ion**. An ion with more protons than electrons has a positive charge and is called a **cation**. An ion with more electrons than protons has a negative charge and is considered an **anion**.

 The attractive and repulsive forces in an atom follow the universal law that "like charges repel and opposite charges attract."

For example, the element oxygen (O) has eight protons and eight electrons. A neutral oxygen atom is represented simply as O. However, if it gains two electrons, it becomes an anion with a charge of −2 and is written as O^{2-}.

All atoms with the same number of protons are the same **element** and cannot be further reduced to a simpler substance by chemical processes. Each element has a symbol, which is a one- or two-letter abbreviation for the element's name. The number of protons in an atom is that atom's **atomic number**.

 Many element symbols are derived from the Latin names for elements. For example, the Latin name for *gold* is *aurum*, and its symbol is Au.

Along with atomic charge, atoms have measurable mass. Protons and neutrons are significantly more massive than electrons (about 1,800 times), so the mass of electrons is not considered when calculating the mass of an atom. Thus, an element's **mass number** is the number of protons and neutrons present in its atoms.

PRACTICE QUESTIONS

1. An atom with five protons and seven electrons has a charge of
    a. −12
    b. −2
    c. 2
    d. 5
    e. 12

    Answer:

    b. is correct. The total charge of an atom is the difference between the number of protons and electrons. Subtract the number of electrons from the number of protons: 5 − 7 = −2.

2. The ion with the greatest number of electrons is
    a. K^+
    b. Cl^-
    c. Ca^+
    d. P^{3-}
    e. S^{2-}

    Answer:

    c. is correct. Calcium has an atomic number of 20 (found on the periodic table), meaning it has twenty protons. For a Ca ion to have a charge of 1+, it must have nineteen electrons. All the other ions have eighteen electrons.

1	2	3	4	5	6	7	8	9	10	11	12	13	14	15	16	17	18
1 H Hydrogen 1.008																	2 He Helium 4.0026
3 Li Lithium 6.941	4 Be Beryllium 9.0122											5 B Boron 10.81	6 C Carbon 12.011	7 N Nitrogen 14.007	8 O Oxygen 15.999	9 F Fluorine 18.998	10 Ne Neon 20.180
11 Na Sodium 22.990	12 Mg Magnesium 24.305											13 Al Aluminum 26.982	14 Si Silicon 28.085	15 P Phosphorus 30.974	16 S Sulfur 32.06	17 Cl Chlorine 35.45	18 Ar Argon 39.948
19 K Potassium 39.098	20 Ca Calcium 40.078	21 Sc Scandium 44.956	22 Ti Titanium 47.867	23 V Vanadium 50.942	24 Cr Chromium 51.996	25 Mn Maganese 54.938	26 Fe Iron 55.845	27 Co Cobalt 58.933	28 Ni Nickel 58.963	29 Cu Copper 63.546	30 Zn Zinc 65.38	31 Ga Gallium 69.723	32 Ge Germanium 72.64	33 Es Arsenic 74.922	34 Se Selenium 78.971	35 Br Bromine 79.904	36 Kr Krypton 83.798
37 Rb Rubidium 85.468	38 Sr Strontium 87.62	39 Y Yttrium 88.906	40 Zr Zirconium 91.224	41 Nb Niobium 92.906	42 Mo Molybdenum 254	43 Tc Technetium 98	44 Ru Ruthenium 101.07	45 Rh Rhodium 102.91	46 Pd Palladium 106.42	47 Ag Silver 107.87	48 Cd Cadmium 112.41	49 In Indium 114.82	50 Sn Tin 118.71	51 Sb Antimony 121.76	52 Te Tellurium 127.60	53 I Iodine 126.90	54 Xe Xenon 121.29
55 Cs Caesium 132.91	56 Ba Barium 137.33	57-71	72 Hf Hafnium 178.49	73 Ta Tantalum 183.84	74 W Tungsten 183.84	75 Re Rhenium 186.21	76 Os Osmium 190.23	77 Ir Iridium 192.22	78 Pt Platinum 195.08	79 Au Gold 196.97	80 Hg Mercury 200.59	81 Tl Thallium 204.38	82 Pb Lead 207.2	83 Bi Bismuth 208.98	84 Po Polonium 209	85 At Astatine 210	86 Rn Radon 222
87 Fr Francium 223.020	88 Ra Radium 226	89-103	104 Rf Rutherfordium 267	105 Db Dubnium 268	106 Sg Seaborgium 271	107 Bh Bohrium 272	108 Hs Hassium 277	109 Mt Meitnerium 276	110 Ds Darmstadtium 281	111 Rg Roentgenium 280	112 Cn Copernicium 285	113 Uut Ununtrium Unknown	114 Fl Flerovium 254	115 Uup Ununpentium Unknown	116 Lv Livermorium 291	117 Uus Ununseptium Unknown	118 Uuo Ununoctium Unknown

Atomic Number
Symbol
Name
Atomic Mass

Lanthanide	57 La Lanthanium 138.905	58 Ce Cerium 140.12	59 Pr Praseodymium 140.91	60 Nd Neodymium 144.24	61 Pm Promethium 144.913	62 Sm Samarium 150.36	63 Eu Europium 151.96	64 Gd Gadolinium 157.25	65 Tb Terbium 158.93	66 Dy Dysprosium 152.50	67 Ho Holmium 154.930	68 Er Erbium 167.259	69 Tm Thulium 168.934	70 Yb Ytterbium 173.065	71 Lu Lutetium 174.967
Actinide	89 Ac Actinium 227.028	90 Th Thorium 232.038	91 Pa Protactinuim 231.036	92 U Uranium 238.029	93 Np Neptunium 237.048	94 Pu Plutonium 244.064	95 Am Americium 243.061	96 Cm Curium 247.070	97 Bk Berkelium 247.070	98 Cf Californium 251.080	99 Es Einsteinium 254	100 Fm Fermium 257.095	101 Md Mendelevium 258.1	102 No Nobelium 259.101	103 Lr Lawrencium 262

Alkaline Metal | Alkaline Earth Metals | Transition Metal | Basic Metal | Metalloid | Nonmetal | Halogen | Noble Gas | Lanthanide | Actinide

Figure 7.2. The Periodic Table of the Elements

The Periodic Table of the Elements

Elements are arranged on the **Periodic Table of the Elements** by their atomic number, which increases from top to bottom and left to right on the table. Hydrogen, the first element on the periodic table, has one proton while helium, the second element, has two, and so on.

The rows of the periodic table are called **periods**, and the vertical columns are called **groups**. Each group contains elements with the same number of valence electrons, meaning the elements have similar chemical properties.

The majority of the elements in the periodic table are metals. Metals have the following properties:

+ They are hard, opaque, and shiny.
+ They are ductile and malleable.
+ They conduct electricity and heat.
+ With the exception of mercury, they are solids.

Metals begin on the left side of the periodic table and span across the middle of the table, almost all the way to the right side. Examples of metals include gold (Au), tin (Sn), and lead (Pb).

Nonmetals are elements that do not conduct electricity and tend to be more reactive than metals. They can be solids, liquids, or gases. The nonmetals are located on the right side of the periodic table. Examples of nonmetals include sulfur (S), hydrogen (H), and oxygen (O).

Metalloids, or semimetals, are elements that possess both metal and nonmetal characteristics. For example, some metalloids are shiny but do not conduct electricity well. Metalloids are located between the metals and nonmetals on the periodic table. Some examples of metalloids are boron (B), silicon (Si), and arsenic (As).

PRACTICE QUESTIONS

3. Bismuth is a
   a. metal
   b. nonmetal
   c. metalloid
   d. transition element
   e. noble gas

   Answer:

   a. is correct. Bismuth is a metal.

4. Fluorine is most likely to form an ionic compound with
   a. nickel (Ni)
   b. beryllium (Be)
   c. sodium (Na)
   d. argon (Ar)
   e. chlorine (Cl)

Chemical Bonds

Chemical bonds are attractions between atoms that create molecules, which are substances consisting of more than one atom. There are three types of bonds: ionic, covalent, and metallic.

In an **ionic bond**, one atom "gives" its electrons to the other, resulting in one positively and one negatively charged atom. The bond is a result of the attraction between the two ions. Ionic bonds form between atoms on the left side of the periodic table (which will lose electrons) and those on the right side (which will gain electrons). Table salt (NaCl) is an example of a molecule held together by an ionic bond.

A **covalent bond** is created by a pair of atoms sharing electrons to fill their valence shells. In a **nonpolar** covalent bond, the electrons are shared evenly. In a **polar** covalent bond, the electrons are shared unevenly. One atom will exert a stronger pull on the shared electrons, giving that atom a slight negative charge. The other atom in the bond will have a slight positive charge. Water (H_2O) is an example of a polar molecule.

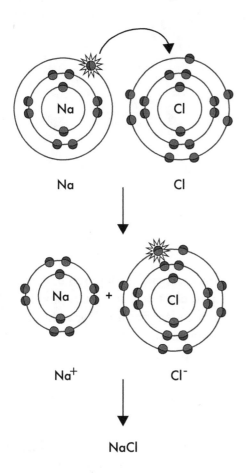

Figure 7.3. The Ionic Bond in Table Salt

The polar nature of water is responsible for many of its unique properties. The small charges within a water molecule cause attraction between the molecules. The molecules then "stick" to each other (cohesion) and to other surfaces (adhesion).

Metals can form tightly packed arrays in which each atom is in close contact with many neighbors. The valence electrons are free to move between atoms and create a "sea" of delocalized charge. Any excitation, such as an electrical current, can cause the electrons to move throughout the array. The high electrical and thermal conductivity of metals is due to this ability of electrons to move throughout the lattice. This type of delocalized bonding is called **metallic bonding**.

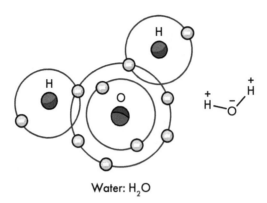

Water: H_2O

Figure 7.4. Polar Covalent Bond

PRACTICE QUESTION

5. A polar covalent bond joins the atoms in the molecule

    a.   LiF

    b. CO_2

    c. H_2

    d.   NaOH

    e. O_2

Answer:

b. is correct. Carbon and oxygen are both nonmetals that combine through a covalent bond. Oxygen has a strong pull on their shared electrons, so CO_2 is polar. In hydrogen and oxygen gases, the identical atoms share electrons equally, so both compounds are nonpolar. Choices a and d are ionic compounds.

Properties of Matter

Matter is any substance that takes up space. The amount of matter in an object is that object's **mass**, which is measured in grams or kilograms. Mass is different from **weight**, which is a measure of the gravitational force exerted on an object. An object's mass never changes, but its weight will change if the gravitational force changes. The **density** of an object is the ratio of an object's mass to its volume.

> Objects weigh less on the moon than on the earth because the pull of gravity on the moon is lower than that on earth. However, the mass of the object is the same no matter where in the universe it goes.

Properties of substances are divided into two categories: physical and chemical. **Physical properties** are those that are measurable and can be seen without changing the chemical makeup of a substance. In contrast, **chemical properties** are those that determine how a substance will behave in a chemical reaction. Chemical properties cannot be identified simply by observing a material. Instead, the material must be engaged in a chemical reaction in order to identify its chemical properties. A **physical change** is a change in a substance's physical properties, and a **chemical change** is a change in its chemical properties.

Table 7.1. Properties of Matter

Physical Properties	Chemical Properties
mass	heat of combustion
temperature	flammability
density	toxicity
color	chemical stability
viscosity	enthalpy of formation

 In both physical and chemical changes, matter is always conserved, meaning it can never be created or destroyed.

Temperature is the name given to the kinetic energy of all the atoms or molecules in a substance. While it might look like matter is not in motion, in fact, its atoms have kinetic energy and are constantly spinning and vibrating. The more energy the atoms have (meaning the more they spin and vibrate) the higher the substance's temperature.

Heat is the movement of energy from one substance to another. Energy will spontaneously move from high-energy (high-temperature) substances to low-energy (low-temperature) substances.

PRACTICE QUESTION

6. A substance that can change shape but not volume is a
   a. solid
   b. liquid
   c. gas
   d. solid or liquid
   e. liquid or gas

Answer:

b. is correct. Liquids can change shape (for instance, when they are poured from one container into another) but not volume.

States of Matter

All matter exists in different **states** (or phases) that depend on the energy of the molecules in the matter. **Solid** matter has densely packed molecules and does not change volume or shape. **Liquids** have more loosely packed molecules and can change shape but not volume. **Gas** molecules are widely dispersed, and gases can change both shape and volume.

Changes in temperature and pressure can cause matter to change states. Generally, adding energy (in the form of heat) changes a substance to a higher energy state (e.g., solid to liquid). Transitions from a high to lower energy state (e.g., liquid to solid) release energy. Each of these changes has a specific name, summarized in the table below.

Table 7.2. Changes in State of Matter

Name	From	To	Occurs At	Enery Change
evaporation	liquid	gas	boiling point	uses energy
condensation	gas	liquid	boiling point	releases energy
melting	solid	liquid	freezing point	uses energy
freezing	liquid	solid	freezing point	releases energy
sublimation	solid	gas	---	uses energy
deposition	gas	solid	---	releases energy

PRACTICE QUESTION

7.   The process that takes place when water reaches its boiling point is called

a.   condensation

b.   evaporation

c.   melting

d.   sublimation

e.   freezing

Answer:

b. is correct. Evaporation is the process of conversion from liquid to gas that occurs at the boiling point.

Chemical Reactions

A **chemical reaction** occurs when one or more substances react to form new substances. **Reactants** are the substances that are consumed or altered in the chemical reaction, and the new substances are **products**. Equations are written with the reactants on the left, the products on the right, and an arrow between them. The state of the chemical compounds are sometimes noted using the labels *s* (solid), *l* (liquid), *g* (gas), or *aq* (aqueous, meaning a solution).

The equation below shows the reaction of hydrogen gas (H_2) and chlorine gas (Cl_2) to form hydrogen chloride (HCl), an acid.

$$H_2\ (g) + Cl_2\ (g) \rightarrow 2HCl\ (aq)$$

Chemical reactions follow the **law of conservation of matter**, which states that matter cannot be created or destroyed. In a reaction, the same types and numbers of atoms that appear on the left side must also appear on the right. To **balance** a chemical equation, coefficients (the numbers before the reactant or product) are added. In the equation above, a coefficient of two is needed on HCl so that two hydrogen and two chlorine atoms appear on each side of the arrow.

There are five main types of chemical reactions; these are summarized in the table below.

Table 7.3. Types of Reactions

Type of Reaction	General Formula	Example Reaction
Synthesis	$A + B \rightarrow C$	$2H_2 + O_2 \rightarrow 2H_2O$
Decomposition	$A \rightarrow B + C$	$2H_2O_2 \rightarrow 2H_2O + O_2$
Single displacement	$AB + C \rightarrow A + BC$	$CH_4 + Cl_2 \rightarrow CH_3Cl + HCl$
Double displacement	$AB + CD \rightarrow AC + BD$	$CuCl_2 + 2AgNo_3 \rightarrow Cu(NO_3)_2 + 2AgCl$
Combustion	$C_xH_y + O_2 \rightarrow CO_2 + H_2O$	$2C_8H_{18} + 25O_2 \rightarrow 16CO_2 + 18H_2O$

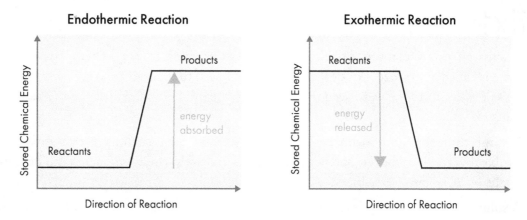

Figure 7.5. Stored Energy in Endothermic and Exothermic Reactions

Energy is required to break chemical bonds, and it is released when bonds form. The total energy absorbed or released during a chemical reaction will depend on the individual bonds being broken and formed. A reaction that releases energy is **exothermic**, and a reaction that absorbs energy is **endothermic**.

PRACTICE QUESTIONS

8. $Pb(NO_3)_2 + K_2CrO_4 \rightarrow PbCrO_4 + 2KNO_3$

The reaction shown above is a

a. combustion reaction

b. decomposition reaction

c. double-displacement reaction

d. single-replacement reaction

e. acid-base neutralization reaction

c. is correct. In the reaction, Pb and K exchange their anions in a double-displacement reaction.

9. An example of a balanced equation is

    a. $KClO_3 \rightarrow KCl + 3O_2$

    b. $2KClO_3 \rightarrow KCl + 2O_2$

    c. $2KClO_3 \rightarrow 2KCl + 3O_2$

    d. $4KClO_3 \rightarrow 2KCl + 2O_2$

    e. $6KClO_3 \rightarrow 6KCl + 3O_2$

Answer:

c. is correct. In this equation, there are equal numbers of each type of atom on both sides (two K atoms, two Cl atoms, and six O atoms).

Mixtures

When substances are combined without a chemical reaction to bond them, the resulting substance is called a **mixture**. Physical changes can be used to separate mixtures. For example, heating salt water until the water evaporates, leaving the salt behind, will separate a salt water solution.

In a mixture, the components can be unevenly distributed, such as in trail mix or soil. These mixtures are described at **heterogeneous**. Alternatively, the components can be **homogeneously**, or uniformly, distributed, as in salt water.

A **solution** is a special type of stable homogeneous mixture. The components of a solution will not separate on their own and cannot be separated using a filter. The substance being dissolved is the **solute**, and the substance acting on the solute, or doing the dissolving, is the **solvent**.

> Solutions can exist as solids, liquids, or gases. For example, carbonated water has a gaseous solute (CO_2) and a liquid solvent (water). A solution formed by combining two solid metals, such as stainless steel, is an **alloy**.

The **solubility** of a solution is the maximum amount of solute that will dissolve in a specific quantity of solvent at a specified temperature. Solutions can be saturated, unsaturated, or supersaturated based on the amount of solute dissolved in the solution.

+ A **saturated** solution has the maximum amount of solute that can be dissolved in the solvent.

+ An **unsaturated** solution contains less solute than a saturated solution would hold.

+ A **supersaturated solution** contains more solvent than a saturated solution. A supersaturated solution can be made by heating the solution to dissolve additional solute and then slowly cooling it down to a specified temperature.

10. A heterogeneous mixture is one in which

a.   the atoms or molecules are distributed unevenly

b.   two substances are in different states

c.   there is a mixture of covalent and ionic compounds

d.   there is a mixture of polar and nonpolar molecules

e.   three or more different molecules are mixed together

Answer:

a. is correct. A heterogeneous mixture is any nonuniform mixture, which means the atoms or molecules are unevenly distributed.

11. A solution in which more solvent can be dissolved is called

a.   unsaturated

b.   saturated

c.   supersaturated

d.   homogeneous

e.   heterogeneous

Answer:

a. is correct. An unsaturated solution has less solute than can be dissolved in the given amount of solvent.

Acids and Bases

Acids and bases are substances that share a distinct set of physical properties. **Acids** are corrosive, sour, and change the color of vegetable dyes like litmus from blue to red. **Bases**, or alkaline solutions, are slippery, bitter, and change the color of litmus from red to blue.

There are a number of different ways to define acids and bases, but generally acids release hydrogen ions (H^+) in solution, while bases release hydroxide (OH^-) ions. For example, hydrochloric acid (HCl) ionizes, or breaks apart, in solution to release H^+ ions:

$$HCl \rightarrow H^+ + Cl$$

The base sodium hydroxide (NaOH) ionizes to release OH^- ions:

$$NaOH \rightarrow Na^+ + OH^-$$

Acids and bases combine in a **neutralization reaction**. During the reaction, the H^+ and OH^- ions join to form water, and the remaining ions combine to form a salt:

$$HCl + NaOH \rightarrow H_2O + NaCl$$

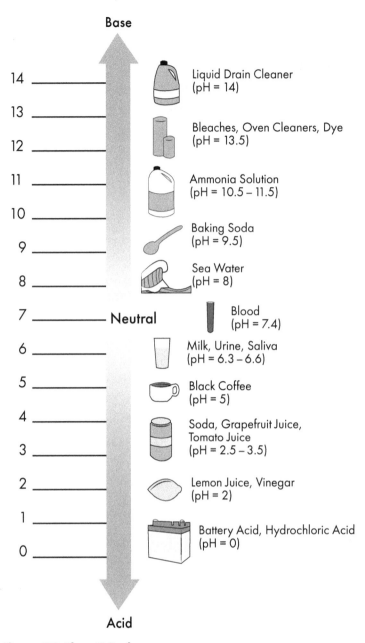

Figure 7.6. The pH Scale

🔍 A **buffer**, or buffer solution, is a solution that resists changes in pH when small quantities of acids or bases are added. A buffer can do this because it contains a weak acid to react with any added base and a weak base to react with any added acid.

The strength of an acid or base is measured on the **pH scale**, which ranges from 1 to 14, with 1 being the strongest acid, 14 being the strongest base, and 7 being neutral. A substance's pH value is a measure of how many hydrogen ions are in the solution. The scale is logarithmic, meaning an acid with a pH of 3 has ten times as many hydrogen ions as an acid with a pH of 4. Water, which separates into equal numbers of H^+ and OH^- ions, has a neutral pH of 7.

12. A neutralization reaction produces

    a. a base

    b. a buffer

    c. hydrogen ions

    d. a salt

    e. an acid

Answer:

d. is correct. A neutralization reaction occurs when an acid and a base combine to form a salt and water.

13. When a nitric acid solution is diluted by a factor of ten, the pH will

    a. go up ten units

    b. go down ten units

    c. go up one unit

    d. go down one unit

    e. stay the same

Answer:

c. is correct. The pH will go up: diluting an acid will decrease the concentration of H^+ ions, and higher pH values represent lower concentrations of H^+ ions. Diluting the acid by a factor of ten will change the pH one unit because the pH scale is logarithmic.

Motion

To study motion, it is necessary to understand the concept of scalars and vectors. **Scalars** are measurements that have a quantity but no direction. **Vectors**, in contrast, have both a quantity and a direction. **Distance** is a scalar: it describes how far an object has traveled along a path. Distance can have values such as 54 m or 16 miles. **Displacement** is a vector: it describes how far an object has traveled from its starting position. A displacement value will indicate direction, such as 54 m east or −16 miles.

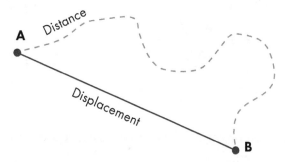

Figure 7.7. Distance versus Displacement

Table 7.4. Physical Science Units

mass	kilograms (kg)
displacement	meters (m)
velocity	meters per second (m/s)
acceleration	meters per second per second (m/s^2)
force	Newtons (N)
work	Joules (J)
energy	Joules (J)
current	amperes (A)
voltage	volts (V)

Speed describes how quickly something is moving. It is found by dividing distance by time, and so is a scalar value. **Velocity** is the rate at which an object changes position. Velocity is found by dividing displacement by time, meaning it is a vector value. An object that travels a certain distance and then returns to its starting point has a velocity of zero because its final position did not change. Its speed, however, can be found by dividing the total distance it traveled by the time it took to make the trip.

Acceleration describes how quickly an object changes velocity. It is also a vector: when acceleration is in the same direction as velocity, the object will move faster. When the acceleration is in the opposite direction of velocity, the object will slow down.

PRACTICE QUESTION

14. A person who starts from rest and increases his velocity to 5 m/s over a time period of 1 second has an acceleration of

   a.   −5 m/s^2

   b.   0 m/s^2

   c.   1 m/s^2

   d.   5 m/s^2

   e.   10 m/s^2

<u>Answer:</u>

d. is correct. Acceleration is the change in velocity over the change in time:

$$a = \frac{v}{t} = \frac{(5 \text{ m/s} - 0 \text{ m/s})}{1 \text{ s}} = \textbf{5 m/s}^2$$

Forces

A push or pull that causes an object to move or change direction is called a **force**. Forces can arise from a number of different sources.

- **Gravity** is the attraction of one mass to another mass. For example, the earth's gravitational field pulls objects toward it, and the sun's gravitational field keeps planets in motion around it.
- **Electrical force** is the creation of a field by charged particles that will cause other charged objects in that field to move.
- **Tension** is found in ropes pulling or holding up an object.
- **Friction** is created by two objects moving against each other.
- **Normal force** occurs when an object is resting on another object.
- **Buoyant force** is the upward force experienced by floating objects.

In 1687, Isaac Newton published **three laws of motion** that describe the behavior of force and mass. Newton's first law is also called the **law of inertia**. It states that an object will maintain its current state of motion unless acted on by an outside force.

Newton's **second law** is an equation, $F = ma$. The equation states that increasing the force on an object will increase its acceleration. In addition, the mass of the object will determine its acceleration: under the same force, a small object will accelerate more quickly than a larger object.

An object in equilibrium is either at rest or is moving at constant velocity; in other words, the object has no acceleration, or $a = 0$. Using Newton's second law, an object is in equilibrium if the net force on the object is 0, or $F = 0$ (this is called the equilibrium condition).

Newton's **third law** states that for every action (force), there will be an equal and opposite reaction (force). For instance, if a person is standing on the floor, there is a force of gravity pulling him toward the earth. However, he is not accelerating toward the earth; he is simply standing at rest on the floor (in equilibrium). So, the floor must provide a force that is equal in magnitude and in the opposite direction to the force of gravity.

PRACTICE QUESTIONS

15. A book resting on a table is prevented from falling on the floor by

   a. gravity

   b. tension

   c. friction

   d. electromagnetic force

   e. normal force

   Answer:

   e. is correct. The normal force pushes up to counterbalance the force of gravity, which points down.

16. An example of an object in equilibrium is
   a.   a parachutist after he jumps from an airplane
   b.   an airplane taking off
   c.   a person sitting still in a chair
   d.   a soccer ball when it is kicked
   e.   the moon orbiting the earth

Answer:

c. is correct. A person sitting in a chair is not accelerating. All the other choices describe objects that are accelerating or changing velocity.

Work

Work is a scalar value that is defined as the application of a force over a distance. It is measured in Joules (J).

A person lifting a book off the ground is an example of someone doing work. The book has a weight because it is being pulled toward the earth. As the person lifts the book, her hand and arm are producing a force that is larger than that weight, causing the book to rise. The higher the person lifts the book, the more work is done.

The sign of the work done is important. In the example of lifting a book, the person's hand is doing positive (+) work on the book. However, gravity is always pulling the book down, which means that during a lift, gravity is doing negative (−) work on the book. If the force and the displacement are in the same direction, then the work is positive (+). If the force and the displacement are in opposite directions, then the work is negative (−). In the case of lifting a book, the net work done on the book is positive.

PRACTICE QUESTION

17. The most work is done on a car when
   a.   pushing on the car, but it does not move
   b.   towing the car up a steep hill for 100 m
   c.   pushing the car 5 m across a parking lot
   d.   painting the car
   e.   driving the car in reverse for 5 m

Answer:

b. A steep hill requires a large force to counter the gravitational force. The large distance will also lead to a large amount of work done. Less work is done in choices c and e, and no work is done in choice a. Choice d is incorrect because painting the car is "work," but not the technical definition of work. The car is not moving while being painted, so no work is done on the car.

Energy

Energy is an abstract concept, but everything in nature has an energy associated with it. Energy is measured in Joules (J). There are many types of energy:

+ mechanical: the energy of motion
+ chemical: the energy in chemical bonds
+ thermal: the energy of an object due to its temperature
+ nuclear: the energy in the nucleus of an atom
+ electric: the energy arising from charged particles
+ magnetic: the energy arising from a magnetic field

There is an energy related to movement called the **kinetic energy (KE)**. Any object that has mass and is moving will have a kinetic energy.

Potential energy (PE) is the energy stored in a system; it can be understood as the potential for an object to gain kinetic energy. There are several types of potential energy.

+ **Electric potential energy** is derived from the interaction between positive and negative charges.
+ Compressing a spring stores **elastic potential energy**.
+ Energy is also stored in chemical bonds as **chemical potential energy**.
+ The energy stored by objects due to their height is **gravitational potential energy**.

Energy can be converted into other forms of energy, but it cannot be created or destroyed. This principle is called the **conservation of energy**. A swing provides a simple example of this principle. Throughout the swing's path, the total energy of the system remains the same. At the highest point of a swing's path, it has potential energy but no kinetic energy (because it has stopped moving momentarily as it changes direction). As the swing drops, that potential energy is converted to kinetic energy, and the swing's velocity increases. At the bottom of its path, all its potential energy has been converted into kinetic energy (meaning its potential energy is

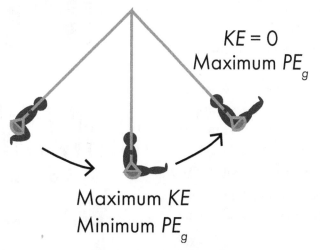

Figure 7.8. Conservation of Energy in a Swing

zero). This process repeats as the swing moves up and down. At any point in the swing's path, the kinetic and potential energies will sum to the same value.

PRACTICE QUESTION

18. The energy stored in a compressed spring is
  a. nuclear energy
  b. mechanical energy
  c. chemical potential energy
  d. gravitational potential energy
  e. elastic potential energy

  <u>Answer:</u>

  e. is correct. Compressing a spring stores elastic potential energy, which is turned into kinetic energy when the spring is released.

Waves

Energy can also be transferred through **waves**, which are repeating pulses of energy. Waves that travel through a medium, like ripples on a pond or compressions in a Slinky, are called **mechanical waves**. Waves that vibrate up and down (like the ripples on a pond) are **transverse waves**, and those that travel through compression (like the Slinky) are **longitudinal waves**. Mechanical waves will travel faster through denser mediums; for example, sound waves will move faster through water than through air.

Waves can be described using a number of different properties. A wave's highest point is called its **crest**, and its lowest point is the **trough**. A wave's **midline** is halfway between the crest and trough; the **amplitude** describes the distance between the midline and the crest (or trough). The distance between crests (or troughs) is the **wavelength**. A wave's **period** is the time it takes for a wave to go through one complete cycle, and the number of cycles a wave goes through in a specific period of time is its **frequency**.

Sound is a special type of longitudinal wave created by vibrations. Our ears are able to interpret these waves as particular sounds. The frequency, or rate, of

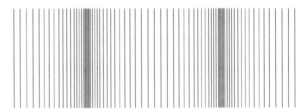
Longitudinal Wave

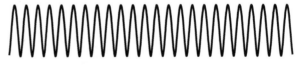
Transverse Wave

Figure 7.9. Types of Waves

the vibration determines the sound's **pitch**. **Loudness** depends on the amplitude, or height, of a sound wave.

The **Doppler effect** is the difference in perceived pitch caused by the motion of the object creating the wave. For example, as an ambulance approaches an observer, the siren's pitch will appear to increase, and then as the ambulance moves away, the siren's pitch will appear to decrease. This occurs because sound waves are compressed as the ambulance approaches the observer and are spread out as the ambulance moves away from the observer.

Electromagnetic waves are composed of oscillating electric and magnetic fields and thus do not require a medium through which to travel. The electromagnetic spectrum classifies the types of electromagnetic waves based on their frequency. These include radio waves, microwaves, X-rays, and visible light.

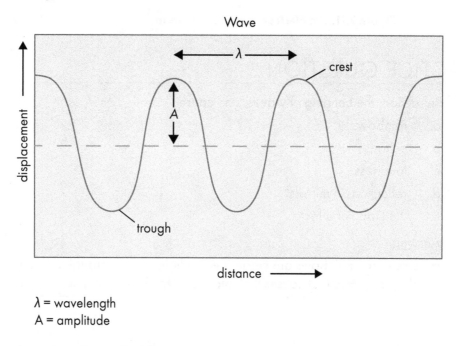

Figure 7.10. Parts of a Wave

The study of light is called **optics**. Because visible light is a wave, it will display properties that are similar to other waves. It will **reflect**, or bounce off, surfaces, which can be observed by shining a flashlight on a mirror. Light will also **refract**, or bend, when it travels between substances. This effect can be seen by placing a pencil in water and observing the apparent bend in the pencil.

Curved pieces of glass called **lenses** can be used to bend light in a way that affects how an image is perceived. Some microscopes, for example, make objects appear larger through the use of specific types of lenses. Eyeglasses also use lenses to correct poor vision.

The frequency of a light wave is responsible for its color, with red/orange colors having a lower frequency than blue/violet colors. White light is a blend of all the frequencies of visible light. Passing white light through a prism will bend each frequency at a slightly different angle, separating the colors and creating a rainbow. Sunlight passing through raindrops can undergo this effect, creating large rainbows in the sky.

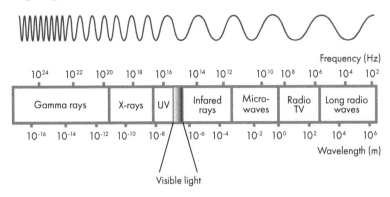

Figure 7.11. The Electromagnetic Spectrum

PRACTICE QUESTION

19. Refraction, the bending of waves, can cause

   a. rainbows

   b. echoes

   c. loudness

   d. reflections in mirrors

   e. the Doppler effect

   Answer:

   a. is correct. Rainbows are created when light passes through an object, such as a raindrop or prism, that causes the colors in light to bend at different angles.

Electricity and Magnetism

Electric charge is created by a difference in the balance of protons and electrons, which creates a positively or negatively charged object. Charged objects create an **electric field** that spreads outward from the object. Other charged objects in that field will experience a force: objects that have opposite charges will be attracted to each other, and objects with the same charge will be repelled, or pushed away, from each other.

Because protons cannot leave the nucleus, charge is created by the movement of electrons. **Static electricity**, or electrostatic charge, occurs when a surface has a buildup of charges. For example, if a student rubs a balloon on her head, the friction will cause electrons to move from her hair to the balloon. This creates a negative charge on the balloon and a positive charge on her hair; the resulting attraction will cause her hair to move toward the balloon.

Electricity is the movement of electrons through a conductor, and an electric circuit is a closed loop through which electricity moves. Circuits include a **voltage** source, which powers the movement of electrons known as **current**. Sources of voltage include batteries, generators, and wall outlets (which are in turn powered by electric power stations). Other elements, such as lights, computers, and microwaves, can then be connected to the circuit and then powered by its electricity.

Magnets are created by the alignment of spinning electrons within a substance. This alignment will occur naturally in some substances, including iron, nickel, and cobalt, all of which can be used to produce permanent magnets. The alignment of electrons creates a magnetic field, which, like an electric or gravitational field, can act on other objects. Magnetic fields have a north and a south pole that act similarly to electric charges: opposite poles will attract, and same poles will repel each other. However, unlike electric charge, which can be either positive or negative, a magnetic field ALWAYS has two poles. If a magnet is cut in half, the result is two magnets, each with a north and a south pole.

Electricity and magnetism are closely related. A moving magnet creates an electric field, and a moving charged particle creates a magnetic field. A specific kind of temporary magnet known as an **electromagnet** can be made by coiling a wire around a metal object and running electricity through it. A magnetic field will be created when the wire contains a current but will disappear when the flow of electricity is stopped.

PRACTICE QUESTION

20. The particles that flow through a circuit to power a light bulb are

    a.   protons

    b.   neutrons

    c.   electrons

    d.   nucleus

    e.   atoms

Answer:

c. is correct. Electrons are negatively charged subatomic particles that exist outside the nucleus of an atom. A power source forces moving electrons through a circuit.

Test Your Knowledge

Read the question, and then choose the most correct answer.

1. Which of the following determines the atomic number of an atom?

    a. the number of electrons orbiting the nucleus

    b. the number of protons in the nucleus

    c. the number of protons and neutrons in the nucleus

    d. the number of protons and electrons in the atom

2. How many neutrons are in an atom of the element $^{88}_{38}Sr$?

    a. 38

    b. 88

    c. 50

    d. 126

3. Refer to the periodic table in Figure 7.2. Which element is a metalloid?

    a. rubidium

    b. vanadium

    c. antimony

    d. iodine

4. Which of the following is NOT a typical property of metals?

    a. Metals have low densities.

    b. Metals are malleable.

    c. Metals are good conductors of electricity and heat.

    d. Metals in solid state consist of ordered structures with tightly packed atoms.

5. Which element has chemical properties most similar to sulfur?

    a. fluorine

    b. argon

    c. phosphorus

    d. oxygen

6. Which of the following groups on the periodic table will typically adopt a charge of +1 when forming ionic compounds?

    a. alkaline earth metals

    b. lanthanides

    c. actinides

    d. alkali metals

7. Match the elements with the type of bond that would occur between them.

Elements	Bond
magnesium and bromine	
carbon and oxygen	
solid copper	

    a. ionic

    b. metallic

    c. covalent

8. Label each compound as polar or nonpolar.

Compound	Polar	Nonpolar
H_2O		
F_2		
HF		

9. How many electrons are included in the double bond between the two oxygen atoms in O_2?

   a. 2
   b. 4
   c. 6
   d. 8

10. Which of the following describes a physical change?

    a. Water becomes ice.
    b. Batter is baked into a cake.
    c. An iron fence rusts.
    d. A firecracker explodes.

11. Which of the following processes produces a gas from a solid?

    a. melting
    b. evaporation
    c. condensation
    d. sublimation

12. Which of the following is a double-replacement reaction?

    a. $HNO_3 (aq) + NaOH (aq) \rightarrow NaNO_3 (aq) + H_2O (l)$
    b. $CS_2 (g) + CO_2 (g) \rightarrow 2COS (g)$
    c. $2N_2O (g) \rightarrow 2N_2 (g) + O_2 (g)$
    d. $BaCl_2 (aq) + H_2SO_4 (aq) \rightarrow 2HCl (aq) + BaSO_4 (s)$

13. Balance the following chemical equation:

    $P_4 + O_2 + H_2O \rightarrow H_3PO_4$

    a. 1:8:6:4
    b. 1:2:2:4
    c. 1:2:6:4
    d. 1:5:6:4

14. Which of the following is NOT a homogeneous mixture?

    a. air
    b. sandy water
    c. brass
    d. salt dissolved in water

15. Which trait defines a saturated solution?

    a. Both the solute and solvent are liquid.
    b. The solute is distributed evenly throughout the solution.
    c. The solute is unevenly distributed throughout the solution.
    d. No more solute can be dissolved in the solution.

16. Which of the following is NOT a definition of an acid?

    a. A substance that contains hydrogen and produces H^+ in water.
    b. A substance that donates protons to a base.
    c. A substance that reacts with a base to form a salt and water.
    d. A substance that accepts protons.

17. A ball is tossed straight into the air with a velocity of 3 m/s. What will its velocity be at its maximum height?

    a. −3 m/s
    b. 0 m/s
    c. 1.5 m/s
    d. 3 m/s

18. How far will a car moving at 40 m/s travel in 2 seconds?

    a. 10 m
    b. 20 m
    c. 40 m
    d. 80 m

19. If a baseball thrown straight up in the air takes 5 seconds to reach its peak, how long will it need to fall back to the player's hand?

    a. 2.5 seconds
    b. 9.8 seconds
    c. 5.0 seconds
    d. 10.0 seconds

20. Which of the following is a measure of the inertia of an object?

    a. mass
    b. speed
    c. acceleration
    d. force

21. A box sliding down a ramp experiences all of the following forces EXCEPT

    a. tension.
    b. friction.
    c. gravitational.
    d. normal.

22. A person with a mass of 80 kg travels to the moon, where the acceleration due to gravity is 1.62 m/s^2. What will her mass be on the moon?

    a. greater than 80 kg
    b. 80 kg
    c. less than 80 kg
    d. The answer cannot be determined without more information.

23. If a force of 300 N is pushing on a block to the right and a force of 400 N is pushing on a block to the left, what is the net force on the block?

    a. 0 N
    b. 100 N to the left
    c. 300 N to the right
    d. 400 N to the left

24. A man is pushing against a heavy rock sitting on a flat plane, and the rock is not moving. The force that holds the rock in place is

    a. friction.
    b. gravity.
    c. normal force.
    d. buoyant force.

25. Which of the following describes what will happen when positive work is done on an object?

    a. The object will gain energy.
    b. The object will lose energy.
    c. The object will increase its temperature.
    d. The object will decrease its temperature.

26. What type of energy is stored in the bond between hydrogen and oxygen in water (H_2O)?

    a. mechanical
    b. chemical
    c. nuclear
    d. electric

27. A microscope makes use of which property of waves to make objects appear larger?

    a. diffraction
    b. amplitude
    c. reflection
    d. refraction

28. Which measurement describes the distance between crests in a wave?

    a. amplitude
    b. wavelength
    c. frequency
    d. period

29. Two negative charges are being held 1 meter apart. What will the charges do when they are released?

a. They will move closer together.

b. They will move farther apart.

c. They will stay 1 meter apart and move in the same direction.

d. They will stay 1 meter apart and not move.

30. The north poles of two magnets are held near each other. At which distance will the magnets experience the most force?

a. 0.1 meters

b. 1 meters

c. 10 meters

d. 100 meters

ANSWER KEY

1. b.

Atomic number is defined as the total number of protons in the nucleus of an atom.

2. c.

Subtracting the atomic number from the mass number gives the number of protons: $A - Z = 88 - 38 = 50$.

3. c.

Antimony is a metalloid. Rubidium is a metal, vanadium is a transition metal, and iodine is a halogen.

4. a.

Because metals tend to consist of ordered, tightly packed atoms, their densities are typically high (not low).

5. d.

Oxygen is in the same group as sulfur and is also a nonmetal.

6. d.

By losing one electron and thereby adopting a +1 charge, alkali metals achieve a noble gas electron configuration, making them more stable.

7.

Elements	Bond
magnesium and bromine	a. is correct. Ionic bonds form between elements on the left side of the periodic table and the right side.
carbon and oxygen	c. is correct. Nonmetals tend to form covalent bonds.
solid copper	b. is correct. Solid metals are held together by metallic bonding.

8.

Com-pound	Polar	Nonpolar
H_2O	O attracts electrons more strongly than H, and H_2O is bent such that the charges on each O do not balance.	
F_2		Because the two atoms are the same, they share electrons equally.
HF	F attracts electrons more strongly than H, creating a polar molecule.	

9. b.

The two oxygen atoms in a covalent double bond share two pairs of electrons, or four total.

10. a.

When water changes form, it does not change the chemical composition of the substance. Once water becomes ice, the ice can easily turn back into water.

11. d.

Sublimation is the phase change in which a material moves directly from the solid phase to the gas phase, bypassing the liquid phase.

12. d.

This reaction is a double-replacement reaction in which the two reactants change partners. Ba^{+2} combines with SO_4^{-2} and H^{+1} combines with Cl^{-1}.

13. d.

$$\_P_4 + \_O_2 + \_H_2O \rightarrow \_H_3PO_4$$

Add a 4 on the right side to balance the four P atoms on the left.

$$\_P_4 + \_O_2 + \_H_2O \rightarrow 4H_3PO_4$$

There are now twelve H atoms on the right, so add a 6 to H_2O on the left.

$$\_P_4 + \_O_2 + 6H_2O \rightarrow 4H_3PO_4$$

There are sixteen O on the right, so add a 5 to O_2 on the left.

$$P_4 + 5O_2 + 6H_2O \rightarrow 4H_3PO_4$$

14. b.

Sandy water is not a homogeneous mixture. Sand and water can be easily separated, making it a heterogeneous mixture.

15. d.

No more solute can be dissolved into a saturated solution.

16. d.

Acids increase the concentration of hydrogen ions in solution and do not accept protons.

17. b.

The velocity of a projectile is zero at its maximum height.

18. d.

Displacement is equal to velocity multiplied by time:

$d = vt = (40 \text{ m/s})(2 \text{ s}) = 80 \text{ m}$

19. c.

The time to the peak and the time to fall back to the original height are equal.

20. a.

Mass is a measure of an object's inertia.

21. a.

Tension is the force that results from objects being pulled or hung.

22. b.

The mass of an object is constant, so the mass would still be 80 kg. (However, the person's weight would be lower on the moon than on the earth.)

23. b.

The total force on an object is found by adding all the individual forces: 300 N + (−400 N) = −100 N (where negative is to the left).

24. a.

When the man pushes on the rock, static friction points opposite the direction of the applied force with the same magnitude. The forces add to zero, so the rock's acceleration is also zero.

25. a.

The object will gain energy.

26. b.

Chemical energy is stored in the bonds between atoms.

27. d.

Lenses refract, or bend, light waves to make objects appear larger.

28. b.

Wavelength is the length of each cycle of the wave, which can be found by measuring between crests.

29. b.

Like charges repel each other, so the two charges will move apart from each other.

30. a.

Magnetic force is inversely proportional to the distance between two objects, so the smallest distance will create the largest force.

EIGHT: EARTH AND SPACE SCIENCE

Astronomy

Astronomy is the study of space. Our planet, **Earth**, is just one out of a group of planets that orbit the sun, which is the star at the center of our solar system. Other planets in our solar system include Mercury, Venus, Mars, Jupiter, Saturn, Uranus, and Neptune. Every planet, except Mercury and Venus, has **moons,** or naturally occurring satellites that orbit a planet. Our solar system also includes **asteroids** and **comets,** small rocky or icy objects that orbit the Sun. Many of these are clustered in the **asteroid belt**, which is located between the orbits of Mars and Jupiter.

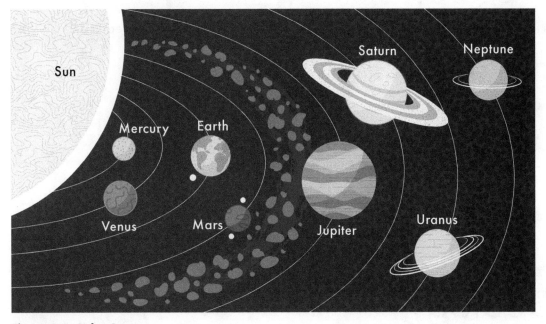

Figure 8.1. Solar System

Our solar system is a small part of a bigger star system called a **galaxy.** (Our galaxy is called the Milky Way.) Galaxies consist of stars, gas, and dust held together by gravity and contain millions of **stars**, which are hot balls of plasma and gases. The universe includes many types of stars, including supergiant stars, white dwarfs, giant stars, and neutron stars. Stars form in **nebulas**, which are large clouds of dust and gas. When very large stars collapse, they create **black holes**, which have a gravitational force so strong that light cannot escape.

Earth, the moon, and the sun interact in a number of ways that impact life on our planet. When the positions of the three align, eclipses occur. A **lunar eclipse** occurs when Earth lines up between the moon and the sun; the moon moves into the shadow of Earth and appears dark in color. A **solar eclipse** occurs when the moon lines up between Earth and the sun; the moon covers the sun, blocking sunlight.

The cycle of day and night and the seasonal cycle are determined by the earth's motion. It takes approximately 365 days, or one **year**, for Earth to revolve around the sun. While Earth is revolving around the sun, it is also rotating on its axis, which takes approximately twenty-four hours, or one **day**. As the planet rotates, different areas alternately face toward the sun and away from the sun, creating night and day.

The earth's axis is not directly perpendicular to its orbit, meaning the planet tilts on its axis. The **seasons** are caused by this tilt. When the Northern Hemisphere is tilted toward the sun, it receives more sunlight and experiences summer. At the same time that the Northern Hemisphere experiences summer, the Southern Hemisphere, which receives less direct sunlight, experiences winter. As the earth revolves, the Northern Hemisphere will tilt away from the sun and move into winter, while the Southern Hemisphere tilts toward the sun and moves into summer.

PRACTICE QUESTION

1. The phenomenon that occurs when the moon moves between the earth and the sun is called a(n)

   a. aurora

   b. lunar eclipse

   c. black hole

   d. solar eclipse

   e. solstice

   Answer:

   d. is correct. When the moon moves between the earth and the sun, a solar eclipse occurs, blocking sunlight from the planet.

Geology

Geology is the study of the minerals and rocks that make up the earth. A **mineral** is a naturally occurring, solid, inorganic substance with a crystalline structure. There are several properties that help identify a mineral, including color, luster, hardness, and density. Examples of minerals include talc, diamonds, and topaz.

Although a **rock** is also a naturally occurring solid, it can be either organic or inorganic and is composed of one or more minerals. Rocks are classified based on their method of formation. The three types of rocks are igneous, sedimentary, and metamorphic. **Igneous rocks** are the result of tectonic processes that bring magma, or melted rock, to the earth's surface; they can form either above or below the surface. **Sedimentary rocks** are formed from the compaction of rock fragments that results from weathering and erosion. Lastly, **metamorphic rocks** form when extreme temperature and pressure cause the structure of pre-existing rocks to change.

The **rock cycle** describes how rocks form and break down. Typically, the cooling and solidification of magma as it rises to the surface creates igneous rocks. These rocks are then subject to **weathering**, the mechanical and/or chemical processes by which rocks break down. During **erosion** the resulting sediment is deposited in a new location. As sediment is deposited, the resulting compaction creates new sedimentary rocks. As new layers are added, rocks and minerals are forced closer to the earth's core where they are subjected to heat and pressure, resulting in metamorphic rock. Eventually, they will reach their melting point and return to magma, starting the cycle over again. This process takes place over hundreds of thousands or even millions of years.

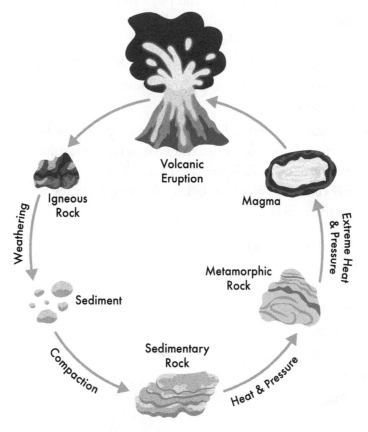

Figure 8.2. The Rock Cycle

Paleontology, the study of the history of life on Earth, is sometimes also considered part of geology. Paleontologists study the rock record, which retains biological history through **fossils**, the preserved remains and traces of ancient life. Fossils can be used to learn about the evolution of life on the planet, particularly bacteria, plants, and animals that have gone extinct. Throughout Earth's history, there have been five documented catastrophic events that caused major extinctions. For each mass extinction, there are several theories about the cause but no definitive answers. Theories about what triggered mass extinctions include climate change, ice ages, asteroid and comet impacts, and volcanic activity.

The surface of the earth is made of large plates that float on the less dense layer beneath them. These **tectonic plates** make up the lithosphere, the planet's surface layer. Over 200 million years ago, the continents were joined together in one giant landmass called **Pangea**. Due to **continental drift**, or the slow movement of tectonic plates, the continents gradually shifted to their current positions.

> The magnitude of an earthquake refers to the amount of energy it releases, measured as the maximum motion during the earthquake. This can indirectly describe how destructive the earthquake was.

The boundaries where plates meet are the locations for many geologic features and events. **Mountains** are formed when plates collide and push land upward, and **trenches** form when one plate is pushed beneath another. In addition, the friction created by plates sliding past each other is responsible for most **earthquakes**.

Volcanoes, which are vents in the earth's crust that allow molten rock to reach the surface, frequently occur along the edges of tectonic plates. However, they can also occur at hotspots located far from plate boundaries.

The outermost layer of the earth, which includes tectonic plates, is called the **lithosphere**. Beneath the lithosphere are, in order, the **asthenosphere**, **mesosphere**, and **core**. The core includes two parts: the **outer core** is a liquid layer, and the **inner core** is composed of solid iron. It is believed the inner core spins at a rate slightly different from the rest of the planet, which creates the earth's magnetic field.

PRACTICE QUESTION

2. Rocks are broken down through the process of
   a. fossilization
   b. compaction
   c. sedimentation
   d. erosion
   e. weathering

   Answer:

   e. is correct. Weathering is the process in which rocks are broken down into smaller pieces by physical or chemical means.

Hydrology

The earth's surface includes many bodies of water that together form the **hydrosphere**. The largest of these are the bodies of salt water called **oceans**. There are five oceans: the Arctic, Atlantic, Indian, Pacific, and Southern. Together, the oceans account for 71 percent of the earth's surface and 97 percent of the earth's water.

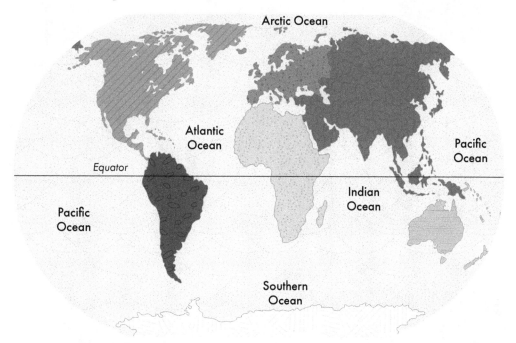

Figure 8.3. The Earth's Oceans

Oceans are subject to cyclic rising and falling water levels at shorelines called **tides**, which are the result of the gravitational pull of the moon and sun. The oceans also experience **waves**, which are caused by the movement of energy through the water.

Other bodies of water include **lakes**, which are usually freshwater, and **seas**, which are usually saltwater. **Rivers** and streams are moving bodies of water that flow into lakes, seas, and oceans. The earth also contains groundwater, or water that is stored underground in rock formations called **aquifers**.

Much of the earth's water is stored as **ice**. The North and South Poles are usually covered in large sheets of ice called polar ice. **Glaciers** are large masses of ice and snow that move. Over long periods of time, they scour Earth's surface, creating features such as lakes and valleys. Large chunks of ice that break off from glaciers are called **icebergs**.

> 97 percent of the water on earth is saltwater. 68 percent of the remaining freshwater is locked up in ice caps and glaciers.

The **water cycle** is the circulation of water throughout the earth's surface, atmosphere, and hydrosphere. Water on the earth's surface evaporates, or changes from a liquid to a gas, and becomes water vapor. Plants also release water vapor through transpiration. Water vapor in the air then comes together to form clouds. When it cools, this water vapor condenses into a liquid and falls from the sky as precipitation, which includes rain, sleet, snow, and hail. Precipitation replenishes groundwater and the water found in features such as lakes and rivers, thus starting the cycle over again.

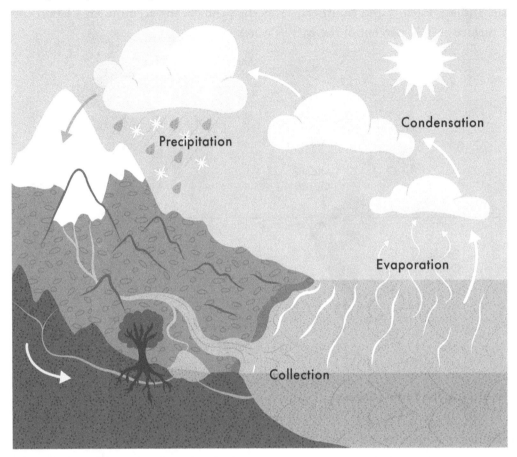

Figure 8.4. The Water Cycle

PRACTICE QUESTION

3. During the water cycle, groundwater is replenished by
    a. transpiration
    b. glaciers
    c. lakes
    d. precipitation
    e. evaporation

    Answer:

    d. is correct. Precipitation such as rain and snow seep into the ground to add to the groundwater supply.

Meteorology

Above the surface of Earth is the mass of gases called the **atmosphere**. The atmosphere includes the **troposphere**, which is closest to the earth, followed by the **stratosphere**, **mesosphere**, and **thermosphere**. The outermost layer of the atmosphere is the **exosphere**, which is located 6,200 miles above the surface. Generally, temperature in the atmosphere decreases with altitude. The **ozone layer**, which captures harmful radiation from the sun, is located in the stratosphere.

> Between each layer, a boundary exists where conditions change. This boundary takes the first part of the name of the previous layer followed by "pause." For example, the boundary between the troposphere and stratosphere is called the tropopause.

The **humidity**, or amount of water vapor in the air, and the **temperature** are two major atmospheric conditions that determine weather, the day-to-day changes in atmospheric conditions. A **warm front** occurs when warm air moves over a cold air mass, causing the air to feel warmer and more humid. A **cold front** occurs when cold air moves under a warm air mass, causing a drop in temperature.

Sometimes, weather turns violent. Tropical cyclones, or hurricanes, originate over warm ocean water. Hurricanes have destructive winds of more than 74 miles per hour and create large storm surges that can cause extensive damage along coastlines. Hurricanes, typhoons, and cyclones are all the same type of storm; they just have different names based on where the storm is located. **Hurricanes** originate in the Atlantic or Eastern Pacific Ocean, **typhoons** in the Western Pacific Ocean, and **cyclones** in the Indian Ocean. **Tornadoes** occur when unstable warm and cold air masses collide and a rotation is created by fast-moving winds.

The long-term weather conditions in a geographic location are called **climate**. A climate zone is a large area that experiences similar average temperature and precipitation. The three major climate zones, based on temperature, are the polar, temperate, and tropical zones. Each climate zone is subdivided into subclimates that have unique characteristics. The **tropical climate zone** (warm temperatures) can be subdivided into tropical wet, tropical wet and dry, semiarid, and arid. The **temperate climate zones** (moderate temperatures) include Mediterranean, humid subtropical, marine West Coast, humid continental, and subarctic. The **polar climate zones** (cold temperatures) include tundra, highlands, nonpermanent ice, and ice cap. Polar climates are cold and experience prolonged, dark winters due to the tilt of the earth's axis.

PRACTICE QUESTION

4. The layer of the atmosphere that absorbs harmful ultraviolet radiation from the sun is the

    a. mesosphere
    b. stratosphere
    c. troposphere
    d. thermosphere
    e. exosphere

Answer:

b. is correct. The stratosphere contains a sublayer called the ozone layer, which absorbs harmful ultraviolet radiation from the sun.

Test Your Knowledge

Read the question, and then choose the most correct answer.

1. Which planet orbits closest to Earth?

   a. Mercury
   b. Venus
   c. Jupiter
   d. Saturn

2. What is the name of the phenomenon when a star suddenly increases in brightness and then disappears from view?

   a. aurora
   b. black hole
   c. eclipse
   d. supernova

3. How long does it take the earth to rotate on its axis?

   a. one hour
   b. one day
   c. one month
   d. one year

4. Which statement about the solar system is true?

   a. Earth is much closer to the sun than it is to other stars.
   b. The moon is closer to Venus than it is to Earth.
   c. At certain times of the year, Jupiter is closer to the sun than Earth is.
   d. Mercury is the closest planet to Earth.

5. When Earth moves between the moon and the sun, it is called a

   a. solar eclipse.
   b. lunar eclipse.
   c. black hole.
   d. supernova.

6. Which planet does not have a moon?

   a. Mercury
   b. Earth
   c. Jupiter
   d. Saturn

7. What is the term for the top layer of the earth's surface?

   a. lithosphere
   b. atmosphere
   c. biosphere
   d. asthenosphere

8. Which action is an example of mechanical weathering?

   a. Calcium carbonate reacts with water to form a cave.
   b. An iron gate rusts.
   c. Tree roots grow under the foundation of a house and cause cracks.
   d. Feldspar turns to clay when exposed to water.

9. Which of the following is caused by geothermal heat?

   a. geysers
   b. tsunamis
   c. tornadoes
   d. hurricanes

10. Which of the following holds the largest percentage of the earth's freshwater?

    a.   glaciers and ice caps

    b.   groundwater

    c.   lakes

    d.   oceans

11. Which of the following best describes how igneous rocks are formed?

    a.   Sediment is compacted by pressure in the earth to form rock.

    b.   Magma comes to the earth's surface and cools to form rock.

    c.   Chemical weathering changes the composition of a rock to form new rock.

    d.   Ancient plant and animal life is calcified to create rock.

12. Which of the following is true as altitude increases in the troposphere?

    a.   Temperature and pressure increase.

    b.   Temperature increases and pressure decreases.

    c.   Temperature and pressure decrease.

    d.   Temperature decreases and pressure increases.

13. Which statement about hurricanes and tornadoes is true?

    a.   Hurricanes and tornadoes spin in opposite directions.

    b.   Tornadoes do not occur in warm climates.

    c.   Tornadoes have a low wind velocity.

    d.   Hurricanes are formed over warm ocean water.

14. Which two properties are used to classify climate zones?

    a.   latitude and temperature

    b.   temperature and precipitation

    c.   elevation and latitude

    d.   precipitation and tilt of Earth's axis

15. Which of the following best describes continental drift?

    a.   The mass extinction of the earth's species that occurred when a meteor struck the earth.

    b.   The spinning of the earth's inner core that creates the earth's magnetic field.

    c.   The formation of land masses from cooled magma.

    d.   The movement of tectonic plates in the lithosphere.

ANSWER KEY

1. b.

Venus's orbit is closest to Earth and is the second planet from the sun.

2. d.

Before a star collapses, the star burns brighter for a period of time and then fades from view. This is a supernova.

3. b.

Earth takes approximately twenty-four hours to rotate on its axis.

4. a.

The sun is about ninety-three million miles from Earth; the next closest star is about twenty-five trillion miles away.

5. b.

A lunar eclipse is when Earth moves between the moon and the sun.

6. a.

Only the first two planets, Mercury and Venus, lack moons.

7. a.

The lithosphere is the top layer of the earth's surface.

8. c.

Mechanical weathering involves breaking a substance down without changing the composition of the substance.

9. a.

Geysers are caused by geothermal heating of water underground.

10. a.

Glaciers and ice caps contain approximately 68.7% of all of Earth's freshwater supply, which is the largest percentage of the resources listed.

11. b.

Igneous rock is formed when magma (melted rock) is brought to the earth's surface and cools.

12. c.

Temperature and pressure both decrease with altitude in the troposphere.

13. d.

Hurricanes require warm ocean water to form.

14. b.

Climate zones are classified by temperature and precipitation.

15. d.

Continental drift is the movement of tectonic plates that lead to the current position of the continents.

NINE: VOCATIONAL ADJUSTMENT INDEX

The ninety questions on the Vocational Adjustment Index assess your personal attitudes, characteristics, and behaviors. Schools will use your score on this section to assess whether your personality is a fit for health care occupations.

Each question is a simple, general statement about personal or professional situations. You will choose to agree or disagree with the statement. You will need to work quickly to answer all the questions.

> **Vocational Adjustment Index Question Format**
>
> *The following statements address certain personal or professional situations. Agreeing or disagreeing with the statements simply reveals how you are likely to think, feel, or act in certain circumstances. If you agree with the statement, select (A) in the corresponding row. If you disagree, select (D). Choose the answer that is most true for you and answer immediately. Work rapidly.*
>
> 1. It is more important to be accurate than to be on time. (A) (D)
> 2. An ideal job includes a flexible schedule. (A) (D)
> 3. People who act like my friends have betrayed me. (A) (D)
> 4. It is difficult to make decisions in stressful situations. (A) (D)
> 5. Many people spend too much time on their phones. (A) (D)

There are no right or wrong answers, so there is no need to waste time deciding what the answer *should* be. Some statements are unflattering or critical, so it might be uncomfortable to select one. That is okay; it is best to answer as honestly as possible. You should also keep in mind that the chosen answers are not meant to be statements of fact. You don't have to select an answer that is necessarily a true statement about yourself, just the one that most generally applies to you.

TEN: Practice Test

ACADEMIC APTITUDE: VERBAL SKILLS

Which word is most different in meaning from the other words?

1. a. distressed   b. worried   c. calm   d. anxious   e. stressed

2. a. tired   b. exhausted   c. lazy   d. weary   e. energetic

3. a. problem   b. complication   c. difficulty   d. certainty   e. obstacle

4. a. mythical   b. ordinary   c. miraculous   d. magical   e. different

5. a. rot   b. wither   c. thrive   d. fail   e. struggle

6. a. attentive   b. thoughtless   c. responsible   d. caring   e. considerate

7. a. complete   b. thorough   c. lacking   d. exhaustive   e. full

8. a. laceration   b. scrape   c. bandage   d. wound   e. sore

9. a. lively   b. dull   c. gloomy   d. somber   e. unhappy

10. a. brief   b. terse   c. concise   d. long   e. sudden

11. a. secretive   b. obscure   c. mysterious   d. cryptic   e. obvious

12. a. gloomy   b. upbeat   c. irritable   d. glum   e. moody

13. a. obsession   b. attraction   c. passion   d. interest   e. indifference

14. a. pleasant   b. amiable   c. kindly   d. cheerful   e. rude

15. a. combine   b. connect   c. join   d. divide   e. unite

16. a. destroy   b. finish   c. create   d. shatter   e. ruin

17. a. cascade   b. drip   c. torrent   d. flood   e. surge

18.   a. calm   b. quiet   c. conflict   d. peace   e. order

19.   a. limited   b. endless   c. eternal   d. lasting   e. constant

20.   a. acquit   b. excuse   c. pardon   d. disapprove   e. absolve

21.   a. arrogance   b. humility   c. vanity   d. narcissism   e. smugness

22.   a. weak   b. defective   c. broken   d. flawed   e. perfect

23.   a. humble   b. bashful   c. timid   d. conceited   e. modest

24.   a. civil   b. polite   c. refined   d. crude   e. gracious

25.   a. absurd   b. playful   c. foolish   d. silly   e. serious

ACADEMIC APTITUDE: ARITHMETIC

Work the problem, and then choose the correct answer.

---

26. Danika bought two packages of ground beef weighing 1.73 lb and 2.17 lb. What was the total weight of the two packages in pounds?

    a. 0.44   b. 1.25   c. 3.81   d. 3.9   e. 4.2

27. Morris went shopping with $80. He spent $24.17 at the hardware store and $32.87 on clothes. How much money did he have left?

    a. $22.96   b. $23.04   c. $42.96   d. $55.83   e. $57.04

28. What is the remainder when 397 is divided by 4?

    a. 0   b. 1   c. 2   d. 3   e. 4

29. A teacher has 50 notebooks to hand out to students. If she has 16 students in her class, and each student receives 2 notebooks, how many notebooks will she have left over?

    a. 2   b. 16   c. 18   d. 32   e. 34

30. Michael is making cupcakes. He plans to give $\frac{1}{2}$ of the cupcakes to a friend and $\frac{1}{3}$ of the cupcakes to his coworkers. If he makes 48 cupcakes, how many will he have left over?

    a. 8   b. 10   c. 12   d. 16   e. 24

31. Which of the following is closest in value to $129,113 + 34,602$?

    a. 162,000   b. 163,000   c. 164,000   d. 165,000   e. 166,000

32. Students board a bus at 7:45 a.m. and arrive at school at 8:20 a.m. For how many minutes are the students on the bus?

    a. 30   b. 35   c. 45   d. 50   e. 65

33. Micah has invited 23 friends to his house and is having pizza for dinner. If each pizza feeds 4 people, how many pizzas should he order?

    a. 4   b. 5   c. 6   d. 7   e. 8

34. Out of 1,560 students at Ward Middle School, 15% want to take French. Which expression represents how many students want to take French?

    a. 1560 ÷ 15   b. 1560 × 15   c. 1560 × 1.51   d. 1560 ÷ 0.15   e. 1560 × 0.15

35. At the grocery store, apples cost $1.89 per pound and oranges cost $2.19 per pound. How much would it cost to purchase 2 lb of apples and 1.5 lb of oranges?

    a. $6.62   b. $7.07   c. $7.14   d. $7.22   e. $7.67

36. Which digit is in the hundredths place when 1.3208 is divided by 5.2?

a. 0   b. 4   c. 5   d. 8   e. 9

37. 17.38 − 19.26 + 14.2 =

a. 12.08   b. 12.32   c. 16.08   d. 16.22   e. 50.84

38. If a person reads 40 pages in 45 minutes, approximately how many minutes will it take her to read 265 pages?

a. 180   b. 202   c. 236   d. 265   e. 298

39. The recommended ratio of nurses to patients in a critical care unit is 1 to 4. How many nurses should be on duty if there are 20 patients in the unit?

a. 4   b. 5   c. 7   d. 8   e. 10

40. Jim is taking care of eight patients during his shift. So far it has taken him 25 minutes to see two patients. At this rate, how many minutes will it take Jim to check in on all eight patients?

a. 50   b. 60   c. 100   d. 120   e. 125

41. Juan is packing a shipment of three books weighing 0.8 lb, 0.49 lb, and 0.89 lb. The maximum weight for the shipping box is 2.5 lb. How much more weight will the box hold in pounds?

a. 0.32   b. 0.48   c. 1.61   d. 2.18   e. 4.68

42. The average rainfall in May for Austin, Texas, is 4.5 in. In July, the average rainfall is 1.67 in. How many more inches of rain fall on average in May than in July?

a. 1.22   b. 2.69   c. 2.83   d. 2.97   e. 6.17

43. If a $285.48 bill will be split evenly between six people, how much will each person pay?

a. $47.58   b. $49.88   c. $225.48   d. $885.46   e. $1,712.88

44. A bridge is 119.7 m long in the summer. In the winter, the metal contracts, and the bridge shrinks by 1.05 m. How many meters long is the bridge in winter?

a. 109.2   b. 118.2   c. 118.65   d. 120.75   e. 130.2

45. Angelica bought a roast weighing 3.2 lb. If the roast cost $25.44, how much did it cost per pound?

a. $5.95   b. $7.44   c. $7.95   d. $8.14   e. $22.24

46. A box of books weighs 6.3 lb. If there are 18 books in the box, how many pounds does each book weigh?

a. 0.35   b. 1.134   c. 3.5   d. 11.34   e. 35

47. Carlos spent $1.68 on bananas. If bananas cost 48 cents per pound, how many pounds of bananas did he buy?

a. 1.2   b. 2.06   c. 2.16   d. 3.5   e. 8.1

48. Sally has $127 in her checking. An automatic draft takes out $150 for her electric bill. What is her balance after the automatic draft?

a. −$277   b. −$123   c. −$23   d. $23   e. $123

49. Five numbers have an average of 16. If the first four numbers have a sum of 68, what is the fifth number?

a. 12   b. 16   c. 52   d. 68   e. 80

50. The recommended dosage of a particular medication is 4 mL per 50 lb of body weight. What is the recommended dosage in milliliters for a person who weighs 175 lb?

a. 14   b. 25   c. 28   d. 44   e. 140

ACADEMIC APTITUDE: NONVERBAL SKILLS

Which shape correctly completes the statement?

51. △ is to ◭ as ◇ is to ?

a. ▽ b. ◈ c. ◈ d. ⊞ e. ◇

52. ⋈ is to ◁ as ◖ is to ?

a. △ b. ◇ c. ◖ d. ◗ e. ◯

53. ⬡ is to ⬢ as △ is to ?

a. ● b. ▲ c. ■ d. ◆ e. ◀

54. ◔ is to ◑ as ◔ is to ?

a. ◖ b. ◕ c. ◔ d. ◑ e. ◔

55. 𝟠 is to 𝟠 as 𝟠 is to ?

a. 𝟠 b. ◯ c. 𝟠 d. 𝟠 e. 𝟠

56. ◿ is to ⋈ as ◸ is to ?

a. ◺ b. ◄ c. ⋈ d. ◿ e. ◿

57. ⠇ is to ⠂ as ⠅ is to ?

a. ⠿ b. ⠐ c. ⠇ d. ⠂ e. ⠇

58. ⊟ is to ⊟ as ⊢ is to ?

a. ▬ b. ▭ c. ⊟ d. •• e. ▬

59. ⫼⫼ is to ⫼⫼ as ⫼⫼ is to ?

a. ⫼⫼ b. ⫼⫼ c. ⫼⫼ d. ⫼⫼ e. ⫼⫼

60. ⊔ is to ⊔ as ⊢ is to ?

a. ⊢ b. ⊟ c. ⊑ d. ⊢ e. ⊑

61. ◗ is to ◗ as ◖ is to ?

a. ◔ b. ◕ c. ◔ d. ◔ e. ◔

62. ⌐ is to ⫟ as ¬ is to ?

a. ⊓ b. ⋔ c. ⊓ d. ⋔ e. ⊓

63. ▯ is to ⊞ as ◺ is to ?

a. ⊠ b. ⊞ c. ▱ d. ⊞ e. ⊠

64. ╱ is to ⌢ as ⌒ is to ?

a. ⬠ b. ⊏ c. ⊏ d. ⊔ e. ⬠

65. ◬◯◯▽ is to ◬◯◯▽ as ◬◯◯▽ is to ?

a. ◬●●▽ b. ◬◯◯▽ c. ◬◯◯▽ d. ◬●●▽ e. ◬◯◯▽

66. ⬚ is to ⬚ as ⬚ is to ?

a. ⬚ b. ⬚ c. ⬚ d. ⬚ e. ⬚

67. ◆◆ is to ◆◆ as ◆◆ is to ?

a. ◆◆   b. ◆◆   c. ◆◆   d. ◆◆   e. ◆◆

68. (x) is to (x) as (x) is to ?

a. (+)   b. (x)   c. (+)   d. (x)   e. (x)

69. ❙❙❙ is to ❙❙❙ as ❙❙❙ is to ?

a. ❙❙❙   b. ❙❙❙   c. ❙❙❙   d. ❙❙❙   e. ❙❙❙

70. ✕ is to ✕ as ✕ is to ?

a. ✕   b. ✕   c. ✕   d. ✕   e. ✕

71. ☐ is to ⊏ as ⌐ is to ?

a. ⊐   b. ⌐   c. =   d. | e. ⊔

72. (x) is to (x) as (x) is to ?

a. (x)   b. (x)   c. (x)   d. (+)   e. (x)

73. ☐ is to ▬ as ◺ is to ?

a. ◢   b. ◣   c. ◢   d. ▲   e. ◹

74. ☐ is to ☐ as ☐ is to ?

a. ☐   b. ☐   c. ☐   d. ☐   e. ☐

75. ⌐ is to ∟ as ⌐ is to ?

a. ∟   b. ⌐   c. ⌐   d. ⌐   e. ⌐

SPELLING

Choose the correct spelling of the word.

1. a. muscle b. muscle c. mucsel
2. a. hormoan b. hormmone c. hormone
3. a. seesure b. seizure c. seazure
4. a. facilitees b. facilitys c. facilities
5. a. decrease b. decreese c. decreace
6. a. transfusion b. transfussion c. transfution
7. a. annatome b. anatomy c. annatomy
8. a. daignoses b. diagnosis c. diegnosis
9. a. equepment b. equipmint c. equipment
10. a. stomach b. stomache c. stomeche
11. a. athritis b. arthritis c. arthritise
12. a. overy b. ovary c. ovarry
13. a. surgical b. surgicle c. sergical
14. a. allerjy b. alerrgy c. allergy
15. a. inflammation b. enflamation c. inflamation
16. a. poisson b. pioson c. poison
17. a. atrophy b. attrophy c. atrophe
18. a. stierile b. sterile c. steerile
19. a. cellular b. celullar c. celluler
20. a. tisue b. tissue c. tissu
21. a. artifitial b. artificial c. artifacial
22. a. immediet b. immidiate c. immediate
23. a. droplat b. dropplet c. droplet
24. a. symptom b. symptome c. simptom
25. a. eleminate b. elemenate c. eliminate
26. a. adhear b. adhere c. adher

27. a. inable   b. enable   c. ennable

28. a. varyous   b. various   c. variouse

29. a. secression   b. secresion   c. secretion

30. a. traumma   b. traumme   c. trauma

31. a. exsessive   b. excesive   c. excessive

32. a. bacteria   b. bactieria   c. bactteria

33. a. funngas   b. funngus   c. fungus

34. a. monetor   b. monitor   c. moniter

35. a. abration   b. abrassion   c. abrasion

36. a. multipal   b. multipple   c. multiple

37. a. tremor   b. tremer   c. tremour

38. a. involvment   b. envolvement   c. involvement

39. a. respiritory   b. resperitory   c. respiratory

40. a. craneal   b. cranial   c. crannial

41. a. dissease   b. diseasse   c. disease

42. a. artery   b. arttery   c. arterie

43. a. vaine   b. vein   c. veine

44. a. cronic   b. chronic   c. chronick

45. a. accute   b. acutte   c. acute

READING COMPREHENSION

Reading Comprehension tests your ability to understand what you have read. Read each passage carefully. Each question is followed by four possible answer choices. Answer each question based on the material contained in each passage.

The greatest changes in sensory, motor, and perceptual development happen in the first two years of life. When babies are first born, most of their senses operate like those of adults. For example, babies are able to hear before they are born; studies show that babies turn toward the sound of their mothers' voices just minutes after being born, indicating they recognize the mother's voice from their time in the womb.

The exception to this rule is vision. A baby's vision changes significantly in the first year of life; initially a baby has a vision range of only 8 – 12 inches and no depth perception. As a result, infants rely primarily on hearing; vision does not become the dominant sense until around the age of twelve months. Babies also prefer faces to other objects. This preference, along with their limited vision range, means that their sight is initially focused on their caregiver.

1. The primary purpose of the passage is to
   a. compare vision in adults to vision in newborns
   b. persuade readers to get their infants' eyes checked
   c. confirm a recent scientific finding about senses
   d. explain how an infant's senses operate and change

2. Vision becomes the dominant sense
   a. at birth
   b. around twelve months of age
   c. when hearing declines
   d. at adulthood

3. Newborns mostly rely on
   a. vision
   b. touch
   c. taste
   d. hearing

4. What is the main idea of this passage?
   a. The senses of babies operate like the senses of adults.
   b. Babies have a limited vision range and rely on hearing for their first months of life.
   c. Babies prefer faces to other objects due to their small range of vision in the early months.
   d. Studies show that babies turn toward the sound of their mothers' voices after being born.

5. What evidence does the author provide to support his claim that babies are able to hear before they are born?
   a. The greatest changes in sensory development happen in the first two years of life.
   b. Vision does not become the dominant sense until around the age of twelve months.
   c. Babies turn toward the sound of their mothers' voices just minutes after being born.
   d. When babies are born, most of their senses operate like those of adults.

In its most basic form, geography is the study of space; more specifically, it studies the physical space of Earth and the ways in which it interacts with, shapes, and is shaped by its habitants. Geographers look at the world from a spatial perspective. This means that at the center of all geographic study is the question *where?* For geographers, the *where* of any interaction, event, or development is a crucial element to understanding it.

This question of *where* can be asked in various fields of study, so there are many subdisciplines of geography. These can be organized into four main categories: (1) regional studies, which examine the characteristics of a particular place; (2) topical studies, which look at a single physical or human feature that impacts the whole world; (3) physical studies, which focus on the physical features of Earth; and (4) human studies, which examine the relationship between human activity and the environment.

6. The subdiscipline of geography that looks at the impact of a single physical or human feature on the world is

   a. regional studies

   b. topical studies

   c. physical studies

   d. human studies

7. Physical studies would most likely examine the

   a. causes of migration during a drought

   b. impact of pollution on human development

   c. height of various mountain ranges around the world

   d. characteristics of a particular region in a country

8. What is the topic of this passage?

   a. human activity

   b. spatial perspective

   c. geography

   d. Earth

9. The center of all geographic study is *where* because

   a. geographers look at the world through a spatial perspective

   b. geography includes the subdiscipline of human studies

   c. it is asked in a variety of fields of study, not just geographic

   d. humans interact with various aspects of their world every day

It could be said that the great battle between the North and South we call the Civil War was a battle for individual identity. The states of the South had their own culture, one based on farming, independence, and the right of both man and state to determine their own paths. Similarly, the North had forged its own identity as a center of centralized commerce and manufacturing. This clash of lifestyles was bound to create tension, and this tension was bound to lead to war. But people who try to sell you this narrative are wrong. The Civil War was not a battle of cultural identities—it was a battle about slavery. All other explanations for the war are either a direct consequence of the South's desire for wealth at the expense of her fellow man or a fanciful invention to cover up this sad portion of our nation's history. And it cannot be denied that this time in our past was very sad indeed.

10. The author believes people say the war was fought because of a clash in cultural identities because they

    a.   want to avoid acknowledging the shameful parts of the United States' history

    b.   do not believe the Civil War was actually fought between the North and the South

    c.   are trying to make a better future for the United States despite its past

    d.   hope to promote the cause of the North instead of the South

11. The author believes that the Civil War was fought because of

    a.   cultural differences

    b.   the South's desire for wealth

    c.   slavery

    d.   individual identity

12. The topic of the passage is

    a.   individual identity

    b.   slavery

    c.   the cause of the Civil War

    d.   desire for wealth

13. The tone of this passage is

    a.   hopeful

    b.   humorous

    c.   cautious

    d.   assertive

14. Based on the information from the passage, a person from the North during the time of the Civil War would most likely

    a.   work in manufacturing

    b.   oppose the Civil War

    c.   be a farmer

    d.   own slaves

Skin coloration and markings have an important role to play in the world of snakes. Those intricate diamonds, stripes, and swirls help the animals hide from predators, but perhaps most importantly (for us humans, anyway), markings can also indicate whether the snake is venomous. While it might seem <u>counterintuitive</u> for a venomous snake to stand out in bright red or blue, that fancy costume tells any nearby predator that approaching it would be a bad idea.

If you see a flashy-looking snake in the woods, though, those markings don't necessarily mean it's venomous: some snakes have found a way to ward off predators without the actual venom. The scarlet kingsnake, for example, has very similar markings to the venomous coral snake with whom it frequently shares a habitat. However, the kingsnake is actually nonvenomous; it's merely pretending to be dangerous to eat. A predatory hawk or eagle, usually hunting from high in the sky, can't tell the difference between the two species, so the kingsnake gets passed over and lives another day.

15. This passage is primarily about

    a.   snake habitats

    b.   predators of snakes

    c.   snake skin coloration and markings

    d.   venomous and nonvenomous snakes

16. The scarlet kingsnake

    a.   is venomous to predators

    b.   often lives in the same areas as the coral snake

    c.   is dangerous to a hawk or eagle

    d.   is difficult to eat

17. According to the passage, venomous snakes can

    a.   have markings that camouflage them from predators

    b.   pretend to be nonvenomous when predators are around

    c.   be a threat to nonvenomous snakes

    d.   be identified by markings on their skin

18. Based on the passage, *counterintuitive* most likely means

    a.   contrary to common belief

    b.   similar in meaning

    c.   difficult to understand

    d.   a wise decision

19. A predatory eagle may pass over a kingsnake because the kingsnake

    a.   is venomous

    b.   can be easily mistaken for a venomous snake

    c.   blends in with its environment

    d.   is not as nutritious to the eagle as other snakes

Taking a person's temperature is one of the most basic and common health care tasks. Everyone from nurses to emergency medical technicians to concerned parents should be able to grab a thermometer and take a patient's or loved one's temperature. But what's the best way to get an accurate reading? The answer depends on the situation.

The most common way people measure body temperature is orally. A simple digital or disposable thermometer is placed under the tongue for a few minutes, and the task is done. There are many situations, however, when measuring temperature orally isn't an option. For example, when a person can't breathe through her nose, she won't be able to keep her mouth closed long enough to get an accurate reading. In these situations, it's often preferable to place the thermometer in the rectum or armpit. Using the rectum also has the added benefit of providing a much more accurate reading than other locations can provide.

It's also often the case that certain people, like agitated patients or fussy babies, won't be able to sit still long enough for an accurate reading. In these situations, it's best to use a thermometer that works much more quickly, such as one that measures temperature in the ear or at the temporal artery. No matter which method is chosen, however, it's important to check the average temperature for each region, as it can vary by several degrees.

20. What is the structure of this text?

    a.   cause and effect

    b.   order and sequence

    c.   problem and solution

    d.   compare and contrast

21. The most common way to take a temperature is

    a.   under the tongue

    b.   in the armpit

    c.   in the ear

    d.   at the temporal artery

22. What is the main idea of this passage?

    a. The best way to take a temperature is by placing the thermometer under the tongue.

    b. Taking a temperature is a very simple task.

    c. Some ways to take a temperature are more beneficial in certain situations.

    d. It is especially difficult to get an accurate temperature reading on children.

23. Why is measuring one's temperature in the ear or at the temporal artery beneficial?

    a. The situation determines the best way to get an accurate temperature reading.

    b. Some patients are not able to sit still long enough for an oral temperature reading.

    c. Everyone should be able to take a patient's or loved one's temperature.

    d. These regions provide a much more accurate reading than other locations.

24. Taking a temperature at the temporal artery

    a. is most accurate when done by a medical doctor

    b. is the best way to get an accurate reading

    c. will result in a different degree reading than from under the tongue

    d. will result in the same degree reading as from the ear

25. According to the text, taking a temperature

    a. is a simple task that most adults should be able to do

    b. can be dangerous if the result is not read correctly

    c. should be left up to medical professionals like nurses

    d. will give consistent results regardless of where it is taken

We've been told for years that the recipe for weight loss is fewer calories in than out. In other words, eat less and exercise more, and your body will take care of the rest. As many who've tried to diet can attest, this <u>edict</u> doesn't always produce results. If you're one of those folks, you might have felt that you just weren't doing it right—that the failure was all your fault.

However, several new studies released this year have suggested that it might not be your fault at all. For example, a study of people who'd lost a high percentage of their body weight (more than 17 percent) in a short period of time found that they could not physically maintain their new weight. Scientists measured their resting metabolic rate and found that they'd need to consume only a few hundred calories a day to meet their metabolic needs. Basically, their bodies were in starvation mode and seemed to desperately hang on to each and every calorie. Eating even a single healthy, well-balanced meal a day would cause these subjects to start packing the pounds back on.

Other studies have shown that factors like intestinal bacteria, distribution of body fat, and hormone levels can affect the manner in which our bodies process calories. There's also the fact that it's actually quite difficult to measure the number of calories consumed during a particular meal and the number used while exercising.

26. This passage is chiefly concerned with

    a. calories

    b. exercise

    c. weight loss

    d. metabolic needs

27. According to the text, hormone levels

    a. can impact a person's ability to lose weight

    b. will change based on a person's diet

    c. make a person think he is losing weight even if he is not

    d. were the subject of a new study released this year

28. Based on the text, *edict* most likely means

    a. hormone

    b. rule

    c. relationship

    d. diet

29. According to the text, people who lose a high percentage of their body weight in a short period of time may

    a. gain more than 17 percent of their body weight back after returning to a normal diet

    b. continue to lose weight if they maintain their normal diet

    c. be susceptible to high levels of intestinal bacteria

    d. start gaining the weight back even with healthy eating habits

30. The author wrote this text to

    a. inform the reader about potential causes of inconsistencies in weight loss

    b. persuade others to practice traditional dieting techniques

    c. warn against losing a high percentage of body weight quickly

    d. compare and contrast the effects of dieting to the effects of exercise

Influenza (also called the flu) has historically been one of the most common, and deadliest, human infections. While many people who contract the virus will recover, many others will not. Over the past 150 years, tens of millions of people have died from the flu, and millions more have been left with lingering complications such as secondary infections.

Although it's a common disease, the flu is not actually highly infectious, meaning it's relatively difficult to contract. The flu can only be transmitted when individuals come into direct contact with bodily fluids of people infected with the flu or when they are exposed to <u>expelled</u> aerosol particles (which result from coughing and sneezing). Because the viruses can only travel short distances as aerosol particles and die within a few hours on hard surfaces, the virus can be contained with fairly simple health measures like hand washing and face masks.

However, the spread of the flu can only be contained when people are aware such measures need to be taken. One of the reasons the flu has historically been so deadly is the amount of time between when people become infectious and when they develop symptoms. Viral shedding—the process by which the body releases viruses that have been successfully reproducing during the infection—takes place two days after infection, while symptoms do not usually develop until the third day of infection. Thus, infected individuals have at least twenty-four hours in which they may unknowingly infect others.

31. The act of releasing viruses that have been reproducing is called

a. contagious

b. viral shedding

c. influenza

d. aerosol particles

32. The primary purpose of the passage is to

a. persuade readers to cover their mouths when they cough

b. argue in favor of the flu vaccine

c. explain why the flu is so common

d. inform readers of the symptoms of the flu so it can be identified

33. In this passage, the word *expelled* most likely means

a. noninfectious

b. ejected

c. harmful

d. hidden

34. Because of the significant amount of time between when people with the flu become infectious and when they develop symptoms,

a. many infected individuals unknowingly infect others

b. millions have been left with lingering complications

c. the infection is not highly contagious

d. viruses can only travel short distances

35. Based on the passage, the flu virus

a. can live on hard surfaces for up to two days

b. is highly infectious and easy to spread to others

c. has killed tens of millions in the past 150 years

d. travels long distances as aerosol particles after a sneeze

GENERAL SCIENCE

Read the question, and then choose the most correct answer.

1.   The inorganic material that makes up bone is

    a. calcium   b. phosphorus   c. collagen   d. potassium   e. actin

2.   An example of a biome is a

    a. beehive   b. cornfield   c. herd of bison d. desert   e. puddle

3.   The planet that is closest to Earth is

    a. Mercury   b. Venus   c. Jupiter   d. Saturn   e. Neptune

4.   The phenomenon when a star suddenly increases in brightness and then disappears from view is a(n)

    a. aurora   b. galaxy   c. black hole d. eclipse   e. supernova

5.   Chloroplasts can be found in the cells of

    a. whales   b. mushrooms c. tulips   d. lizards   e. fish

6.   Isotopes of an element will have the same number of

    a. electrons   b. neutrons   c. protons   d. atoms   e. ions

7.   An electrocardiogram (EKG) can be used to diagnose

    a. diabetes   b. torn ligaments c. cancer   d. tachycardia e. influenza

8.   The number of nucleotides in a codon is

    a. 3   b. 4   c. 6   d. 22   e. 64

9.   The negatively charged atoms inside an atom are called

    a. protons   b. neutrons   c. electrons   d. ions   e. nucleus

10.   A box sliding down a ramp experiences all of the following forces EXCEPT

    a. tension   b. friction   c. gravity   d. normal   e. buoyant

11. An example of an organism that decomposes organic matter is a(n)

    a. apple tree   b. mushroom   c. goat   d. lion   e. vulture

12. An example of an organism that regulates its body temperature externally is a

    a. pelican   b. dolphin   c. whale   d. lobster   e. leopard

13. Which part of the body is affected by a right tibia fracture?

    a. upper arm   b. lower arm   c. upper leg   d. lower leg   e. head

14. The digestive enzymes produced by the pancreas pass into the

    a. stomach   b. gallbladder   c. esophagus   d. large intestine   e. small intestine

15. An example of a physical change is

    a. freezing water   b. baking a cake   c. a rusting fence   d. an exploding firecracker   e. neutralizing an acid

16. A nonrenewable energy source is

    a. water   b. wind   c. coal   d. sunlight   e. geothermal

17. The top layer of the earth's surface is called the

    a. exosphere   b. lithosphere   c. atmosphere   d. biosphere   e. asthenosphere

18. Skeletal muscle is attached to bone by

    a. ligaments   b. cartilage   c. tendons   d. nerves   e. fascia

19. During digestion, food passes through the

    a. esophagus   b. gallbladder   c. trachea   d. pancreas   e. liver

20. The earth rotates on its axis in

    a. one hour   b. one day   c. one month   d. one year   e. one hundred years

21. The process that uses carbon dioxide to produce sugars is called

    a. digestion   b. chloroplast   c. decomposition   d. photosynthesis   e. cellular respiration

22. $2C_6H_{14} + 19O_2 \rightarrow 12CO_2 + 14H_2O$

The reaction shown above is a(n)

a. substitution reaction

b. acid-base reaction

c. decomposition reaction

d. combustion reaction

e. synthesis reaction

23. The abiotic factor in an ecosystem could include

a. producers

b. consumers

c. predators

d. decomposers

e. water

24. In a food web, fungi are

a. producers

b. primary consumers

c. secondary consumers

d. tertiary consumers

e. decomposers

25. The mechanism of evolution is

a. gene flow

b. genetic drift

c. mutation

d. sexual selection

e. natural selection

26. The muscular organ that processes food material into smaller pieces and helps mix it with saliva is the

a. pharynx

b. tongue

c. diaphragm

d. stomach

e. esophagus

27. A strong acid will

a. completely ionize in water

b. donate more than one proton

c. have a pH close to 7

d. not ionize

e. have at least one metal atom

28. The largest bone in the human body is the

a. tibia

b. humerus

c. scapula

d. femur

e. ulna

29. When skin is exposed to the sunlight, it produces

a. vitamin A

b. vitamin E

c. vitamin K

d. vitamin D

e. vitamin B

30. The light reactions of photosynthesis occur in the

a. mitochondria

b. chloroplast

c. cytoplasm

d. vacuole

e. nucleus

31. The exchange of nutrients, gases, and cellular waste happens in the

    a. veins   b. arteries   c. capillaries   d. venules   e. arterioles

32. The incus, stapes, and malleus play an important role in

    a. vision   b. taste   c. hearing   d. smell   e. touch

33. The adrenal glands are located near the

    a. brain   b. thyroid   c. kidneys   d. bladder   e. heart

34. Wind speed is measured using

    a. a thermometer b. a wind vane c. an anemometer d. a rain gauge e. a barometer

35. One milliliter is equivalent to

    a. 1 g   b. 1 pt   c. 1 lb   d. 1 m^2 e. 1 cm^3

36. Mature sperm is stored in the

    a. testes   b. bladder   c. vas deferens   d. epididymis   e. penis

37. The meninges protect the

    a. brain   b. heart   c. stomach   d. uterus   e. testes

38. Organic molecules must contain

    a. carbon   b. phosphorous c. nitrogen   d. oxygen   e. helium

39. DNA and RNA are built from monomers called

    a. amino acids   b. sugars   c. lipids   d. polymerases e. nucleotides

40. The nucleotide found in RNA but not DNA is

    a. adenine   b. cytosine   c. thymine   d. uracil   e. guanine

41. An organism with 16 total chromosomes will produce gametes with a chromosome number of

    a. 4   b. 8   c. 16   d. 32   e. 64

42. An example of a wedge is a(n)

    a. wagon   b. ramp   c. ax   d. seesaw   e. car axle

43. The number of electrons needed by a noble gas to fill its outermost electron shell is

    a. 0   b. 1   c. 2   d. 3   e. 4

44. Photosynthesis takes place in the

    a. roots   b. stem   c. bark   d. flower   e. leaves

45. The process that occurs when water vapor becomes a solid is

    a. condensation   b. sublimation   c. evaporation   d. deposition   e. freezing

46. Orange juice, which is primarily composed of citric acid and malic acid, likely has a pH of

    a. 4   b. 7   c. 9   d. 13   e. 14

47. The mass of an object is measured with a

    a. thermometer   b. graduated cylinder   c. ruler   d. barometer   e. balance

48. The resistance to motion caused by one object rubbing against another object is

    a. inertia   b. friction   c. velocity   d. gravity   e. acceleration

49. The rock formed when lava cools and solidifies is called

    a. igneous   b. sedimentary   c. metamorphic   d. sandstone   e. mineral

50. An example of a longitudinal wave is a

    a. surface wave   b. light wave   c. sound wave   d. radio wave   e. microwave

51. The gas found in the largest quantity in Earth's atmosphere is

    a. carbon monoxide   b. bromine   c. nitrogen   d. fluorine   e. oxygen

52. All atoms of an element contain the same number of

    a. electrons   b. molecules   c. protons   d. ions   e. neutrons

53. The most common element in the universe is

   a. carbon   b. lithium   c. potassium   d. titanium   e. hydrogen

54. The storm LEAST likely to form over ocean water is a

   a. hurricane   b. typhoon   c. cyclone   d. tornado   e. squall

55. To neutralize an acid spill, use

   a. baking soda   b. lemon juice   c. cat litter   d. water   e. vinegar

56. The force that attracts a body toward the center of the earth is

   a. friction   b. gravity   c. pull   d. tension   e. buoyancy

57. Energy that is stored and is waiting to work is called

   a. kinetic   b. thermal   c. mechanical   d. chemical   e. potential

58. An example of a translucent object is a

   a. book   b. glass of water   c. T-shirt   d. car window   e. door

59. An example of an electrical insulator is a

   a. spoon   b. key   c. marble   d. penny   e. wire

60. Stratus clouds can be described as

   a. often gray   b. big and tall   c. high in the sky   d. puffy   e. usually wispy

VOCATIONAL ADJUSTMENT INDEX

The following statements address certain personal or professional situations. Agreeing or disagreeing with the statements simply reveals how you are likely to think, feel, or act in certain circumstances. If you agree with the statement, select (A) in the corresponding row. If you disagree, select (D). Choose the answer that is most true for you and answer immediately. *Work rapidly.*

1. People spend too much time focusing on their careers.   1.   (A)   (D)

2. Most people are too competitive.   2.   (A)   (D)

3. It is important to be a lifelong learner.   3.   (A)   (D)

4. Collaboration is key to the success of any organization.   4.   (A)   (D)

5. Most workplace evaluations are unfair.   5.   (A)   (D)

6. Most older coworkers are out of touch.   6.   (A)   (D)

7. People usually have the best intentions.   7.   (A)   (D)

8. Working with others rather than alone is preferable.   8.   (A)   (D)

9. It is important to take risks.   9.   (A)   (D)

10. Efficiency is better than quality.   10.   (A)   (D)

11. Kind hearts are for weak leaders.   11.   (A)   (D)

12. A job is just a paycheck.   12.   (A)   (D)

13. Conflict can be avoided through active listening.   13.   (A)   (D)

14. Working with others is difficult.   14.   (A)   (D)

15. Making rules is better than following rules.   15.   (A)   (D)

16. Most coworkers are helpful.   16.   (A)   (D)

17. Helping the elderly is rewarding.   17.   (A)   (D)

18. Multitasking is difficult in collaborative settings.   18.   (A)   (D)

19. Quiet environments are best for productivity.   19.   (A)   (D)

20. Happiness is more important than financial stability.   20.   (A)   (D)

21. You have to work for what you want.   21.   (A)   (D)

22. Working with children is inspiring.   22.   (A)   (D)

23. It is acceptable to be selfish in life.   23.   (A)   (D)

24. Society is overly competitive.   24.   (A)   (D)

25. Perfection is achievable.   25.   (A)   (D)

26. An ideal job would be one without a strong workplace culture.   26.   (A)   (D)

27.	It is important to separate business and friendship in the workplace.	27.	Ⓐ	Ⓓ
28.	It is difficult to make new friends.	28.	Ⓐ	Ⓓ
29.	Success is more important than relationships.	29.	Ⓐ	Ⓓ
30.	It is never acceptable to fail or lose.	30.	Ⓐ	Ⓓ
31.	Social events are more exciting than alone time.	31.	Ⓐ	Ⓓ
32.	Most supervisors are compassionate.	32.	Ⓐ	Ⓓ
33.	It is more important to highlight someone's strengths than point out their weaknesses.	33.	Ⓐ	Ⓓ
34.	Being radically candid is important.	34.	Ⓐ	Ⓓ
35.	Unity is much more important than diversity.	35.	Ⓐ	Ⓓ
36.	Most young people are clueless about the world.	36.	Ⓐ	Ⓓ
37.	Everybody has the right to their own opinions.	37.	Ⓐ	Ⓓ
38.	It is better to be vocal than to be submissive.	38.	Ⓐ	Ⓓ
39.	It is better to be respected than feared.	39.	Ⓐ	Ⓓ
40.	The best supervisors know how to delegate tasks to their workers.	40.	Ⓐ	Ⓓ
41.	Seniority is more important than performance.	41.	Ⓐ	Ⓓ
42.	The best workers are self-motivated.	42.	Ⓐ	Ⓓ
43.	Discrimination does not really exist.	43.	Ⓐ	Ⓓ
44.	It is important to make a list of daily tasks.	44.	Ⓐ	Ⓓ
45.	An authority figure should never be contradicted.	45.	Ⓐ	Ⓓ
46.	Some rules are meant to be broken.	46.	Ⓐ	Ⓓ
47.	Employees should be fired if they make a mistake.	47.	Ⓐ	Ⓓ
48.	People who complain are weak.	48.	Ⓐ	Ⓓ
49.	Customers are normally difficult to work with.	49.	Ⓐ	Ⓓ
50.	All leaders should be charismatic.	50.	Ⓐ	Ⓓ
51.	Stress is hard to handle in the workplace.	51.	Ⓐ	Ⓓ
52.	Teamwork is key to organizational success.	52.	Ⓐ	Ⓓ
53.	There is one right path in life and many wrong paths.	53.	Ⓐ	Ⓓ
54.	Money is the root of all evil.	54.	Ⓐ	Ⓓ
55.	All people should be treated with dignity.	55.	Ⓐ	Ⓓ
56.	Friendships with colleagues should be avoided.	56.	Ⓐ	Ⓓ
57.	It feels good to be the center of attention.	57.	Ⓐ	Ⓓ
58.	Most tasks at work are dehumanizing.	58.	Ⓐ	Ⓓ

59. Employee values should align in the workplace.   59. (A) (D)

60. Most jobs consume too much time.   60. (A) (D)

61. More elderly people need to retire earlier in life.   61. (A) (D)

62. Disagreement is uncomfortable.   62. (A) (D)

63. Sacrifice is important for team success.   63. (A) (D)

64. Most police officers and security guards are uptight.   64. (A) (D)

65. An ideal supervisor would be one who is direct and honest.   65. (A) (D)

66. An ideal supervisor would be one who focuses on the details.   66. (A) (D)

67. Most people foolishly just follow the rules.   67. (A) (D)

68. Customer service is an important part of any job.   68. (A) (D)

69. Cheating on an exam is never acceptable.   69. (A) (D)

70. Many young people have all the best intentions.   70. (A) (D)

71. The most stimulating environments are calm.   71. (A) (D)

72. Large events are intimidating.   72. (A) (D)

73. Sometimes it is necessary to take an unsanctioned break at work.   73. (A) (D)

74. It is easy to reinvent yourself in new environments.   74. (A) (D)

75. Conversation with strangers is quite easy.   75. (A) (D)

76. Self-created goals are better than those created by others.   76. (A) (D)

77. Flexibility is more important than structure.   77. (A) (D)

78. Isolated work at a computer is better than collaborative work at a conference table.   78. (A) (D)

79. Teachers often cater too much to student needs.   79. (A) (D)

80. Variety is necessary for happiness.   80. (A) (D)

81. Too many people are looking for a handout in this world.   81. (A) (D)

82. People who have trouble choosing a career cannot be trusted as employees.   82. (A) (D)

83. People who question norms are more likely to succeed in the workforce.   83. (A) (D)

84. Every employee must always be on time, no matter the circumstance.   84. (A) (D)

85. Every person deserves access to high-quality medical care.   85. (A) (D)

86. It is unfair to break a promise to a colleague.   86. (A) (D)

87. It is okay to give up when overwhelmed.   87. (A) (D)

88. It is better to lie than hurt someone's feelings.   88. (A) (D)

89. Silence is a sign of insecurity.   89. (A) (D)

90. A series of smaller projects is preferable to one large project.   90. (A) (D)

ANSWER KEY

Academic Aptitude: Verbal Skills

1. c.

Calm means "at ease or peaceful," and the other four words describe the feeling of being upset.

2. e.

Energetic means "wide awake or perky," and the other four words describe the need for rest.

3. d.

Certainty means "without a doubt," and the other four words describe issues or situations that need to be solved.

4. b.

Ordinary means "common or regular," and the other four words mean something strange or extraordinary.

5. c.

Thrive means "to grow in a positive way," and the other four words describe the inability to grow or the absence of growth.

6. b.

Thoughtless means "inconsiderate"; the other four words describe someone considerate and caring.

7. c.

Lacking means "missing or incomplete," and the other four words describe something that is complete or has all its parts.

8. c.

Bandage means "a covering for an injury," and the other four words are types of injuries.

9. a.

Lively means "upbeat or energetic," and the other four words refer to something lacking in positive energy.

10. d.

Long means "lengthy"; the other four words refer to something short or abrupt.

11. e.

Obvious means "understandable or apparent," and the other four words refer to something unknown, mysterious, or puzzling.

12. b.

Upbeat means "having a positive attitude," and the other four words refer to having a negative emotional state.

13. e.

Indifference means "disinterested"; the other four words refer to having an affection or liking for something.

14. e.

Rude means "showing a lack of manners or consideration," and the other four words refer to being friendly or agreeable.

15. d.

Divide means to "separate or disconnect," and the other four words refer to joining things together.

16. c.

Create means "to make something," and the other four words refer to destroying something.

17. b.

Drip means "trickle or drop," and the other four words refer to a heavy flow—usually of water or blood.

18. c.

Conflict means "a competition or lack of agreement," and the other four words describe a state of peace or harmony.

19. a.

Limited means "having defined boundaries," and the other four words refer to something that is never-ending.

20. d.

Disapprove means "condemn"; the other four words refer to forgiveness or approval.

21. b.

Humility means "modesty"; the other four words refer to being conceited.

22. e.

Perfect means "flawless"; the other four words refer to something flawed or defective.

23. d.

Conceited means "snobbish or arrogant," and the other four words refer to modesty and humbleness.

24. d.

Crude means "vulgar or rude," and the other four words refer to being well mannered.

25. e.

Serious means "thoughtful and sober," and the other four words refer to something ridiculous.

Academic Aptitude: Arithmetic

26. d.

Line up the decimals and add.

$$\begin{array}{r} 1.73 \\ +\ 2.17 \\ \hline \mathbf{3.90} \end{array}$$

27. a.

$24.17 + $32.87 = $57.04

$80.00 − $57.04 = **$22.96**

28. b.

Find the highest possible multiple of 4 that is less than or equal to 397, and then subtract to find the remainder.

99 × 4 = 396

397 − 396 = **1**

29. c.

If each student receives 2 notebooks, the teacher will need 16 × 2 = 32 notebooks. After handing out the notebooks, she will have 50 − 32 = **18 notebooks left**.

30. a.

Add the number of cupcakes he will give to his friend and to his coworkers, then subtract that value from 48.

# of cupcakes for his friend:

$\frac{1}{2} \times 48 = 24$

# of cupcakes for his coworkers:

$\frac{1}{3} \times 48 = 16$

48 − (24 + 16) = **8**

31. c.

Round each value and add.

129,113 ≈ 129,000

34,602 ≈ 35,000

129,000 + 35,000 = **164,000**

32. b.

There are 15 minutes between 7:45 a.m. and 8:00 a.m. and 20 minutes between 8:00 a.m. and 8:20 a.m.

15 minutes + 20 minutes = **35 minutes**

33. c.

23 ÷ 4 = 5.75 pizzas

Round up to **6 pizzas**.

34. e.

Use the formula for finding percentages. Express the percentage as a decimal.

part = *whole* × *percentage* = **1560 × 0.15**

35. b.

Multiply the cost per pound by the number of pounds purchased to find the cost of each fruit.

apples: 2(1.89) = 3.78

oranges: 1.5(2.19) = 3.285

3.78 + 3.285 = 7.065 = **$7.07**

36. c.

Divide 1.3208 by 5.2.

```
      .254
52 ) 13.208
      104
      280
      260
      208
      208
        0
```

37. b.

Align the decimals and add/subtract from left to right.

$$17.38 - 19.26 + 14.2$$
$$= (-1.88) + 14.2 = \mathbf{12.32}$$

38. e.

Write a proportion and then solve for x.

$$\frac{40}{45} = \frac{265}{x}$$
$$40x = 11{,}925$$
$$x = 298.125 \approx \mathbf{298}$$

39. b.

$$\frac{1}{4} = \frac{x}{20}$$
$$4x = 20$$
$$x = \mathbf{5}$$

40. c.

$$\frac{25}{2} = \frac{x}{8}$$
$$2x = 200$$
$$x = \mathbf{100}$$

41. a.

$$0.8 + 0.49 + 0.89 = 2.18$$
$$2.5 - 2.18 = \mathbf{0.32}$$

42. c.

Line up the decimals and subtract.

```
  4.50
- 1.67
  2.83
```

43. a.

$\$285.48 \div 6 = \mathbf{\$47.58}$

44. c.

Line up the decimals and subtract.

```
 119.70
-  1.05
 118.65
```

45. c.

$\$25.44 \div 3.2 = \mathbf{\$7.95}$

46. a.

$6.3 \div 18 = \mathbf{0.35\ lb}$

47. d.

48 cents = $0.48

$\$1.68 \div \$0.48 = \mathbf{3.5}$

48. c.

$127 - 150 = 127 + (-150) = \mathbf{-23}$

49. a.

The average of five numbers is the sum of the numbers divided by 5. Multiply the average by 5 to find the sum; subtract to find the fifth number.

$$\frac{sum}{5} = 16$$
$$sum = 16 \times 5 = 80$$
$$80 - 68 = \mathbf{12}$$

50. a.

$$\frac{4}{50} = \frac{x}{175}$$
$$50x = 700$$
$$x = \mathbf{14\ mL}$$

Academic Aptitude: Nonverbal Skills

51.	b.	**64.**	a.
52.	a.	**65.**	a.
53.	e.	**66.**	b.
54.	a.	**67.**	c.
55.	c.	**68.**	d.
56.	e.	**69.**	a.
57.	d.	**70.**	b.
58.	c.	**71.**	d.
59.	c.	**72.**	b.
60.	a.	**73.**	c.
61.	a.	**74.**	e.
62.	c.	**75.**	c.
63.	e.		

Spelling

1.	a. muscle	**24.**	a. symptom
2.	c. hormone	**25.**	c. eliminate
3.	b. seizure	**26.**	b. adhere
4.	c. facilities	**27.**	b. enable
5.	a. decrease	**28.**	b. various
6.	a. transfusion	**29.**	c. secretion
7.	b. anatomy	**30.**	c. trauma
8.	b. diagnosis	**31.**	c. excessive
9.	c. equipment	**32.**	a. bacteria
10.	a. stomach	**33.**	c. fungus
11.	b. arthritis	**34.**	b. monitor
12.	b. ovary	**35.**	c. abrasion
13.	a. surgical	**36.**	c. multiple
14.	c. allergy	**37.**	a. tremor
15.	a. inflammation	**38.**	c. involvement
16.	c. poison	**39.**	c. respiratory
17.	a. atrophy	**40.**	b. cranial
18.	b. sterile	**41.**	c. disease
19.	a. cellular	**42.**	a. artery
20.	b. tissue	**43.**	b. vein
21.	b. artificial	**44.**	b. chronic
22.	c. immediate	**45.**	c. acute
23.	c. droplet		

1. d.

    The passage explains how an infant's senses operate while specifically detailing the changes experienced with vision.

2. b.

    The passage states that vision does not become the dominant sense until around the age of twelve months.

3. d.

    The passage explains that infants rely primarily on hearing because vision does not become a dominant sense until around the age of twelve months.

4. b.

    The passage specifically explains the changes an infant experiences in vision and that because of this late development, hearing is a dominant sense at first.

5. c.

    The author explains that studies show that babies turn toward the sound of their mothers' voices just minutes after being born, indicating that an infant recognizes the mother's voice from their time in the womb. This evidence supports the claim that babies are able to hear before they are born.

6. b.

    The author states that topical studies look at a single physical or human feature that impacts the whole world.

7. c.

    Physical studies focus on the physical features (mountain ranges) of Earth.

8. c.

    This passage focuses on geography and its purpose.

9. a.

    Geography is the study of space, which means it looks at the world through a spatial perspective, answering the question of *where* something is located.

10. a.

    The author says that any explanation for the cause of the Civil War that does not involve slavery is just a fanciful invention to cover up this sad portion of our nation's history. This implies that people do not want to admit something so shameful happened.

11. c.

    The author says, "The Civil War was not a battle of cultural identities—it was a battle about slavery."

12. c.

    The passage explores proposed causes of the Civil War, which are represented in the other answer choices.

13. d.

    The author writes this passage to correct misinformation on the topic of the causes of the Civil War. He writes with an assertive, or self-confident, tone, insisting that his interpretation of this historical event is accurate while the others are wrong. For example, he says, "People who try to sell you this narrative are wrong," showing his confidence in his position and his disdain for others' opinions on this topic.

14. a.

    The text explains that the North had "forged its own identity as the center of centralized commerce and manufacturing."

15. c.

    This passage explains how the snake's coloration and markings help it hide from predators while also warning humans and predators that it may be venomous.

16. b.

    The author explains that the scarlet kingsnake and coral snake frequently share a habitat.

17. d.

    The author explains that the markings on a snake can indicate whether a snake is venomous.

18. a.

The text says, "[I]t might seem counterintuitive for a venomous snake to stand out in bright red or blue," meaning that it seems like a venomous snake would want to stay hidden from predators. However, the text continues by explaining that venomous snakes actually can have vivid skin colors and prints to ward off predators, so *counterintuitive* means "contrary to common belief."

19. b.

The author explains that the markings of a kingsnake are very similar to those of a venomous coral snake. The coral snake is dangerous to a predatory eagle, so the eagle avoids eating the kingsnake for fear it is a coral snake.

20. d.

In this text, the various methods of measuring temperatures are being compared and contrasted to answer the question, "What is the best way to get an accurate reading?"

21. a.

The text states that the most common way people take someone's temperature is orally, and the author goes on to clarify that the correct location of the oral thermometer is under the tongue.

22. c.

The article explains the many ways a temperature can be taken. It also tells which methods are most useful and reliable in various situations.

23. b.

The author explains that while taking a temperature orally is most common, many patients are not able to sit still for the length of time it takes to get an accurate reading. Using one's ear or temporal artery is quicker and therefore beneficial in these situations.

24. c.

The author explains that it is important to check the average temperature for each region, as it can vary by several degrees.

25. a.

The first paragraph of the text explains that taking a temperature is a basic medical procedure that can be done by nearly anyone, including a parent.

26. c.

The passage explains weight loss and how each of the other answer choices impact one's ability to lose weight.

27. a.

The text says that hormone levels can affect the manner in which our bodies process calories, which impacts a person's ability to lose weight.

28. b.

The text uses the word *edict* to refer to the commonly understood rule of dieting that says an individual must burn more calories than he or she takes in.

29. d.

The text says that in some cases people who lose a high percentage of their body weight in a short period of time cannot physically maintain their new weight, and as a result, their body will desperately hang on to calories resulting in weight gain even with a healthy diet.

30. a.

The text explains that following a traditional model for calorie intake may not always produce results because of several factors that may interfere with the weight loss process.

31. b.

The process of the body releasing viruses that have been successfully reproducing during the infection is called viral shedding.

32. c.

The topic sentence explains that the flu has historically been one of the most common human infections, and the rest of the passage explains why that is, despite the fact that it is relatively difficult to contract.

33. b.

Because these aerosol particles result from coughing or sneezing, *expelled* means ejected, or forced out.

34. a.

Many infected with the flu unknowingly infect others because their symptoms are undetected for at least twenty-four hours.

35. c.

The passage explains in the first paragraph that the flu is very deadly and has killed tens of millions in the past 150 years.

General Science

1. a.

Calcium is the most abundant mineral found in bones, as well as in the entire body.

2. d.

A biome is a large ecological community that includes specific plants and animals; a desert is one example.

3. b.

Venus's orbit is closest to Earth. Venus is the second planet from the sun, and Earth is the third planet from the sun.

4. e.

Before a star collapses, the star burns brighter for a period of time and then fades from view. This is a supernova.

5. c.

Tulips are plants, meaning they have chloroplasts to perform photosynthesis.

6. c.

Isotopes are atoms of the same element with the same number of protons but different numbers of neutrons.

7. d.

Tachycardia is an abnormally fast heart rate, and electrocardiograms show the electrical activity of the heart.

8. a.

Each codon contains three nucleotides.

9. c.

Electrons are negatively charged particles in an atom; electrons orbit the nucleus.

10. a.

Tension is the force that results from objects being pulled or hung.

11. b.

Mushrooms are fungi. Fungi break down organic material left by dead animals and plants, making them decomposers.

12. d.

The metabolic rate of crustaceans, such as lobsters, is too low to regulate their temperature. Crustaceans use behavioral techniques, such as moving to shallow water, to maintain body temperature.

13. d.

The tibia is a lower leg bone.

14. e.

The digestive enzymes produced by the pancreas pass into the small intestine.

15. a.

When water changes form, it does not change the chemical composition of the substance. Once water becomes ice, the ice can easily turn back into water.

16. c.

Coal is nonrenewable because once coal is burned, it cannot be quickly replaced.

17. b.

The lithosphere is the top layer of the earth's surface.

18. c.

The skeletal muscles and the bone are attached by the tendons.

19. a.

The esophagus is the muscular passageway through which food travels on its way from the mouth to the stomach.

20. b.

Earth takes approximately twenty-four hours to rotate on its axis.

21. d.

Photosynthesis is the process by which plants convert the energy of the sun into stored chemical energy (glucose).

22. d.

Combustion is defined as a reaction in which a hydrocarbon reacts with O_2 to produce CO_2 and H_2O.

23. e.

Nonliving things in an ecosystem, like air and water, are abiotic factors.

24. e.

Most fungi derive their energy by breaking down dead plant and animal matter.

25. e.

The mechanism of natural selection is rooted in the idea that there is variation in inherited traits among a population of organisms, resulting in differential reproduction.

26. b.

The tongue is the muscle that helps break apart food, mix it with saliva, and direct it toward the esophagus.

27. a.

When placed in water, strong acids immediately break apart into their constituent ions.

28. d.

The femur is the largest bone of the human body.

29. d.

Sunlight helps the skin produce vitamin D.

30. b.

The light reactions of photosynthesis occur in the chloroplast. Each chloroplast has stacks of membranes called thylakoids where enzymes convert light energy into chemical energy.

31. c.

Capillaries enable exchange of cellular waste, gases, and nutrients on the cellular level.

32. c.

The incus, stapes, and malleus are bones connected to the skull that play an important role in the sense of hearing.

33. c.

Adrenal glands sit on top of each kidney.

34. c.

An anemometer measures wind speed.

35. e.

$1 \text{ ml} = 1 \text{ cm}^3$

36. d.

Mature sperm are stored in the epididymis.

37. a.

Meninges are present only in the dorsal cavity that holds the spinal cord and brain.

38. a.

Organic compounds may contain phosphorous, nitrogen, or oxygen, but they *must* contain carbon.

39. e.

Nucleic acids (DNA and RNA) are composed of nucleotides. Each nucleotide is composed of a five-carbon sugar, a nitrogenous base, and a phosphate group.

40. d.

Uracil is found in RNA but not in DNA.

41. b.

Gametes (sperm and egg) have half the number of chromosomes contained in an organism's somatic cells.

42. c.

An ax is an example of a wedge.

43. a.

The valence shell of the noble gases (group 18) is full, so these gases do not need to add electrons.

44. e.

Through photosynthesis, leaves use the sun's energy to convert carbon dioxide into glucose.

45. d.

Deposition occurs when a gas becomes a solid.

46. a.

Acids have a pH between 0 and 7.

47. e.

A balance measures mass.

48. b.

Friction occurs when motion is impeded because one object is rubbing against another object.

49. a.

Igneous rocks form when liquid rock cools and solidifies.

50. c.

Sound waves are longitudinal waves because the vibrations travel in the same direction as the energy.

51. c.

Nitrogen makes up 78 percent of Earth's atmosphere.

52. c.

All atoms of the same element contain the same number of protons.

53. e.

Hydrogen is the most common element in the universe.

54. d.

Tornadoes occur when warm air masses collide with cold air masses over land.

55. a.

Baking soda (sodium bicarbonate) is a base, which will neutralize an acid.

56. b.

Gravity is a force that attracts objects to the center of the earth or toward other objects having mass.

57. e.

Potential energy is energy that is stored and waiting to work.

58. c.

A T-shirt is translucent; it lets some light pass through.

59. c.

A marble is an example of an electrical insulator—it stops the transfer of electrical energy. The other choices are all electrical conductors.

60. a.

Stratus clouds are often gray.

Vocational Adjustment Index

There is no "right" answer to the questions on the Vocational Adjustment Index. Every school will interpret your score differently, so just focus on answering the questions quickly and honestly.

Follow the link below to take your second PSB RNSAE practice test:

www.ascenciatestprep.com/psb-rnsae-online-resources